Positional Therapy in Obstructive Sleep Apnea

Nico de Vries • Madeline Ravesloot
J. Peter van Maanen
Editors

Positional Therapy in Obstructive Sleep Apnea

Springer

Editors
Nico de Vries
Department of Otolaryngology
Sint Lucas Andreas Ziekenhuis
Amsterdam, The Netherlands

Madeline Ravesloot
Department of Otorhinolaryngology
Sint Lucas Andreas Ziekenhuis
Amsterdam, The Netherlands

J. Peter van Maanen
Department of Otolaryngology
Sint Lucas Andreas Ziekenhuis
Amsterdam, The Netherlands

ISBN 978-3-319-34280-1 ISBN 978-3-319-09626-1 (eBook)
DOI 10.1007/978-3-319-09626-1
Springer Cham Heidelberg New York Dordrecht London

Printed on acid-free paper

Springer is part of Springer Science+Business Media (www.springer.com)

Contents

Part VI Treatment of Positional OSA

Contributors

Linda B.L. Benoist, M.D. Ear Nose and Throat, Sint Lucas Andreas Ziekenhuis, Amsterdam, The Netherlands

Matt T. Bianchi, M.D., Ph.D. Neurology Department, Massachusetts General Hospital, Boston, MA, USA

Marc J. Braem, D.D.S., Ph.D. Department of Special Care Dentistry, Antwerp University Hospital, University of Antwerp, Edegem, Antwerp, Belgium

Naricha Chirakalwasan, M.D. Division of Pulmonary and Critical Care Medicine, Department of Medicine, Faculty of Medicine, Chulalongkorn University, Bangkok, Thailand

Excellence Center for Sleep Disorders, King Chulalongkorn Memorial Hospital, Thai Red Cross Society, Bangkok, Thailand

Ji Ho Choi, M.D., Ph.D. Department of Otorhinolaryngology-Head and Neck Surgery, Korea University Ansan Hospital, Korea University College of Medicine, Gyeonggi-do, Republic of Korea

Wilfried A. de Backer, M.D., Ph.D. Department of Pulmonary Medicine, Antwerp University Hospital, Antwerp, Belgium

Multidisciplinary Sleep Disorders Centre, Antwerp University Hospital, Antwerp, Belgium

Jan de Lange, D.M.D., M.D., Ph.D. Department of Oral and Maxillofacial Surgery, Academic Medical Centre, University of Amsterdam, Amsterdam, The Netherlands

Maurits H.T. de Ruiter, D.D.S. Department of Oral and Maxillofacial Surgery, Academic Medical Center, Amsterdam, The Netherlands

Nico de Vries, M.D., Ph.D. Department of Otolaryngology, Sint Lucas Andreas Ziekenhuis, Amsterdam, The Netherlands

Department of Otolaryngology, University Hospital Antwerp, Antwerp, Belgium

Marijke Dieltjens, M.B.S. Department of Special Care Dentistry, Antwerp University Hospital, University of Antwerp, Edegam, Antwerp, Belgium

Lideke N. Dun, M.Sc. Department of Otolaryngology/Head and Neck Surgery, Saint Lucas Andreas Hospital, Amsterdam, The Netherlands

Aida Dynia, M.A. Fleischman Unit for the Study of Disability, Loewenstein Hospital – Rehabilitation Center, Raanana, Israel

Edith Eitan Sleep Disorders Unit, Loewenstein Hospital – Rehabilitation Center, Raanana, Israel

Michaël H. Frank, D.M.D., M.D. Department of Oral and Maxillofacial Surgery, Academic Medical Centre, University of Amsterdam, Amsterdam, The Netherlands

Natan Gadoth, M.D. Sleep Disorders Unit, Loewenstein Hospital – Rehabilitation Center, Raanana, Israel

Vlada Goizman Sleep Disorders Unit, Loewenstein Hospital – Rehabilitation Center, Raanana, Israel

Martijn Grijseels Department of Otolaryngology/Head Neck Surgery, Leiden University Medical Centre, University of Amsterdam, Amsterdam, The Netherlands

Brenda Hermsen, M.D. Department of Gynecology, Sint Lucas Andreas Ziekenhuis, Amsterdam, The Netherlands

Anthony A.J. Hilgevoord, M.D., Ph.D. Department of Neurology and Clinical Neurophysiology, St. Lucas Andreas Hospital, Amsterdam, The Netherlands

Zhang Huankang, M.S. Department of Otorhinolaryngology-Head and Neck Surgery, Fudan University, Eye, Ear, Nose and Throat Hospital, Shanghai, China

Amal Isaiah, M.D., D.Phil. Department of Otorhinolaryngology-HNS, University of Maryland, Baltimore, MD, USA

Hennie Janssen, M.D., Ph.D. Sleep Medicine Centre, Kempenhaeghe, Heeze, The Netherlands

Huang Jingjing, M.S. Department of Otorhinolaryngology-Head and Neck Surgery, Fudan University, Eye, Ear, Nose and Throat Hospital, Shanghai, China

Ioannis Koutsourelakis, M.D., Ph.D. Department of Otolaryngology/Head and Neck Surgery, Saint Lucas Andreas Hospital, Amsterdam, The Netherlands

Samuel Krachman, D.O. Division of Pulmonary, Critical Care and Sleep Medicine, Temple University School of Medicine, Philadelphia, PA, USA

Xiao Kuanlin, M.D. Department of Otorhinolaryngology-Head and Neck Surgery, Fudan University, Eye, Ear, Nose and Throat Hospital, Shanghai, China

D. Martin Laman, M.D., Ph.D. Department of Clinical Neurophysiology, St. Lucas Andreas Hospital, Amsterdam, The Netherlands

Chul Hee Lee, M.D., Ph.D. Department of Otorhinolaryngology, Seoul National University Bundang Hospital, Bundang-gu, Seongnam-si, South Korea

Seung Hoon Lee, M.D., Ph.D. Department of Otorhinolaryngology-Head and Neck Surgery, Korea University Ansan Hospital, Korea University College of Medicine, Gyeonggi-do, Republic of Korea

M. Jeffery Mador, M.D. Division of Pulmonary, Critical Care and Sleep Medicine, University at Buffalo, Buffalo, NY, USA

Western New York Veteran Affairs Healthcare System, Buffalo, NY, USA

Joachim T. Maurer, M.D. Department of Otorhinolaryngology, Head & Neck Surgery, Sleep Disorders Center, University Hospital Mannheim, Mannheim, Germany

Kristel A.W. Meester, B.Sc. Department of Clinical Neurophysiology, St. Lucas Andreas Hospital, Amsterdam, The Netherlands

Sharon Morong, M.D., M.Sc., F.R.C.S.C. Department of Otolaryngology, Sint Lucas Andreas Ziekenhuis, Amsterdam, The Netherlands

Khitam Nasser, P.S.G.T. Sleep Disorders Unit, Loewenstein Hospital – Rehabilitation Center, Raanana, Israel

Arie Oksenberg, Ph.D. Sleep Disorders Unit, Loewenstein Hospital – Rehabilitation Center, Raanana, Israel

Sebastiaan Overeem, M.D., Ph.D. Sleep Medicine Centre, Kempenhaeghe, Heeze, The Netherlands

Kevin D. Pereira, M.D., M.S. University of Maryland School of Medicine, Baltimore, MD, USA

Dirk Pevernagie, M.D., Ph.D. Sleep Medicine Centre, Kempenhaeghe, Heeze, The Netherlands

Madeline Ravesloot, M.D., Ph.D. Department of Otorhinolaryngology, Sint Lucas Andreas Ziekenhuis, Amsterdam, The Netherlands

Chae-Seo Rhee, M.D., Ph.D. Department of Otorhinolaryngology, Seoul National University Bundang Hospital, Bundang-gu, Seongnam-si, South Korea

Wietske Richard, M.D., Ph.D. Department of Otolaryngology/Head and Neck Surgery, Saint Lucas Andreas Hospital, Amsterdam, The Netherlands

Faiza Safiruddin, M.D. Department of Otolaryngology/Head and Neck Surgery, Saint Lucas Andreas Hospital, Amsterdam, The Netherlands

Mahesh Shetty, M.D. Department of Pulmonary, Critical Care and Sleep Medicine, University at Buffalo, Buffalo, NY, USA

Irene Swift, M.D. Division of Pulmonary, Critical Care and Sleep Medicine, Temple University School of Medicine, Philadelphia, PA, USA

Eline C. Vrijland van Beest, M.Sc., M.B.I. NightBalance B.V., Delft, The Netherlands

Paul H. van de Heyning, M.D., Ph.D. ENT Department and Head and Neck Surgery, Antwerp University Hospital, University of Antwerp, Edegem, Antwerp, Belgium

Arjan van der Star, M.Sc. NightBalance B.V., Delft, The Netherlands

Ellen R. van Kesteren, B.Sc. Department of Neurology and Clinical Neurophysiology, St. Lucas Andreas Hospital, Amsterdam, The Netherlands

Marjolein A.J. van Looij, M.D., Ph.D. Ear Nose and Throat Surgery, Sint Lucas Andreas Ziekenhuis, Amsterdam, The Netherlands

J. Peter van Maanen, M.D. Department of Otolaryngology, Sint Lucas Andreas Ziekenhuis, Amsterdam, The Netherlands

Piet-Heijn J.M. van Mechelen, M.Sc. ApneuVereniging (Dutch Apnea Association), Heemstede, The Netherlands

Olivier M. Vanderveken, M.D., Ph.D. ENT Department and Head and Neck Surgery, Antwerp University Hospital, University of Antwerp, Edegem, Antwerp, Belgium

Maria Elena Vega, M.D. Division of Pulmonary, Critical Care and Sleep Medicine, Temple University School of Medicine, Philadephia, PA, USA

Johan A. Verbraecken, M.D., Ph.D. Department of Pulmonary Medicine, Antwerp University Hospital, Antwerp, Belgium

Multidisciplinary Sleep Disorders Centre, Antwerp University Hospital, Antwerp, Belgium

Annelies E. Verbruggen, M.D. ENT Department and Head and Neck Surgery, Antwerp University Hospital, University of Antwerp, Edegem, Antwerp, Belgium

E.A. Verhagen, Ph.D. Department of Public and Occupational Health, EMGO Institute for Health and Care Research, VU Medical Center, Amsterdam, The Netherlands

Anneclaire V. Vroegop, M.D., Ph.D. ENT Department and Head and Neck Surgery, Antwerp University Hospital, Edegem, Antwerp, Belgium

Saint Lucas Andreas Hospital, Amsterdam, The Netherlands

Marc Willemen Multidisciplinary Sleep Disorders Centre, University of Antwerp, Antwerp, Belgium

Birgit I. Witte, M.Sc., Ph.D. Department of Epidemiology and Biostatistics, VU University Medical Centre, Amsterdam, The Netherlands

Tae-Bin Won, M.D., Ph.D. Department of Otorhinolaryngology, Seoul National University College of Medicine, Seoul National University Hospital, Seongnam, Korea

Hou Xiaolin, M.S. Department of Otorhinolaryngology-Head and Neck Surgery, Xinhua Hospital, Shanghai Jiaotong University, Shanghai, China

Part I
General

Introduction

Nico de Vries

Why This Book?

This book aims to bring the reader to the revelation that body position is important in the aetiology of sleep-disordered breathing. This aspect of its aetiology has been neglected and overlooked for too long. Positional-dependent obstructive sleep apnea (OSA) can be treated effectively with new forms of positional therapy. I hope the reader will recognize that there is much room for improvement in diagnosis and treatment of OSA. This book will provide the reader with the tools to implement positional therapy in clinical practice. I hope it will serve as motivation for fantastic presentations and inspiring manuscripts on well-conducted research.

Commonly, OSA is described as a disease that is caused by a combination of certain anatomical features, neuromuscular drive and muscle tone. It is well known that the prevalence of OSA increases with age and body weight and that OSA occurs more frequently in men. Other important risk factors include sedative and alcohol use. It seems that sleep position, despite being an important risk factor for OSA and an essential feature of the aetiology of (beginning) OSA, is not always recognized and even overlooked.

Over the years I have started to recognize that the role of gravity and body position is much more important than many of us realize, in particular in early disease. I have the impression that due to the absence of successful therapy, specified to treat position dependence, we have been misled to conclude that there is little to gain in this subgroup of patients with OSA, even though more than half of patients with

N. de Vries, M.D., Ph.D. (✉)
Department of Otolaryngology, Sint Lucas Andreas Ziekenhuis,
Jan Tooropstraat 164, Amsterdam 1061AE, The Netherlands

Department of Otolaryngology, University Hospital Antwerp,
Wikrijkstraat 10, Antwerp 2650, Belgium
e-mail: n.vries@slaz.nl

N. de Vries et al. (eds.), *Positional Therapy in Obstructive Sleep Apnea*,
DOI 10.1007/978-3-319-09626-1_1

OSA are position dependent. Many guidelines, for example, do not advocate the registration of body position during polysomnographies. With the introduction of efficacious positional therapy, I am of the opinion that the role of body position has been undervalued, underdiagnosed and undertreated.

About Me

One of the great aspects of being a surgeon participating in research is the stimulating, developing and innovative environment. During the past years, I have been fortunate to have the opportunity to participate in various (inter)national meetings, congresses, workshops, (live) surgeries, animal laboratory science experiments, cadaver dissections, writing committees of position papers and guideline committees on sleep-disordered breathing in general and obstructive sleep apnea in particular. Not only have I had the privilege of working with and for professionals but also with patients and patient societies. I have witnessed many eloquent speakers deliver fantastic presentations and inspiring manuscripts on well-conducted research covering all aspects of OSA, from expert opinions to evidence-based practice and from background questions such as genetics, inflammatory cells in the upper airway, pharyngeal anatomy/collapsibility and epidemiology to foreground questions. (This list is so extensive that I have placed it in a footnote.[1]) Additionally, working in such an international environment is enriched by discussions concerning international differences in guidelines regarding diagnostic work-up and treatment and international differences in reimbursement of diagnosis and treatment of OSA. In my opinion, positional OSA and positional therapy, however, so far do not gain the attention that they deserve.

Strengths of the Book

Treatment of OSA is steadily moving away from a CPAP-centred, "one-size-fits-all" approach towards individualized medicine. The keyword is treatment diversification. Next to CPAP, oral devices—and in selected patients, surgery—are

[1] This list includes: the value of different types of sleep studies, imaging, computerized fluid dynamics, evaluation of pharyngeal shape and size using anatomical coherence tomography, Pcrit measurements, ventilatory response-to-disturbance ratio (loop gain), ability of the upper airway to stiffen/dilate in response to an increase in ventilatory drive, arousal threshold, general examination and specific assessment of the upper airway—including drug-induced sleep endoscopy—health consequences and health economics of untreated OSA, cost-effectiveness of treatment, treatment with continuous positive airway pressure (CPAP), AutoPAP, BIPAP, compliance of CPAP, oral devices, anatomy, neuromuscular drive, obstructive vs. mixed and central OSA, OSA and obesity and vice versa, bariatric surgery, OSA and driving, OSA and general anaesthesia, various forms of palatal and base of tongue surgery, multimodality treatment, multilevel surgery, bimaxillary osteotomies, experimental procedures such as implants (Apneon, Aspire, Pillars, Pavad, ReVent), transoral robotic surgery, transcervical approaches, stimulation of the hypoglossal nerve (upper airway stimulation, neuromodulation) and so on and so forth.

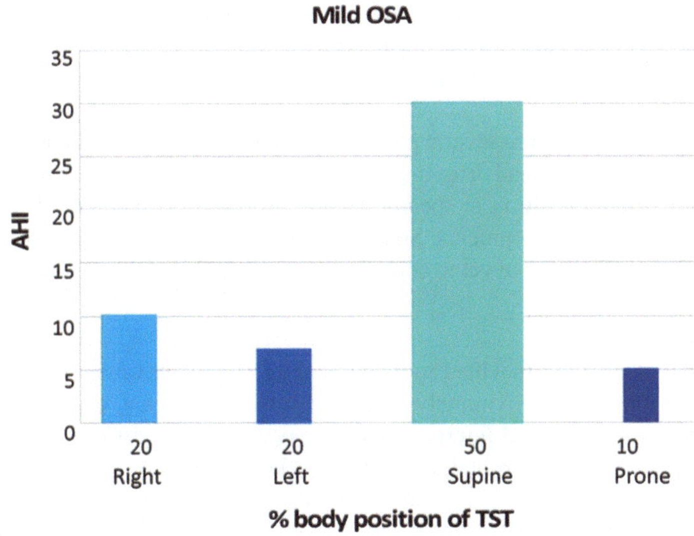

Fig. 1 Percentage of the total sleeping time (TST) spent in supine position and an apnea-hypopnea index (AHI) of a patient with mild OSA

gaining momentum. In my view, the most promising new development particularly in mild to moderate disease however is positional therapy. We are leaving tennis ball therapy behind and starting a new era with new-generation devices such as the sleep position trainer. More than 50 % of patients with mild OSA are positional, defined as at least twice as many events during sleep in supine position as in the other sleeping positions. In fact, in more than half of patients, mild OSA and positional OSA are synonymous (Fig. 1; for animation, see www.positionalosas.com).

Figure 1 depicts a very archetypal patient with mild OSA, who sleeps 50 % of the total sleeping time on his/her back. In this sleeping position, the AHI is 30, while the average AHI in non-supine position is less than 10. This 50 % of the total sleeping in supine position is not unusual. In one of the studies reported in this book, the average percentage slept in supine position before treatment was exactly 50 %. Positional therapy is nothing more than elimination of the supine position.

Published and ongoing studies show that the new-generation positional therapy is effective and patient friendly, has no side effects, does not change sleep quality or may even improve it and is reversible, with good compliance, and this all with acceptable costs. Positional therapy can be a stand-alone therapy or can be combined with other treatments such as oral device therapy or surgery. It can be used for patients with habitual snoring as well as in patients with OSA. Its role in several other specific patient populations is currently investigated, such as will be shown in this book. Devices such as the sleep position trainer have the potential to become "game changers".

We have tried to put a book together that can be read as a whole, but that can also be consumed per separate chapter. Such a product implicates that there is some overlap and therefore some basic principles and introductions come back from time to time.

Some authors comment on the same problem from a different angle. This is inevitable, and not necessarily negative, while not all is proved yet. The upside is that if one wants to read one specific chapter only, it is not necessary to read all the preceding chapters first.

The book is divided into several parts: (1) an introductory general part, (2) a part on work-up (sleep study and drug-induced sedated endoscopy, and a general part on work-up), (3) sleep position in specific patient groups, (4) treatment of positional OSA and (5) future developments. Some studies have been concluded, while others are ongoing, and some have yet to start. There could not be a better moment to publish this book.

Acknowledgements I am indebted to many people. This book was possible without the support of my young, extremely smart and enthusiastic team: my residents, former residents, national and international fellows and the great sleep laboratory of the Sint Lucas Andreas Hospital, Amsterdam, The Netherlands.

In particular I want to thank my co-editors Madeline Ravesloot, Peter van Maanen, but also Linda Benoist, Faiza Safiruddin, Sharon Morong, Marjolein van Looij, Eline van Beest, Arjan van der Star, Yiannis Koutsourelakis, Martin Laman, Ton Hilgevoord, Vincent van Ammers, Ellen van Kesteren, Ellen Beekman and Hans Moinat. I thank my partners Peter van Rijn and Joep Tan for allowing me to do what I like most. It's a privilege to work with you all.

Nico de Vries

OSAS: The Magnitude of the Problem

Johan A. Verbraecken

Introduction

Obstructive sleep apnea syndrome (OSAS) is very common [1, 2] and represents an increasing part of clinical (respiratory) practice in developed countries. OSAS is currently recognised to be one of the most common chronic respiratory disorders, with only asthma and possibly COPD having a similar prevalence [3–5]. Questions regarding risks, diagnosis and therapeutical options are of importance to both clinicians and healthcare policymakers. As the medical community and the general public have become more aware of the relationships among snoring, excessive daytime sleepiness, cardiovascular disease and OSAS, doctors are seeing an increasing number of patients with such problems. Excessive daytime sleepiness is one of the cardinal symptoms [6]. Untreated OSAS has substantial health consequences [7]. Moderate to severe OSAS is associated with an increased risk of death from any cause in middle-aged adults, especially men. They are closely related to increases in body weight and, as a result, the tendency to develop upper airway collapse during sleep. It is obvious that OSAS has different phenotypes and that there are relevant gender differences and important aging effects [8–10]. Moreover, the condition carries significant morbidity and is associated with an increased risk of stroke, myocardial infarction, arrhythmias, hypertension and metabolic and neurobehavioural consequences [11].

J.A. Verbraecken, M.D., Ph.D. (✉)
Department of Pulmonary Medicine, Antwerp University Hospital,
Wilrijkstraat 10, Edegem, Antwerp 2650, Belgium

Multidisciplinary Sleep Disorders Centre, Antwerp University Hospital,
Wilrijkstraat 10, Edegem, Antwerp 2650, Belgium
e-mail: johan.verbraecken@uza.be

N. de Vries et al. (eds.), *Positional Therapy in Obstructive Sleep Apnea*,
DOI 10.1007/978-3-319-09626-1_2

Definitions

Obstructive sleep apnea syndrome is part of a spectrum of respiratory disturbances that occur during sleep, described with a widely used term as sleep-disordered breathing (SDB) [12]. The International Classification of Sleep Disorders (ICSD-3) has defined four major categories of SDB: obstructive sleep apnea disorders (including obstructive sleep apnea hypopnea syndrome or OSAS), central sleep apnea syndrome (CSA), sleep-related hypoventilation disorders and sleep -related hypoxemia disorders [13]. The fundamental difference between the first two major categories is the pathophysiological mechanism which causes the respiratory disturbance [14]. In OSAS, the upper airway occlusion is most often caused by abnormal anatomy and/or abnormal control of the muscles that maintain the patency of the upper airway. In CSA, dysfunctional ventilatory control in the central neurons is involved, finally resulting in loss of ventilatory effort. Central and obstructive apneas are rarely seen in isolation in a single patient, which suggests that the mechanisms responsible for the different types of apnea must overlap. It was more preferable to discuss each of these separately, although they could be placed under the common denominator of "sleep-disordered breathing syndrome" [14]. An obstructive apnea-hypopnea can be defined as an event that lasts for at least 10 s and is characterised by a transient reduction in (hypopnea) or complete cessation (apnea) of breathing [12]. Based on the AASM criteria from 1999, a hypopnea can be defined as a decrease from baseline in the amplitude of a valid measure of breathing during sleep that either reaches >50 % with an oxygen desaturation of 3 % or an arousal or alternatively a 30 % reduction with 4 % oxygen desaturation [12]. Recently, the AASM adopted a simplified hypopnea definition which considers a hypopnea if the peak signal excursions drop by ≥3 % of pre-event baseline using nasal cannula, with a duration of ≥10 s, and ≥3 % oxygen desaturation from pre-event baseline or the event is associated with an arousal [15].

Central sleep apnea refers to the cessation of ventilation lasting for at least 10 s (in adults) due to transient loss of neural output to the respiratory muscles [12]. The degree of severity is defined on the basis of the number of apneas and hypopneas occurring during 1 h of sleep (apnea-hypopnea index or AHI) and the severity of daytime symptoms. According to ICSD-3, the presence of criteria A and B, or C satisfies the diagnosis of a clinically significant obstructive sleep apnea-hypopnea syndrome (see Table 1) [12]. The severity of OSAS can be defined as mild for an AHI≥5 and <15, moderate for an AHI≥15 and ≤30 and severe for an AHI>30 [16]. Based on these criteria, sleep apnea occurs in 4 % of men and 2 % of women who are 30–60 years old [1]. The definition of OSAS, using two components, breathing pattern disturbances during sleep and daytime symptoms, indicates that there are also subjects who present with sleep apnea without symptoms. These cases are referred to as OSAS and have an even higher prevalence, recently estimated to be 20 % for OSAS in a Spanish population [10]. OSAS can be subdivided into adult type and paediatric type, since the diagnostic criteria and clinical presentation for abnormal breathing during sleep are different for adult cases and paediatric ones [15]. Obstructive breathing events may include apneas, hypopneas and respiratory

Table 1 ICSD-3 Criteria for the diagnosis of a clinically significant obstructive sleep apnea-hypopnea syndrome

A → The presence of one or more of the following applies:
i. The patient complains of sleepiness, nonrestorative sleep, fatigue, or insomnia symptoms.
ii. The patient wakes with breath holding, gasping, or choking
iii. The bed partner or other observer reports loud snoring, breathing interruptions, or both during the patient's sleep
iv. The patient has been diagnosed with hypertension, a mood disorder, cognitive dysfunction, coronary artery disease, stroke, congestive heart failure, atrial fibrillation, or type 2 diabetes mellitus
B → Polysomnographic (PSG) of ambulatory polygraphic (PG) recording shows the following:
i. Five or more scoreable predominantly obstructive respiratory events (obstructive and mixed apneas, hypopneas, or RERA's) per hour of sleep during a PSG or per hour of monitoring (PG)
OR
C. Polysomnographic recording shows the following:
i. Fifteen or more predominantly obstructive respiratory events (apneas, hypopneas, or RERAs) per hour of sleep during a PSG or per hour of monitoring (PG)

effort-related arousals (RERAs) [17]. A RERA can be defined as a sequence of breaths characterised by increasing respiratory effort leading to arousal from sleep, but not fulfilling the criteria for apnea or hypopnea [15, 17]. Moreover, these events present with a pattern of progressively more negative esophageal pressures, terminated by an abrupt change in pressure to a less negative level and an arousal. Esophageal pressure is still recommended as the method of choice [15, 18], but the flattening of the flow curve obtained by nasal pressure is explicitly mentioned, together with induction plethysmography, as feasible alternatives [15]. In daily practice, nasal pressure is the method of choice for most sleep laboratories. These events also last 10 s or more. If a definition for hypopnea is used which requires an associated desaturation OR arousal, then there are relatively few events scored as RERAs. Upper airway resistance syndrome (UARS) is characterised by increased upper airway resistance, followed by repetitive arousals, finally resulting in daytime sleepiness [19, 20]. The essential polysomnographic features are the absence of obstructive sleep apneas, an AHI<5 and a lack of significant oxygen desaturation, which differ from the laboratory findings of OSAS [15]. Currently, the term UARS is no longer used as an independent disease, but is subsumed under the diagnosis of OSAS because the pathophysiology does not significantly differ from that of OSAS.

The diagnosis of CSA is made by criteria recommended by the ICSD-3 manual as well [13]. Patients with primary central sleep apnea present with (1) sleepiness or difficulty initiating or maintaining sleep, frequent awakenings, or non restorative sleep or awakening, short of breath or snoring or witnessed apneas. PSG demonstrates five or more central apneas and/or hypopneas per hour of sleep (PSG). The number of central apneas and/or central hypopneas is > 50 % of the total number of apneas and hypopneas, with absence of Cheyne-Stokes breathing. There is no evidence of daytime or nocturnal hypoventilation. All these criteria must be met (2) repetitive nocturnal arousals and awakenings during sleep or insomnia complaints or (3) awakening short of breath, combined with five or more central apneas per hour of sleep. The disorder is not better explained by another current sleep disorder, medication use (e.g. opioids) or substance use disorder. Very often, many patients with CSA have mild hypocapnia or normocapnia, but rarely hypercapnia and hypoventilation are also observed. A periodic pattern of waxing and waning of ventilation with periods of hyperventilation alternating with central apnea-hypopnea is defined as central sleep apnea with Cheyne-Stokes breathing (CSB). According to ICSD-3 manual, CSB can be considered if (A) presence of one or more of the following: (1) sleepiness, (2) difficulty initiating or maintaining sleep, frequent awakenings, or nonrestorative sleep, (3) awakening short of breath, (4) snoring, or (5) witnessed apneas. (B) The presence of atrial fibrillation/flutter, congestive heart failure, or a neurological disorder. (C) PSG (during diagnostic or positive airway pressure titration) shows all of the following: (1) Five or more central apneas and/or central hypopneas per hour of sleep. (2) The total number of central apneas and/or hypopneas is > 50 % of the total number of apneas and hypopneas. (3) The pattern of ventilation meets criteria for Cheyne-Stokes breathing. (D) The disorder is not better explained by another current sleep disorder, medication use (e.g. opioids), or substance use disorder.

Although symptoms are not mandatory to make the final diagnosis, patients often report excessive daytime sleepiness, repetitive arousals and awakenings during sleep, insomnia complaints or awakening short of breath [13].

A third patient group in the spectrum of SDB is termed sleep-related hypoventilation/hypoxemic syndrome. Sleep-induced hypoventilation is characterised by arterial carbon dioxide tension ($PaCO_2$) >45 mmHg or disproportionately increased levels while asleep relative to levels during wakefulness [12]. This group encompasses obesity hypoventilation syndrome, congenital central alveolar hypoventilation syndrome, late onset central hypoventilation with hypothalamic dysfunction, idiopathic central alveolar hypoventilation, sleep related hypoventilation due to a medication or substance and sleep related hypoventilation due to a medical disorder [13]. Obesity hypoventilation syndrome (OHS) is probably the most prevalent clinical presentation of this syndrome. OHS is defined as the association of obesity (BMI > 30 kg/m^2) and hypercapnia ($PaCO_2$ > 45 mmHg) that is not primarily due to lung parenchymal or airway disease, pulmonary vascular pathology, chest wall disorder (other than mass loading from obesity), medication use, neurologic disorder, muscle weakness, or a known congenital or idiopathic central alveolar hypoventilation syndrome [21–24]. There is however not a commonly accepted definition for OHS. A last patient group is defined as sleep related hypoxemia disorder and is characterised by significant hypoxemia during sleep, and believed to be secondary to a medical or neurological disorder. PSG, PG or nocturnal oximetry shows the arterial oxygen saturation during sleep of <= 88 % in adults for >= 5 min. Sleep hypoventilation has not been documented.

Different definitions have been proposed by the AASM for the different entities of sleep-disordered breathing (ICSD-3 versus scoring manual), which may complicate the understanding of the problem [13–18].

Epidemiology of Obstructive Sleep Apnea

Epidemiological studies investigating the prevalence of SDB are all biased by the lack of a uniform definition [1, 10]. The prevalence of an AHI>5 in the general population has previously been estimated to be 24 % in males, without symptoms of sleepiness taken into account [1]. When symptoms of sleepiness were also included, the prevalence decreased to 4 % in males and 2 % in females. Using a more restrictive definition including only symptomatic subjects with a fair amount of respiratory events that warrant CPAP therapy, the prevalence is about 0.5 % for middle-aged men with a normal BMI and 1.5 % for the same group with an increased BMI [25, 26]. The growing prevalence of SDB is in parallel with the growing prevalence of obesity. Most of the cases are however unsuspected, since the two most important complaints of loud snoring and a tendency to fall asleep during daytime are often considered normal variants, and patients frequently do not seek medical attention [27]. Unfortunately, many patients who do seek medical attention are dismissed as having no significant disturbance, without formal assessment, and it is very common for patients who have been suffering for many years to present to sleep clinics. Snoring is the hallmark of relevant OSAS, with a prevalence based on epidemiological studies of 9–50 % in men and 4–17 % in women. In a multicentre study performed in Iceland, Belgium and Sweden, asking for snoring at least 3 nights a week, very similar results were found [28]. Several population-based studies have reported an increase in snoring with age, followed by a decrease after the age of 50–60 years in both males and females [26, 28–32]. Some cross-sectional epidemiological surveys have found significant associations between cigarette smoking and snoring, linked to airway inflammation and nocturnal nicotine withdrawal [33].

Common risk factors for OSAS are obesity, gender, aging, race, smoking and alcohol use, besides co-morbidities as enlarged tonsils, adenoids and craniofacial abnormalities.

Obesity

About 80 % of OSAS patients are obese and obesity is an established risk factor for OSAS. A very tight relationship has been observed between body weight change and AHI: a 10 % weight gain has been shown to predict an approximate 32 % increase in the AHI, a 10 % weight loss predicts a 26 % decrease in the AHI, and a 10 % weight gain predicts a sixfold increase in the odds of developing moderate to severe OSAS [34]. Obesity causes upper airway narrowing as a result of excess fat in the (peri- and para)pharyngeal tissues [35]. Despite the strong relationship with obesity, it is important to remember that not all subjects who are obese or have a large neck circumference suffer from relevant sleep apnea and that one-third of OSAS patients are not obese [36, 37].

Age

Several papers have shown a higher prevalence of OSAS in the elderly. In the Sleep Heart Health Study, it was shown that 25 % of males and 11 % of females in the age group 40–98 years had an AHI of higher than 15 events per hour [38]. However, daytime symptoms may be less common with advancing age [39]. The influence of male gender and BMI on OSAS tends to wane with age, and the overall prevalence of symptomatic OSAS seems to stabilise after age 65 years, while the age distribution of OSAS seems to increase regardless of age [9]. On the other hand, the age distribution of patients first diagnosed with OSAS generally peaks at the age of 50. Anyway, the high prevalence of sleep apnea in the elderly has led to a debate regarding its causes and consequences in older people [40, 41]. It could be suggested that older OSAS patients may be habituated to the added disease-related sleep disruption of OSAS and, therefore, do not suffer symptoms of daytime sleepiness in the same way as younger patients.

Gender

Epidemiological studies have reported that OSAS is much more prevalent in males. Possible explanations include the effects of hormonal influences affecting upper airway musculature and its ability to collapse, differences in body fat distribution and sex differences in pharyngeal structure and function [36].

A referral bias and gender differences in clinical presentation may have resulted in more males than females being diagnosed [42]. Males with OSAS are more likely to have symptoms of loud snoring, witnessed apneas or sleepiness.

Symptoms expressed by female OSAS patients are less typical and encompass insomnia, fatigue, morning headache and depression, while male bed partners are less likely to report snoring and apneas to their family physician as compared to their female counterpart. Therefore, female OSAS patients are less likely to be diagnosed and treated as compared to their male counterpart. Currently, there is increasing recognition that the disease is also prevalent in females, particularly after the menopause, and that the clinical manifestations may differ from those in males [43, 44].

Smoking and Alcohol Use

The role of smoking as an established risk factor for OSAS remains controversial. Wetter et al. found a dose-response relationship between smoking and AHI, while smokers in the Sleep Heart Health Study displayed less sleep apnea than nonsmokers [45, 46]. These discrepancies remain unexplained, and there is a need to unravel the link between tobacco consumption and OSAS. Solid epidemiological studies related to chronic alcohol intake and sleep apnea are missing, due to a lack of reliable instruments for estimating alcohol use. Some population-based cross-sectional studies have reported a significant association between chronic alcohol intake and OSAS, whereas other cross-sectional or longitudinal studies did not [30, 47].

Race

Although data are scarce, African-Americans and Asians appear to be at higher risk of developing OSAS than Caucasians [48]. This finding could at least partly be explained by differences in craniofacial structure [49].

Symptoms and Signs

Symptoms of OSAS can be divided in symptoms experienced by the patient himself and symptoms recognised by the bed partner [50, 51].

Snoring

Obstructive sleep apnea is mainly characterised clinically by loud snoring. It is often more cumbersome for the bed partner than for the patient himself and is often existing for a long time. Four or five loud snores followed by a silence (apnea) and another series of loud snores is a very suggestive description of a subject with obstructive apnea. The resumption of ventilation can be associated with loud stridorous breathing ("gasping"). Typically, these symptoms are more prominent in the supine position or after alcohol consumption. Occasionally, however, snoring may not be so obvious even in the presence of severe sleep apnea [52]. There is also a growing body of evidence that snoring might cause daytime sleepiness in the absence of OSAS [1]. This might be explained by the upper airway resistance syndrome that is characterised by episodes of increased respiratory effort followed by arousals and daytime sleepiness or by upper airway inflammation due to snoring-induced vibrations within the pharynx [53, 54].

Sleepiness

Pathological daytime sleepiness is the second key symptom in the diagnosis of sleep apnea [51, 55, 56]. It is caused by loss of deep sleep, which presents 20 % of total sleep time in young subjects. The obstruction of the upper airways leads to the activation of the central nervous system, the so-called arousal, with sleep fragmentation as a consequence. A more fragmented sleep will result in a more sleepy patient during daytime. In general, patient and environment will not take much attention towards this daytime sleepiness, as far as it does not lead to repetitive car accidents or occupational accidents. Extreme sleepiness is characterised by falling asleep inadvertently during motor activity (talking, eating). Unequivocal sleepiness means falling asleep at rest, or while driving. The extension of normal diurnal sleepiness is considered as mild sleepiness. Tests have been developed to measure sleepiness more objectively [57]. The multiple sleep latency test (MSLT), maintenance of wakefulness test (MWT) and vigilance tests are used for this purpose. The use of the self-administered questionnaire, the Epworth Sleepiness Scale (ESS), which was validated with MSLT, enhances the accessibility of the quantification of EDS. There is however some controversy, since the ESS does not correlate well with the MSLT and other vigilance tests. Also the AHI only weakly correlates with quantified measures of sleepiness, which indicates that some individuals cope better with sleep fragmentation than others, or could be related to brain susceptibility and subjective perception of the consequences of hypoxemia [58]. Using a cut-off value of 18 events per hour including all apneas, hypopneas and flow limitation events, a sensitivity of 71 % and a specificity of 60 % for identifying subjects with excessive daytime sleepiness were obtained. When flow limitations are not taken into account, the sensitivity/specificity is even far worse [59]. Hence, for clinical purposes, it must be clear that the respiratory disturbance index is a more reliable parameter, but even then, its correlation with daytime symptoms also remains suboptimal.

In the Sleep Heart Health Study, also a weak correlation between the AHI and sleepiness was reported: the ESS only rose from 7.2 to 9.3 when the AHI changed from less than 5 to more than 30 [6]. It is however important to decide whether CPAP therapy should be instituted to treat daytime sleepiness. In case of sleep apnea, MSLT and vigilance testing are most often restricted to patients with persistent hypersomnolence despite adequate continuous positive airway pressure (CPAP) therapy or surgical or oral device therapy. On the other hand, routine use of these tests could be recommended for medicolegal reasons [60]. While tasks arising at regular intervals can even be performed at decreased levels of vigilance, fulfilling the criteria of light sleep, this is not the case for unexpected tasks and events. Therefore, up to 9 % of all traffic accidents are ascribed to sleepiness. In those car accidents in which sleepiness was the obvious cause, the rate of deaths was three times as high as in other accidents. Falling asleep while driving seems to be the cause of 3 % of the accidents causing material damage, 20 % of the accidents causing injuries and 50 % of the accidents causing death [61]. Not rarely, a recent accident can give occasion to consult a physician. A polysomnographic study revealed that socially disturbing loud snoring is associated with OSAS (AHI > 10) in 20 % of the patients referred to exclude sleep apnea. The combination of loud snoring with excessive daytime sleepiness reveals OSAS in 35 % of the referred patients [62]. The difficulty particularly in moderately severe OSAS is to identify EDS resulting from causes other than sleep apnea. Depression and mood disturbance are among the most important confounding factors [63–65]. Obesity alone may also interfere through adipokines and chemokines being activated even in the absence of OSAS. In OSAS, stress activation involving both the HPA axis and the sympathetic system may also play some role.

Other Symptoms at Night

Abnormal motor activity, problems with maintaining sleep and awakening too early in the morning, nightmares, nocturnal dyspnea, nocturnal suffocation and nycturia are often reported. OSAS patients often sleep restless and turn and toss. Apneas are often associated with movements, which can sometimes be limited to mild movements, but abrupt more pronounced arm and leg movements with involuntary kicking and beating of the bed partner can occur [66]. Due to this nocturnal motor activity, OSAS patients often suffer from severe nocturnal transpiration. Nevertheless, the patient is often convinced that he/she is sleeping well at night and is unconscious of the breathing disturbances.

Other Daytime Symptoms

Detailed history taking of patient and bed partner can unravel the association between main symptoms and the sleep apnea syndrome: matinal headache (due to nocturnal CO_2 retention), being not refreshed in the morning, behaviour changes, decreased intellectual performance, depression, anxiety, automatic behaviour, social problems, marital problems, impotence (men), decreased libido, unexplained muscle discomfort and—last but not least—decreased quality of life. The absence of symptoms does not exclude OSAS. On the other hand, it is remarkable that, despite these typical symptoms, the interval between the first symptoms and the final diagnosis can often take some years.

Gender and Age Bias

It should be kept in mind that most studies have been performed in middle-aged subjects (range 50–60 years), clearly overweight male subjects with moderate to severe OSAS. Hence, the symptoms and neurobehavioural as well as cardiovascular and metabolic sequelae in OSAS mainly apply to this cohort. Nevertheless, OSAS can also have a large impact on daytime sleepiness and quality of life in the elderly (>70 years old). Surprisingly, history and daytime symptoms can be less specific in this age category [67]. A gender bias also takes place in the OSAS population, as discussed earlier.

Morbidity and Mortality

Cardiovascular Morbidity

OSAS is a serious health hazard being recognised as an independent risk factor for arterial hypertension, stroke, cardiac arrhythmias and coronary artery disease [7, 68, 69].

Arterial Hypertension

Elevated blood pressure can be present during sleep as a consequence of OSAS [70]. Moreover, hypertension during wakefulness may be related to OSAS. 45 % of patients with OSAS have hypertension. In OSAS, hypoxia increases sympathetic tone via chemo- and baroreflex activation, thus increasing blood pressure [70, 71]. Increased negative intrathoracic pressure (causing increased venous return) and arousal from sleep, both in association with apnoeic events, also contribute to the rise in blood pressure seen in OSAS [72–74]. The absence in OSAS patients of the normal decrease in BP during sleep, termed as "non-dipping", may be the earliest sign of OSAS-related hypertension and an independent risk factor for developing coronary artery disease [75, 76], as well as heart failure, especially heart failure with preserved ejection fraction and a strong risk factor for stroke. The Wisconsin Sleep Cohort Study, a large population-based study ($n=1{,}060$), reported a dose-response relationship between OSAS and hypertension. After correction for known risk factors of hypertension, this relationship was still present [77]. Also the Sleep Heart Health Study ($n=6{,}424$) identified OSAS as an independent risk factor for hypertension [78]. In the 4-year follow-up period, the odds ratio of developing hypertension increased linearly with increasing AHI [79].

Stroke

Evidence from a variety of studies has suggested a link between stroke and OSAS. OSAS patients have an increased risk of stroke [80–82], with the 10-year predicted occurrence of stroke being 14 % [83]. Vice versa, a high prevalence of OSAS was also demonstrated in patients with stroke [84–87].

Central apneas and Cheyne-Stokes respiration have been shown to occur quite commonly in the acute phase of stroke but spontaneously resolve with time and seldom need treatment.

Intermittent hypoxia is probably the most critical factor in the cerebrovascular abnormalities predisposing OSAS patients to stroke. Moreover, impaired cerebrovascular response to hypoxia has been reported in OSAS patients, which is consistent with underlying abnormal endothelial function. Overall, fluctuations in blood pressure, reduction in cerebral blood flow, altered cerebral autoregulation, endothelial dysfunction, accelerated atherogenesis and pro-thrombotic and pro-inflammatory states are mechanisms implicated in the increased risk for stroke in OSAS [88]. Studies have found a direct relationship between nocturnal oxygen desaturations, intima-media thickness and atherosclerotic plaques in the carotid artery, independent of the presence of hypertension, and thereby support a causal relation between OSAS, atherosclerosis and subsequent stroke [89, 90]. Another correlation was found between increased severity of OSAS and incidence of stroke and death in a cohort of OSAS patients after a median follow-up of 3.4 years [80]. Consequently, increased mortality was reported in patients with severe OSAS (AHI > 30) after stroke [85, 91], and cross-sectional data from the Sleep Heart Health Study have shown greater odds for stroke in the highest quartile (AHI > 11) (1.58 [95 % CI 1.02–2.46]) than in the lower quartile (AHI 4.4–11) (1.42 [75 % CI 0.91–2.21]) [82]. Another group showed an odds ratio of 4.33 (95 % CI 1.32–14.24) for prevalent stroke in moderate to severe OSAS (AHI ≥ 20), independent of other risk factors, compared to patients without OSAS. After 4 years of follow-up, an AHI ≥ 20 at baseline was associated with an increased risk of incident stroke after adjustment for age and sex, but not for body mass index (OR 4.48 [95 % CI 1.31–5.33]). However, after adjustment for age, sex and BMI, the OR was still elevated but no longer statistically significant (OR 3.08 [95 % CI 0.74–12.81]) [81].

Cardiac Arrhythmias

Different types of cardiac arrhythmias have been observed and associated with OSAS. The most common arrhythmias during sleep include non-sustained tachycardia, sinus arrest, second-degree atrioventricular conduction block and premature ventricular contractions. Their prevalence and complexity increase with the severity of the OSAS and the associated hypoxemia [92–94]. The Sleep Heart Health Study suggested that patients with OSAS had increased likelihood of atrial fibrillation (OR 4.02 [95 % CI 1.03–15.74]), non-sustained tachycardia (OR 3.40 [95 % CI 1.03–11.20]) and complex ventricular ectopy (OR 1.75 [95 % CI 1.11–2.74]) [95]. The mechanisms by which OSAS induces ventricular arrhythmias are uncertain, but hypoxia, bradyarrhythmias and sympathetic activation induced by apneic events may play an important role. It has been shown that ventricular premature beats decreased by 58 % after 1 month of CPAP treatment in OSAS patients with congestive heart failure (CHF) [96]. The Sleep Heart Health Study assessed a fourfold increase in the prevalence of atrial fibrillation in subjects with an AHI ≥ 30 [95]. Hypoxemia, sympathetic activation, blood pressure changes, transmural pressure surges and systemic inflammation may be mechanisms that predispose to the development of atrial fibrillation. The relationship between OSAS and atrial fibrillation may also contribute to the increased risk of stroke observed in patients with OSAS.

Coronary Artery Disease

Some studies suggest an independent association between OSAS and coronary artery disease (CAD) in middle-aged males and females [97]. One study assessed not only the association between coronary artery calcification (CAC) and OSAS but also highlighted the association between CAC and increasing OSAS severity. The odds ratio for CAC increased with OSAS severity: mild (OR 2.1 [50 % CI 0.8–5.4]), moderate (OR 2.4 [75 % CI 1.0–6.4]) and severe OSAS (OR 3.3 [95 % CI 1.2–9.4]) [98]. The frequency of nocturnal oxygen desaturation correlated with the extent of coronary lesions and explained 13.4 % of their variance, suggesting a pathogenetic role of OSAS in coronary atherosclerosis [99]. The chronic effects of OSAS, such as systemic inflammation, oxidative stress, vascular smooth cell activation, lymphocyte activation, increased lipid levels, lowering in macrophages, lipid peroxidation, high-density lipoprotein dysfunction and endothelial dysfunction, potentially trigger the formation of atherosclerotic plaques. Plaque rupture can be provoked by the acute effects of OSAS, such as intermittent hypoxemia, acidosis, increased BP and systemic vasoconstriction, in conjunction with simultaneous changes in intrathoracic and transmural pressure [88]. Hence, the increased oxygen demand and reduced oxygen supply at night in OSAS patients may trigger an attack of myocardial ischemia and nocturnal angina. Nocturnal angina and ST depression have been described in OSAS patients, which may be diminished after CPAP treatment [100, 101]. However, another study did not find evidence of nocturnal myocardial injury detectable by measurements of cardiac troponin T in patients with established CAD and moderate/severe OSAS [102]. In addition, observations of the occurrence of myocardial infarction (MI) in OSAS patients assessed an altered time interval of nocturnal sudden death compared to the general population. In general, the likelihood of onset of MI is between 06:00 and 11.00 h. In contrast, almost half of OSAS patients have their onset of MI during the sleep hours, between 22:00 and 06:00 h. This may implicate that OSAS may precipitate nocturnal MI [103, 104].

Subclinical Cardiocirculatory Impairment

One of the recent major clinical findings in the past years is the occurrence of atherosclerosis in OSAS patients free of any cardiovascular morbidity and of other cardiovascular risk factors [89, 105]. This is part of the subclinical cardiocirculatory impairment described in OSAS, together with masked hypertension [106], increase in arterial stiffness [107], diastolic dysfunction [108, 109] and left but also right ventricle hypertrophy [110]. Some of these early cardiovascular changes have been correlated with systemic inflammation [111], related to intermittent hypoxemia [112]. About half of the cases presenting with the clinical syndrome of heart failure have a normal left ventricular ejection fraction (so-called heart failure with preserved ejection fraction), and left ventricular diastolic dysfunction is considered to be a common underlying pathology [113]. Studies have shown that the impairment of left ventricular diastolic function is common in OSAS patients, suggesting subclinical myocardial disease that may account for the risk of heart failure [114–116] and also suggesting a role of OSAS in pulmonary hypertension. OSAS appears to be associated with cardiac remodelling and altered diastolic function and to exert an additive effect to that of increased blood pressure in patients with both hypertension and OSAS [108]. Cross-sectional data from the Sleep Heart Health Study have shown a strong association of SDB in moderate and severe OSAS with heart failure (OR 2.38 [95 % CI 1.22–4.62]) and a less strong association for mild OSAS (OR 1.95 [75 % CI 0.99–3.83]) [117].

Cardiovascular Mortality

Observational cohort studies indicate that untreated patients with OSAS have an increased risk of fatal and nonfatal cardiovascular events, an increased risk of sudden cardiac death during the sleeping hours and a higher risk of stroke or death from any cause [7, 68]. According to He et al., the probability of cumulative 8-year survival was 0.96 for patients with an apnea index <20 and 0.63 for those with an apnea index >20. Difference in mortality related to apnea index was particularly true in the patients less than 50 years of age, in whom mortality from other causes is uncommon [118]. In the study of Marin et al., multivariate analysis, adjusted for potential confounders, showed that untreated severe OSAS significantly increased the risk of fatal (OR 2.87 [95 % CI 1.17–7.51]) cardiovascular events compared with healthy participants [7]. Treatment with tracheostomy or CPAP attenuated this risk [7, 118].

Since the group treated with CPAP received more intensive follow-up during the first year after diagnosis (two additional visits), outcome could be improved in this group independently of the CPAP treatment. Moreover, these results were only applicable to men. In patients with coronary artery disease but also in stroke, the occurrence of OSAS was a significant predictor of (early) death [119, 120]. These studies have the inherent limitation of lacking a randomised controlled design, which clearly limits the evidence level. In one prospective study, it was found that the apnea index was a predictor of excess mortality in the fourth and fifth decade, but not in the elderly [121]. In some population-based cohorts, a decrease in survival was reported with increasing OSAS severity, with an OR of 3.0 (95 % CI 1.4–6.3) (Wisconsin) and 1.46 (1.14–1.86) (Sleep Heart Health Study) in subjects with an AHI ≥ 30 compared with those with an AHI < 5 [122, 123]. However, after stratification by age and gender in the Sleep Heart Health Study, the OR remained only significant in males aged <70 years. Lavie et al. proposed a survival advantage in moderate OSAS, suggesting, as a potential mechanism, that chronic intermittent hypoxia during sleep may activate adaptive pathways in the elderly [124]. For example, older subjects have a reduced acute cardiovascular response to arousal from sleep, compared with younger people [125]. Hence, the poorer cardiovascular reactivity of older adults may, paradoxically, reduce the impact of arousals from sleep and protect against cardiovascular morbidity and mortality. However, it has to be reminded that the cardiovascular consequences of sleep apnea in older people may also be influenced by survival bias, as middle-aged, hypertensive OSAS patients may not survive into old age. Discrepancies among studies could potentially be explained by the heterogeneity of the patients included in the elderly populations.

Metabolic Consequences

A number of OSAS metabolic consequences have been identified. Some studies found increased insulin resistance and impaired glucose tolerance in OSAS patients, independent of body weight [126–128], and a worsening of insulin resistance with increasing AHI [129]. However, other investigations failed to demonstrate an independent effect of AHI owing to the major impact of obesity [130]. In cohort of the general population, both the Wisconsin Cohort Study and the Sleep Heart Health Study have identified OSAS as an independent risk factor for insulin resistance, after adjustment for potential confounding variables, such as age, sex and BMI [131, 132]. However, subjects with an AHI ≥ 15 did not differ significantly from those with an AHI < 5 when it came to the risk of developing diabetes over a 4-year period (OR 1.62 [95 % CI 0.7–3.6]), after adjustment for age, sex and BMI [132]. Intermittent hypoxia and sleep fragmentation are thought to play a key role in the development of metabolic disturbances through the activation of the sympathetic nervous system and pro-inflammatory pathways. It was shown that even lower-grade desaturations are strongly linked with glycaemic status abnormalities [133]. Furthermore, the increase in risk for developing diabetes overtime is increased in OSAS independent of the decrease in arterial oxygen saturation [134]. Sleep fragmentation due to cortical and automatic arousals accounts for alterations in sympathetic/parasympathetic activity, and the simultaneous presence of metabolic syndrome and OSAS further increases sympathetic activity and worsens glycaemic control, even after adjustment for body mass index [135]. Alteration in glucose metabolism and sympathovagal balance has been observed previously in normal subjects following two nights of experimental sleep fragmentation [136].

Cognitive Deficits

It comes as no surprise that OSAS with the consecutive sleep disturbance has detrimental effects on cerebral function. Memory, attention and learning ability have been reported to be abnormal in some OSAS patients [137–140]. Both "lower-level" processes (arousal and alertness) and "higher-level" cognitive processes (e.g. executive attention) have been disturbed, including the ability to inhibit inappropriate behaviours and thoughts, regulate attention and plan and organise for the future [50, 141, 142]. Specific cognitive impairments (like thinking, perception, memory, communication or the ability to learn new information) are present in 76 % of OSAS patients [143]. Studies using functional MRI or PET indicate sleep loss as the primary cause of neurocognitive deficits, mainly a basal slowing in information processing, more so than hypoxemia [142]. Whether there are not only functional but also anatomical sequels of OSAS is more difficult to evaluate, since the profound effects of decreased alertness on higher cognitive functioning mimic cerebral damage due to hypoxia. OSAS can promote axonal dysfunction or loss, as well as myelin metabolism impairment in the frontal periventricular white matter, which causes cognitive executive dysfunction [144]. A therapeutic challenge with CPAP can learn that not all cognitive function alterations reverse, and they may represent neuronal damage. Moreover, when cognitive function is preserved in OSAS patients, functional brain imaging has revealed that brain activation is increased, compared with the activation that occurs in healthy controls performing the same task. The association between preserved cognitive function and greater activation in OSAS patients suggests that increased cerebral recruitment (overrecruitment) is required to maintain cognitive performance [145, 146]. Currently, it is also well established that cognitive and attentional deficits may occur in OSAS in the absence of perceived subjective EDS [147]. It questions the sensitivity of the tools used for evaluating EDS. Moreover, attentional deficits may occur without objective EDS [147]. Reaction time and sustained and divided attention tasks may be altered in the absence of sleepiness. It should further be studied whether these attentional deficits may impair driving ability and other social and professional abilities. If confirmed, it raises the question of who should be treated, since the absence of perceived sleepiness would then not be required for treating OSAS.

Associations

Epidemiological studies provide strong evidence that OSAS is highly prevalent in patients with obesity [34, 148], diabetes mellitus [36, 51, 149], arterial hypertension [88, 150], metabolic syndrome [151], cardiovascular disease [152–155] and endocrinopathies [51, 156]. Often, patients with OSAS suffer from sleepiness during daytime, but other symptoms can be present as well, while others remain asymptomatic. In the presence of other disorders, symptoms in OSAS may not conform to the typical history and physical findings. Moreover, sleepiness is a frequently reported symptom in the absence of OSAS and is thereby not a useful clinical symptom to suggest the diagnosis of OSAS in these patients. On the other hand, patients with medical disorders often express fatigue, tiredness or lack of energy rather than sleepiness itself, which can be related to the medical disturbance but can also be the cardinal symptom of an underlying OSAS [12, 157–159] or any other sleep disorder. Their negative effects are more frequent, rapid and intensive if patients suffering from medical disorders also suffer from OSAS. Due to this coincidence of OSAS and disorders of other systems, their consequences are mutually increased [160].

Comorbid OSAS in Obesity

Obesity is linked with OSAS. According to various data, the simultaneous occurrence of obesity and OSAS is approximately 35 %, and their mutual relationship is reciprocal. Deposition of fat even in the neck area, especially in men with central type of obesity, contributes to upper airway obstruction and to easier development of apneas during sleep.

Controversy remains as to whether specific anthropometric indices of body habitus, such as neck or waist circumference, are better predictors of OSAS as compared with BMI alone [36, 149].

However, despite the strong relationship with obesity, it is important to remember that not all subjects who are obese or have a large neck circumference suffer from sleep apnea and that some one-third of OSAS patients are not obese [36].

Comorbid OSAS in Arterial Hypertension

Several large population-based cross-sectional studies have reported an independent link between arterial hypertension and OSAS, when controlling for multiple potential confounding variables. OSAS and systemic hypertension commonly coexist: OSAS is present in at least 30 % of hypertensive patients, while about half of OSAS patients suffer from systemic hypertension [88]. In patients with refractory hypertension, up to 85 % has OSAS. Currently, OSAS is also considered a risk factor in the hypertension management guidelines [150, 161].

Comorbid OSAS in Congestive Heart Failure

Studies have suggested an increased prevalence of OSAS as well as CSA in patients with CHF, even in patients with asymptomatic left ventricular dysfunction, between 20 and 50 % [152]. A failing heart with reduced left ventricular ejection fraction, diastolic dysfunction and increased filling pressures is more vulnerable to stressors such as increased blood pressure (afterload) or sympathetic activation as compared with a healthy heart. It explains why OSAS is particularly detrimental in patients with established heart failure. These data imply that strategies to recognise sleep apnea are highly warranted in CHF patients. Predictive factors for the presence of CSA were male gender, the presence of atrial fibrillation, daytime hypocapnia or age >60 years. The predictive factors for OSAS include an increased BMI (BMI > 35 kg/m^2) in men and age >60 in women [162]. Surprisingly, the majority of patients with CHF and comorbid OSAS do not complain of excessive daytime sleepiness, possibly owing to chronically elevated sympathetic activity [163].

Comorbid OSAS in Atrial Fibrillation

In a study comparing patients with atrial fibrillation (AF) ($n=151$) to patients with no history of AF in a general cardiology practice ($n=312$), Gami et al. demonstrated that the proportion of patients with OSAS was significantly higher in the patients with AF than in the patients without AF (49 % vs. 32 %, $p=0.0004$) [154]. The adjusted OR for AF was 2.19 in OSAS subjects ($p=0.0006$). In a multivariate analysis, BMI, neck circumference, hypertension, diabetes mellitus and AF remained significantly associated with OSAS, and the OR was largest for AF. A higher recurrence of atrial fibrillation after cardioversion has also been reported in those with untreated OSAS compared to those without OSAS [164]. Therefore, patients referred for the evaluation of significant tachyarrhythmia or bradyarrhythmia should be questioned about symptoms of sleep apnea.

Comorbid OSAS in Coronary Artery Disease

There is a high prevalence of OSAS among patients with angiographically proven coronary artery disease and an increased incidence of coronary artery disease in patients free of coronary symptoms at the time of OSAS diagnosis [155]. Data suggest that patients with coronary artery disease should be particularly questioned for symptoms and signs of sleep apnea. If there is even the slightest suspicion of sleep apnea, the patients should undergo a polysomnography [162].

Comorbid OSAS in Endocrine and Metabolic Disorders

OSAS is common in many endocrine and metabolic conditions, like insulin resistance, type 2 diabetes and the metabolic syndrome [51, 156, 165]. Given the high prevalence of OSAS among these patient categories, specialists treating metabolic disorders and abnormalities should consider investigation for OSAS in their patients.

Hypothyroidism

OSAS has been reported to occur frequently in patients with untreated hypothyroidism (50–100 %), especially when myxoedema (dry skin and hair, loss of mental and physical vigour) is present [166]. However, there are no conclusive studies since an association could largely be explained by coexisting obesity and male sex. No large prospective studies investigating the prevalence of OSAS in patients with hypothyroidism are available. However, patients with hypothyroidism, especially when clinical signs are present, should be screened for the presence of OSAS. Symptoms of OSAS in patients with comorbid hypothyroidism do not substantially differ from those with normal thyroid function [51, 165].

Pathogenesis appears to involve both myopathy and upper airway edema [167]. Both maximal and median apnea duration and maximum oxyhaemoglobin saturation are significantly correlated with thyroxin levels and improve with substitution therapy. Hormone therapy also significantly improves apnea index and arousal index. Some studies report persisting apneas despite adequate replacement therapy, which supports the view of a chance rather than causal association. In these circumstances, such patients continue to require regular nasal CPAP.

Acromegaly

OSAS is common in acromegaly, a condition resulting from excessive growth hormone, with prevalence rates ranging from 12 % to 75 % in unselected patients with acromegaly [168]. Sleep apnea is more likely to occur with increased severity of acromegaly, higher age, greater neck circumference, greater initial tongue volume, presence of alterations in craniofacial dimensions (predominantly of the mandible) and upper airway narrowing due to changes in pharyngeal soft tissues [169]. Other factors involved are facial bone deformity, mucosal edema, hypertrophy of the pharyngeal and laryngeal cartilages and the presence of nasal polyps. Increases in BMI in acromegaly may be due to increased muscle mass rather than the increased body fat typically seen in obesity, and BMI is often normal [170]. There appears to be no relationship between OSAS and biochemical parameters of disease activity such as growth hormone and IGF-1 levels. OSAS may still persist despite normalisation of growth hormone levels during therapy. CSA is also common and is associated with higher random growth hormone and IGF-1 levels than in OSAS. Possible mechanisms for the development of central apneas in patients with acromegaly include reflex inhibition of the respiratory centre as a result of the narrowing of the upper airways or due to an increase in the ventilatory response of the respiratory centre to CO_2. At present, it is not known what proportion of patients with both sleep apnea and acromegaly will have complete resolution of their sleep apnea after cure of acromegaly. Nevertheless, it is clear that sleep apnea does occur in cured acromegaly, due to coincidence, slow resolution of the effects of acromegaly, or maybe permanent effects on upper airway function or sleep-related regulation [156, 165].

Cushing's Syndrome

Patients with Cushing's syndrome (CS) have an excess of adrenocorticosteroid hormones. Sleep complaints are common, including an increased incidence of OSAS of approximately 18–32 % in patients with CS (in those with pituitary disease) [171]. In one study all CS patients had an AHI of at least 5. Fat accumulation in the parapharyngeal area may be important in the pathogenesis of OSAS [172]. Patients with CS can also present with steroid-induced changes in sleep architecture including more fragmented sleep, poorer sleep continuity, shortened REM latency, a decrease in delta sleep and an increased REM density, which may explain the insomnia and fatigue and possibly some of the psychiatric symptoms. These features can be aggravated by concomitant OSAS [12, 51, 156, 173].

OSAS and Diabetes Mellitus

Both type 2 diabetes mellitus and OSAS have a prevalence of 3–5 % of the general population and occur with increased frequency in the obese [174]. Therefore, it is not surprising that a significant number of patients suffer from both conditions. Recent reports have indicated that many patients with type 2 diabetes have OSAS, but the relationship between OSAS and metabolic disturbance is most likely bidirectional and at least partially independent of adiposity [175]. In type 2 diabetic patients with OSAS, several studies have assessed the impact of CPAP treatment on glycaemic control [176]. Recent observational studies using continuous glucose monitoring techniques have reported positive effects of CPAP on glycaemic control, already present during the first night of treatment, as variability of glycaemic values decreased compared with baseline conditions [177]. The reduction in HbA1c level was significantly correlated with CPAP use. Hence, screening for OSAS in diabetes may help to improve glycaemic control, especially in insufficiently controlled type 2 diabetic patients. In diabetic patients with autonomic neuropathy, OSAS is also more prevalent (26 %) than in those without, and diabetic neuropathy appears to be directly linked to OSAS [178].

OSAS and Metabolic Syndrome

According to clinical and epidemiological studies, the cluster of risk factors known as the metabolic syndrome is associated with increased risk of diabetes, cardiovascular events and mortality in the general population [179]. Insulin resistance is considered as the major metabolic abnormality and is usually associated with an increased amount of visceral fat [180, 181]. A very high prevalence of severe OSAS (82 %) was reported in metabolic syndrome patients [151]. Prevalence of the metabolic syndrome is also higher in patients with OSAS than in the European general population (15–20 %) or in obese subjects without OSAS [182]. This indicates a bidirectional association between OSAS and metabolic syndrome. Indeed, visceral obesity and the cluster of the metabolic risk factors may lead to OSAS, which in turn may accelerate these metabolic abnormalities, possibly through the induction of inflammation and oxidative stress [151]. Co-occurrence of these two conditions increases remarkably the risk of cardiovascular events and mortality, with higher blood pressure and sympathetic activity, compared with patients with metabolic syndrome without OSAS. The need for screening of metabolic syndrome patients for OSAS is furthermore highlighted by several studies demonstrating improvements in insulin sensitivity in patients with metabolic syndrome after successful treatment of comorbid OSAS by CPAP [183].

OSAS in COPD

Patients with COPD sleep poorly compared to healthy subjects [184]. By coincidence they have a high prevalence of OSAS. The incidence of sleep complaints is related to the rates of respiratory symptoms in COPD patients [184, 185]. However, compared with patients who only have COPD, those suffering also from OSAS have higher ESS scores, lower total sleep time, lower sleep efficiency and higher arousal index [186]. The coexistence of COPD and OSAS favors the presence of daytime hypoxemia and can lead to earlier development of hypercapnia relative to the COPD severity class. Arousals may or may not be related to hypoxemia [165, 187].

OSAS in Chronic Renal Failure and End-Stage Renal Disease

OSAS is ten times more prevalent in patients with end-stage renal disease than in the normal population and is improved by haemodialysis [188]. The pathophysiology of OSAS in this population is mainly related to metabolic disturbances including uraemia, fluid overload, dialysis treatments (with accompanying changes in serum electrolytes, osmolarity and acid-base balance) and the production of somnogenic substances such as IL-1 and TNF-α during dialysis. Patients with end-stage renal disease do not often conform to the stereotypical presentation of OSAS and are generally not obese [189, 190]. Patients with end-stage renal disease often have multiple sleep disturbances, which may complicate the interpretation of signs and symptoms of OSAS and may result in underdiagnosis of OSAS in this population [51, 189].

OSAS and Polycythaemia

Hypoxemic states are frequently associated with increased haematocrit levels [191]. In OSAS, it is thought that this hypoxic stress might lead to secondary polycythaemia. The evidence is largely anecdotal, and there have been few studies that systematically examined this phenomenon [192, 193]. However, after controlling for possible confounding variables, haematocrit is only modestly increased (just 2–3 %) in patients with severe OSAS, compared to controls, and still within the clinically accepted normal range. Hence, OSAS does not lead to clinically significant polycythaemia. On the other hand, the search for the origin of unexplained polycythaemia anecdotally reveals the presence of OSAS.

Moreover, the observation that successful treatment of OSAS with nasal CPAP decreases haematocrit after 1 night indicates a causal relationship between polycythaemia and OSAS [194]. An association with OSAS will more often be found in the presence of other comorbid respiratory conditions, with hypoventilation and chronic nocturnal hypoxemia, as present in obesity hypoventilation [21].

Economical Burden of Untreated OSAS

OSAS gives rise to several complications like motor vehicle accidents (MVAs) and occupational accidents secondary to hypersomnolence, cardiovascular complications and metabolic disturbances like insulin resistance and lipid disturbances. Patients with OSAS have not only more accidents but very often also repeated accidents [195]. It may therefore also represent a health hazard for unaffected individuals who happen to cross the road in front of these patients. There is no doubt that medical consumption in OSAS is also significantly increased: there are more hospitalisations, more ambulatory contacts and a higher consumption of drugs [196]. In 2000, the costs related to car accidents in the USA due to OSAS were estimated at more than 15 billion dollars [197]. A very effective method to document the additional cost of OSAS is the comparison of the costs before and after treatment. In a retrospective study, the hospitalisation duration was evaluated 2 years before and 2 years after the start of CPAP therapy [198]. 88 patients were studied and the number of hospitalisation days decreased (from 413 in the 2 years before the therapy to 54 in the 2 years following the start of the therapy), which is a very convincing effect. Several studies have also demonstrated the effect of CPAP therapy on the costs related to accidents due to OSAS. In a study in 547 OSAS patients looking at the incidence of accidents before and after the start of CPAP therapy, it was shown that the number of effective accidents decreased from 1.6 to 1.1 per patient and the number of near-miss accidents from 4.5 to 1.8 per patient [199]. The number of hospitalisation days related to accidents decreased from 885 days to 84 days. It has to be remarked that not only MVAs were taken into account but also occupational and domestic accidents. Sassani et al. calculated that this could reduce the cost of 15 billion dollars to almost 3 billion dollars [197]. Although these data originate from the USA, there is no reason to believe that this data would be different in Europe. The cost per QALY related to MVAs amounts for only 3,354 dollars [200, 201]. These values compare very favourably with other publicly funded therapies and are lower than the cost per QALY for coronary reperfusion in ischaemic heart disease (18,000 dollars), the use of inhalation corticoids in COPD (19,000 dollars) [202] or the use of cholesterol-lowering therapy (54,000 dollars to 1.4 million dollars) [203]. Moreover, the overall medical consumption seems to decrease after the start of an efficient therapy [204], while medical consumption is increasing gradually in patients with untreated OSAS. After the diagnostic assessment and start of therapy, there was a decrease of 1.95 visits per year versus an increase of 0.48 visits in the control group. Of course, the correct and efficient performance of tasks in an occupational setting has also a great economic impact, although it is hard to measure this directly. In an older study excessive daytime sleepiness at work was evaluated in workers with and without complaints of snoring. Those with snoring had four times more sleepiness than those without. Also the ability to concentrate on new tasks and to learn and execute them was significantly worse [205]. Therefore, it is not surprising that economic models have clearly demonstrated the cost-effectiveness of interventions for OSAS [200, 206, 207].

Meanwhile, it has also become clear that this cost-effectivity is not only related to the effects in males [208]. Also in women a decrease in medical consumption could be achieved after the start of CPAP therapy. Again, also in women a gradual increase in medical consumption in the 2 years before diagnosis and a significant decrease in the 2 following years took place [209]. Altogether, there is enough evidence that demonstrates that SDB, particularly OSAS, is associated with a strong increase in medical consumption. On the one hand, this is the consequence of the co-morbidities but on the other hand also due to excessive daytime sleepiness-related accidents on the road or at work. Several studies have also indicated that an efficient treatment, predominantly CPAP, can significantly decrease this increased medical consumption. Economic models show a very favourable cost per QALY for CPAP therapy. Therefore, screening and treatment of OSAS is one of the better cost-effective interventions.

Conclusions

OSAS is a highly prevalent disorder and characterised by considerable cardiovascular, metabolic and neurocognitive morbidity. Untreated patients with OSAS also have an increased risk of fatal cardiovascular events and death from any cause. Loud snoring is the most prominent symptom. There is still no final agreement on the definitions to be used to describe patients with OSAS. OSAS is also very often associated in common medical disorders.

Patients with OSAS have increased utilisation of health resources, related to the severity of the disease and the associated co-morbidities. These costs increase over time until diagnosis and decrease after the administration of an effective treatment. Moreover, OSAS represents a serious hazard on the road. Therefore, early identification of abnormalities is warranted and may reduce end-organ damage and economic burden.

References

1. Young T, Palta M, Dempsey J, Skatrud J, Weber S, Badr S. The occurrence of sleep-disordered breathing among middle-aged adults. N Engl J Med. 1993;328(17):1230–5.
2. Young T, Peppard PE, Gottlieb DJ. Epidemiology of obstructive sleep apnea. A population health perspective. Am J Respir Crit Care Med. 2002;165:1217–39.
3. Mannino DM, Homa DM, Akinbami LJ, Ford ES, Redd SC. Chronic obstructive pulmonary disease surveillance – United States, 1971–2000. MMWR. 2002;51:1–16.
4. Lindberg A, Jonsson AC, Rönmark E, et al. Prevalence of chronic obstructive pulmonary disease according to BTS, ERS, GOLD and ATS criteria in relation to doctor's diagnosis, symptoms, age, gender, and smoking habits. Respiration. 2005;72:471–9.
5. Von Mutius E, Martinez FD, Fritzsch C, Nicolai T, Roell G, Thiemann H. Prevalence of asthma and atopy in two areas of West and East Germany. Am J Respir Crit Care Med. 1994;149:358–64.

6. Gottlieb DJ, Whitney CW, Bonekat WH, et al. Relation of sleepiness to respiratory disturbance index: the Sleep Heart Health Study. Am J Respir Crit Care Med. 1999;159:502–7.
7. Marin JM, Crrizo SJ, Vicente E, et al. Long-term cardiovascular outcomes in men with obstructive sleep apnoea-hypopnoea with or without treatment with continuous positive airway pressure: an observational study. Lancet. 2005;365(9464):1046–53.
8. Valipour A, Lothaller H, Rauscher H, Zwick H, Burghuber OC, Lavie P. Gender-related differences in symptoms of patients with suspected breathing disorders in sleep: a clinical population study using the sleep disorders questionnaire. Sleep. 2007;30(3):312–9.
9. Bixler EO, Vgontzas AN, Ten Havre T, et al. Effects of age on sleep apnea in men: prevalence and severity. Am J Respir Crit Care Med. 1998;157:144–8.
10. Durán J, Esnaola S, Rubio R, Iztueta A. Obstructive sleep apnea-hypopnea and related clinical features in a population-based sample of subjects aged 30 to 70 yr. Am J Respir Crit Care Med. 2001;163:685–9.
11. McNicholas WT, Bonsignore MR. Sleep apnoea as an independent risk factor for cardiovascular disease: current evidence, basic mechanisms and research priorities. Eur Respir J. 2007;29:156–78.
12. Report of a Task Force of the American Academy of Sleep Medicine. Sleep-related breathing disorders in adults: recommendations for syndrome definition and measurement techniques in clinical research. Sleep. 1999;22:667–89.
13. American Academy of Sleep Medicine. International classification of sleep disorders, 3rd ed. Darien, IL: American Academy of Sleep Medicine; 2014.
14. Verbraecken J, De Backer W. Upper airway mechanics. Respiration. 2009;78:121–33.
15. Berry RB, Budhiraja R, Gottlieb DJ, et al. Rules for scoring respiratory events in sleep. Update of the 2007 AASM Manual for the scoring of sleep and associated events. J Clin Sleep Med. 2012;8(5):597–619.
16. Epstein LJ, Kristo D, Strollo Jr PJ, et al. Clinical guidelines for the evaluation, management and long-term care of obstructive sleep apnea in adults. J Clin Sleep Med. 2009;5:263–76.
17. Ayappa I, Norman RG, Krieger AC, Rosen A, O'malley RL, Rapoport DM. Non-Invasive detection of respiratory effort-related arousals (REras) by a nasal cannula/pressure transducer system. Sleep. 2000;23(6):763–71.
18. Iber C, Ancoli-Israel S, Chesson AL, et al. The AASM Manual for the scoring of sleep and associated events: rules, terminology and technical specifications. AASM Manual for scoring sleep. AASM, Westchester, IL, USA. 2007.
19. Gold AR, et al. The symptoms and signs of upper airway resistance syndrome. A link to the functional somatic syndromes. Chest. 2003;123:87–95.
20. Bao G, Guilleminault C. Upper airway resistance syndrome – one decade later. Curr Opin Pulm Med. 2004;10:461–7.
21. Piper AJ. Nocturnal hypoventilation – identifying and treating syndromes. Indian J Med Res. 2010;131:350–65.
22. Mokhlesi B. Obesity hypoventilation syndrome: a state-of-the-art review. Respir Care. 2010;55:1347–65.
23. Berger KI, Goldring RM, Rapoport DM. Obesity hypoventilation syndrome. Semin Respir Crit Care Med. 2009;30:253–61.
24. Berger KI, Ayappa I, Chatr-Amontri B, et al. Obesity hypoventilation syndrome as a spectrum of respiratory disturbances during sleep. Chest. 2001;120:1231–8.
25. Stradling JR, Davies RJ. Sleep. 1: Obstructive sleep apnoea/hypopnoea syndrome: definitions, epidemiology, and natural history. Thorax. 2004;59:73–8.
26. Stradling JR, Barbour C, Glennon J, Langford BA, Crosby JH. Prevalence of sleepiness and its relation to autonomic evidence of arousals and increased inspiratory effort in a community based population of men and women. J Sleep Res. 2000;9:381–8.
27. McNicholas WT, Bonsignore MR. Obstructive sleep apnoea. Introduction. Eur Respir Mon. 2010;50:vii–ix.
28. Janson C, Gislason T, De Backer W, et al. Daytime sleepiness, snoring and gastro-oesophageal reflux amongst young adults in three European countries. J Intern Med. 1995;237:277–85.

29. Schmidt-Nowara WW, Coultas DB, Wiggins C, et al. Snoring in a Hispanic-American population. Risk factors and association with hypertension and other morbidity. Arch Intern Med. 1990;150:597–601.
30. Lindberg E, Taube A, Janson C, et al. A 10-year follow-up of snoring in men. Chest. 1998;114:1048–55.
31. Svensson M, Lindberg E, Naessen T, et al. Risk factors associated with snoring in women with special emphasis on body mass index: a population-based study. Chest. 2006;129:933–41.
32. Cirignotta F, D'Alessandro R, Partinen M, et al. Prevalence of every night snoring and obstructive sleep apnoeas among 30-69-year-old men in Bologna, Italy. Acta Psychiatr Scand. 1989;79:366–72.
33. Franklin KA, Gislason T, Omenaas E, et al. The influence of active and passive smoking on habitual snoring. Am J Respir Crit Care Med. 2004;170:799–803.
34. Peppard PE, Young T, Palta M, Dempsey J, Skatrud J. Longitudinal study of moderate weight change and sleep-disordered breathing. JAMA. 2000;284(23):3015–21.
35. Schwab RJ, Gupta KB, Gefter WB, Metzger LJ, Hoffman EA, Pack AI. Upper airway and soft tissue anatomy in normal subjects and patients with sleep-disordered breathing. Significance of the lateral pharyngeal walls. Am J Respir Crit Care Med. 1995;152:1673–89.
36. Lindberg E. Epidemiology of OSA. Eur Respir Mon. 2010;50:51–68.
37. Lecube A, Sampol G, Lloberes P, et al. Asymptomatic sleep-disordered breathing in premenopausal women awaiting bariatric surgery. Obes Surg. 2010;20:454–61.
38. Young T, Shahar E, Nieto FJ, et al. Sleep Heart Health Study Research Group. Predictors of sleep-disordered breathing in community-dwelling adults: the sleep Heart Health Study. Arch Intern Med 2002;162(8):893–900.
39. Young T. Sleep-disordered breathing in older adults: is it a condition distinct from that in middle-aged adults? Sleep. 1996;19(7):529–30.
40. Lévy P, Pépin JL, Malauzat D, et al. Is sleep apnea syndrome in the elderly a specific entity? Sleep. 1996;19:S29–38.
41. Lavie P, Lavie L, Herer P. All-cause mortality in males with sleep apnoea syndrome: declining mortality rates with age. Eur Respir J. 2005;25:514–20.
42. Young T, Hutton R, Finn L, et al. The gender bias in sleep apnea diagnosis. Are women missed because they have different symptoms? Arch Intern Med. 1996;156(21):2445–51.
43. Ye L, Pien GW, Weaver TE. Gender differences in the clinical manifestation of obstructive sleep apnea. Sleep Med. 2009;10:1075–84.
44. Hader C, Schroeder A, Hinz M, et al. Sleep disordered breathing in the elderly: comparison of women and men. J Physiol Pharmacol. 2005;56 Suppl 4:85–91.
45. Wetter DW, Young TB, Bidwell TR, et al. Smoking as a risk factor for sleep-disordered breathing. Arch Intern Med. 1994;154:2219–24.
46. Newman AB, Nieto FJ, Guidry U, et al. Relation of sleep-disordered breathing to cardiovascular disease risk factors: the Sleep Heart Health Study. Am J Epidemiol. 2001;154:50–9.
47. Peppard PE, Austin D, Brown RL. Association of alcohol consumption and sleep disordered breathing in men and women. J Clin Sleep Med. 2007;3:265–70.
48. Villaneuva AT, Buchanan PR, Yee BJ, Grunstein RR. Ethnicity and obstructive sleep apnoea. Sleep Med Rev. 2005;9:419–36.
49. Lee RW, Vasudavan S, Hui DS, Prvan T, Petocz P, Darendeliler MA, Cistulli PA. Differences in craniofacial structures and obesity in Caucasian and Chinese patients with obstructive sleep apnea. Sleep. 2010;33:1075–80.
50. Banno K, Kryger MH. Sleep apnea: clinical investigations in humans. Sleep Med. 2007;8:400–26.
51. Tkacova R, Dorkova Z. Clinical presentations of OSA in adults. Eur Respir Mon. 2010;50:86–103.
52. Peter JH, Koehler U, Grote L, Podszus T. Manifestations and consequences of obstructive sleep apnoea. Eur Respir J. 1995;8:1572–83.

53. Guilleminault C, Stoohs R, Clerk A, et al. A cause of excessive daytime sleepiness. The upper airway resistance syndrome. Chest. 1993;104:781–7.
54. Vgontzas AN, Zoumakis E, Lin HM, et al. Marked decrease in sleepiness in patients with sleep apnea by etanercept, a tumor necrosis factor-alpha antagonist. J Clin Endocrinol Metab. 2004;89:4409–13.
55. Ohayon MM. Epidemiology of excessive daytime sleepiness. Sleep Med Clin. 2006;1:9–16.
56. Hirshkowitz M, Gast H. Sleep-related breathing disorders and sleepiness. Sleep Med Clin. 2006;1:491–8.
57. Silber MH. The investigation of sleepiness. Sleep Med Clin. 2006;1:1–7.
58. Martin SE, Engleman HM, Kingshott RN, Douglas NJ. Microarousals in patients with sleep apnoea/hypopnoea syndrome. J Sleep Res. 1997;6(4):276–80.
59. Hosselet J, Ayappa I, Norman RG, Krieger AC, Rapoport DM. Classification of sleep-disordered breathing. Am J Respir Crit Care Med. 2001;163:398–405.
60. Arand D, Bonnet M, Hurwitz T, Milter M, Rosa R, Sangal RB. The clinical use of the MSLT and MWT. Sleep. 2005;28:123–44.
61. Krieger J, McNicholas WT, Levy P, et al. Public health and medicolegal implications of sleep apnoea. Eur Respir J. 2002;20:1594–609.
62. Boudewyns A, Willemen M, De Cock W, et al. Does socially disturbing snoring and/or excessive daytime sleepiness warrant polysomnography? Clin Otolaryngol. 1997;22:403–7.
63. Koutsourelakis I, Perraki E, Economou NT, et al. Predictors of residual sleepiness in adequately treated obstructive sleep apnoea patients. Eur Respir J. 2009;34:687–93.
64. Stradling JR, Smith D, Croby J. Post-CPAP sleepiness – a specific syndrome? J Sleep Res. 2007;16:436–8.
65. Pépin JL, Viot-Blanc V, Escourrou P, et al. Prevalence of residual excessive sleepiness in CPAP-treated sleep apnoea patients: the French multicentre study. Eur Respir J. 2009;33: 1062–7.
66. Walters AS. Clinical identification of the simple sleep-related movement disorders. Chest. 2007;131:1260–6.
67. Bonsignore MR, McNicholas WT. Sleep-disordered breathing in the elderly. Eur Respir Mon. 2009;43:179–204.
68. Gami AS, Howard DE, Olson EJ, et al. Day-night pattern of sudden death in obstructive sleep apnea. N Engl J Med. 2005;353(12):1206–14.
69. Artz M, Young T, Finn L, et al. Association of sleep-disordered breathing and the occurrence of stroke. Am J Respir Crit Care Med. 2005;172:1447–51.
70. Duran-Cantolla J, Aizpuru F, Martinez-Null C, Barbé-Illa F. Obstructive sleep apnea/hypopnea and systemic hypertension. Sleep Med Rev. 2009;13:323–31.
71. Veale D, Pepin JL, Levy PA. Autonomic stress tests in obstructive sleep apnea syndrome and snoring. Sleep. 1992;15:505–13.
72. Peker Y, Hedner J, Norum J, Kraiczi H, Carlson J. Increased incidence of cardiovascular disease in middle-aged men with obstructive sleep apnea: a 7-year follow-up. Am J Respir Crit Care Med. 2002;166(2):159–65.
73. Silverberg DS, Oksenberg A. Are sleep-related breathing disorders important contributing factors to the production of essential hypertension? Curr Hypertens Rep. 2001;3(3):209–15.
74. Hedner J, Bengtsson-Bostrom K, Peker Y, Grote L, Rastam L, Lindblad U. Hypertension prevalence in obstructive sleep apnoea and sex: a population-based case-control study. Eur Respir J. 2006;27(3):564–70.
75. Suzuki M, Guilleminault C, Otsuka K, Shiomi T. Blood pressure "dipping" and "non-dipping" in obstructive sleep apnea syndrome patients. Sleep. 1996;19(5):382–7.
76. Davies CW, Crosby JH, Mullins RL, Barbour C, Davies RJ, Stradling JR. Case-control study of 24 hour ambulatory blood pressure in patients with obstructive sleep apnoea and normal matched control subjects. Thorax. 2000;55(9):736–40.
77. Young T, Peppard P, Palta M, Hla KM, Finn L, Morgan B, Skatrud J. Population-based study of sleep-disordered breathing as a risk factor for hypertension. Arch Intern Med. 1997; 157(15):1746–52.

78. Nieto FJ, Young TB, Lind BK, et al. Association of sleep-disordered breathing, sleep apnea, and hypertension in a large community-based study. Sleep heart health study. JAMA. 2000;283(14):1829–36.
79. Peppard PE, Young T, Palta M, Skatrud J. Prospective study of the association between sleep-disordered breathing and hypertension. N Engl J Med. 2000;342(19):1378–84.
80. Yaggi HK, Concato J, Kernan WN, Lichtman JH, Brass LM, Mohsenin V. Obstructive sleep apnea as a risk factor for stroke and death. N Engl J Med. 2005;353(19):2034–41.
81. Arzt M, Young T, Finn L, Skatrud JB, Bradley TD. Association of sleep-disordered breathing and the occurrence of stroke. Am J Respir Crit Care Med. 2005;172(11):1447–51.
82. Redline S, Yenokyan G, Gottlieb DJ, et al. Obstructive sleep apnea-hypopnea and incident stroke: the Sleep Heart Health Study. Am J Respir Crit Care Med. 2010;182:269–77.
83. Kiely J, McNicholas W. Cardiovascular risk factors in patients with obstructive sleep apnoea syndrome. Eur Respir J. 2000;16:128–33.
84. Good D, Henkle J, Gelber D, Welsh J, Verhulst S. Sleep-disordered breathing and poor functional outcome after stroke. Stroke. 1996;27(2):252–9.
85. Bassetti C, Milanova M, Grugger M. Sleep-disordered breathing and acute ischemic stroke: diagnosis, risk factors, treatment, evolution, and long-term clinical outcome. Stroke. 2006;37(4):967–72.
86. Bassetti C, Aldrich MS, Chervin RD, Quint D. Sleep apnea in patients with transient ischemic attack and stroke: a prospective study of 59 patients. Neurology. 1996;47(5):1167–73.
87. Wessendorf TE, Teschler H, Wang YM, Konietzko N, Thilmann AF. Sleep-disordered breathing among patients with first-ever stroke. J Neurol. 2000;247(1):41–7.
88. Somers VK, White DP, Amin R, et al. Sleep apnea and cardiovascular disease: An American Heart Association/American College of Cardiology Foundation Scientific Statement from the American Heart Association Council for High Blood Pressure Research Professional Education Committee, Council on Clinical Cardiology, Stroke Council, and Council on Cardiovascular Nursing. In Collaboration with the National Heart, Lung, and Blood Institute National Center on Sleep Disorders Research (National Institutes of Health). Circulation. 2008;118:1080–111.
89. Baguet JP, Hammer L, Levy P, Pierre H, Launois S, Mallion JM, Pepin JL. The severity of oxygen desaturation is predictive of carotid wall thickening and plaque occurrence. Chest. 2005;128(5):3407–12.
90. Suzuki T, Nakano H, Maekawa J, Okamoto Y, Ohnishi Y, Yamauchi M, Kimura H. Obstructive sleep apnea and carotid-artery intima-media thickness. Sleep. 2004;27(1):129–33.
91. Parra O, Arboix A, Montserrat JM, Quinto L, Bechich S, Garcia-Eroles L. Sleep-related breathing disorders: impact on mortality of cerebrovascular disease. Eur Respir J. 2004;24(2):267–72.
92. Liston R, Deegan P, McCreery C, McNicholas W. Role of respiratory sleep disorders in the pathogenesis of nocturnal angina and arrhythmias. Postgrad Med J. 1994;70(822):275–80.
93. Koehler U, Schafer H. Is obstructive sleep apnea (OSA) a risk factor for myocardial infarction and cardiac arrhythmias in patients with coronary heart disease (CHD)? Sleep. 1996;19(4):283–6.
94. Shepard Jr JW. Hypertension, cardiac arrhythmias, myocardial infarction, and stroke in relation to obstructive sleep apnea. Clin Chest Med. 1992;13(3):437–58.
95. Mehra R, Benjamin EJ, Shahar E, Gottlieb DJ, Nawabit R, Kirchner HL, Sahadevan J, Redline S. Association of nocturnal arrhythmias with sleep-disordered breathing: the Sleep Heart Health Study. Am J Respir Crit Care Med. 2006;173(8):910–6.
96. Ryan CM, Usui K, Floras JS, Bradley TD. Effect of continuous positive airway pressure on ventricular ectopy in heart failure patients with obstructive sleep apnoea. Thorax. 2005;60(9):781–5.
97. Peker Y, Kraiczi H, Hedner J, Loth S, Johansson A, Bende M. An independent association between obstructive sleep apnoea and coronary artery disease. Eur Respir J. 1999;14(1):179–84.

98. Sorajja D, Gami AS, Somers VK, Behrenbeck TR, Garcia-Touchard A, Lopez-Jimenez F. Independent association between obstructive sleep apnea and subclinical coronary artery disease. Chest. 2008;133(4):927–33.
99. Hayashi M, Fujimoto K, Urushibata K, Uchikawa S, Imamura H, Kubo K. Nocturnal oxygen desaturation correlates with the severity of coronary atherosclerosis in coronary artery disease. Chest. 2003;124(3):936–41.
100. Franklin KA, Nilsson JB, Sahlin C, Naslund U. Sleep apnoea and nocturnal angina. Lancet. 1995;345(8957):1085–7.
101. Peled N, Abinader EG, Pillar G, Sharif D, Lavie P. Nocturnal ischemic events in patients with obstructive sleep apnea syndrome and ischemic heart disease: effects of continuous positive air pressure treatment. J Am Coll Cardiol. 1999;34(6):1744–9.
102. Gami AS, Svatikova A, Wolk R, Olson EJ, Duenwald CJ, Jaffe AS, Somers VK. Cardiac troponin T in obstructive sleep apnea. Chest. 2004;125(6):2097–100.
103. Narkiewicz K, Montano N, Cogliati C, van de Borne PJ, Dyken ME, Somers VK. Altered cardiovascular variability in obstructive sleep apnea. Circulation. 1998;98(11):1071–7.
104. Kuniyoshi FH, Garcia-Touchard A, Gami AS, et al. Day-night variation of acute myocardial infarction in obstructive sleep apnea. J Am Coll Cardiol. 2008;52(5):343–6.
105. Drager LF, Bortolotto LA, Lorenzi MC, et al. Early signs of atherosclerosis in obstructive sleep apnea. Am J Respir Crit Care Med. 2005;172(5):613–8.
106. Baguet JP, Hammer L, Levy P, et al. Night-time and diastolic hypertension are common and underestimated conditions in newly diagnosed apnoeic patients. J Hypertens. 2005;23(3):521–7.
107. Tsioufis C, Thomopoulos K, Dimitriadis K, et al. The incremental effect of obstructive sleep apnoea syndrome on arterial stiffness in newly diagnosed essential hypertensive subjects. J Hypertens. 2007;25(1):141–6.
108. Drager LF, et al. Obstructive sleep apnea, hypertension, and their interaction on arterial stiffness and heart remodeling. Chest. 2007;131:1379–86.
109. Alchanatis M, Tourkohoriti G, Kosmas EN, et al. Evidence for left ventricular dysfunction in patients with obstructive sleep apnoea syndrome. Eur Respir J. 2002;20(5):1239–45.
110. Shivalkar B, Van de Heyning C, Kerremans M, et al. Obstructive sleep apnea syndrome: more insights on structural and functional cardiac alterations, and the effects of treatment with continuous positive airway pressure. J Am Coll Cardiol. 2006;47:1433–9.
111. Minoguchi K, Yokoe T, Tazaki T, et al. Increased carotid intima-media thickness and serum inflammatory markers in obstructive sleep apnea. Am J Respir Crit Care Med. 2005;172(5):625–30.
112. Lavie L. Obstructive sleep apnoea syndrome – an oxidative stress disorder. Sleep Med Rev. 2003;7(1):35–51.
113. Aurigemma GP, Gaasch WH. Diastolic heart failure. N Engl J Med. 2004;351(11):1097–105.
114. Chan J, Sanderson J, Chan W, Lai C, Choy D, Ho A, Leung R. Prevalence of sleep-disordered breathing in diastolic heart failure. Chest. 1997;111(6):1488–93.
115. Fung JW, Li TS, Choy DK, et al. Severe obstructive sleep apnea is associated with left ventricular diastolic dysfunction. Chest. 2002;121(2):422–9.
116. Arias MA, Garcia-Rio F, Alonso-Fernandez A, Mediano O, Martinez I, Villamor J. Obstructive sleep apnea syndrome affects left ventricular diastolic function: effects of nasal continuous positive airway pressure in men. Circulation. 2005;112(3):375–83.
117. Shahar E, Whitney CRS. Sleep-disordered breathing and cardiovascular disease: cross-sectional results of the Sleep Heart Health Study. Am J Respir Crit Care Med. 2001;163(1):19–25.
118. He J, Kryger MH, Zorick FJ, Conway W, Roth T. Mortality and apnea index in obstructive sleep apnea. Chest. 1988;94:9–14.
119. Sahlin C, Sandberg O, Gustafson Y, et al. Obstructive sleep apnea is a risk factor for death in patients with stroke: a 10-year follow-up. Arch Intern Med. 2008;168:297–301.

120. Peker Y, Hedner J, Kraiczi H, et al. Respiratory disturbance index: an independent predictor of mortality in coronary artery disease. Am J Respir Crit Care Med. 2000;162:81–6.
121. Lavie P, Herer P, Peled R, et al. Mortality in sleep apnea patients: a multivariate analysis of risk factors. Sleep. 1995;18:149–57.
122. Young T, Finn L, Peppard PE, et al. Sleep disordered breathing and mortality: eighteen-year follow-up of the Wisconsin sleep cohort. Sleep. 2008;31:1071–8.
123. Punjabi N, Caffo BS, Goodwin JL, et al. Sleep disordered breathing and mortality: a prospective cohort study. PLoS Med. 2009;6:1–9.
124. Lavie P, Lavie L. Unexpected survival advantage in elderly people with moderate sleep apnoea. J Sleep Res. 2009;18:397–403.
125. Goff EA, O'Driscoll DM, Simmonds AK, et al. The cardiovascular response to arousal from sleep decreases with age in healthy adults. Sleep. 2008;31:1009–17.
126. Strohl KP, Novak RD, Singer W, et al. Insulin levels, blood pressure and sleep apnea. Sleep. 1994;17(7):614–8.
127. Ip MS, Lam B, Ng MM, et al. Obstructive sleep apnea is independently associated with insulin resistance. Am J Respir Crit Care Med. 2002;165(5):670–6.
128. Vgontzas AN, Papanicolaou DA, Bixler EO, et al. Sleep apnea and daytime sleepiness and fatigue: relation to visceral obesity, insulin resistance, and hypercytokinemia. J Clin Endocrinol Metab. 2000;85(3):1151–8.
129. Punjabi NM, Sorkin JD, Katzel LI, et al. Sleep-disordered breathing and insulin resistance in middle-aged and overweight men. Am J Respir Crit Care Med. 2002;165(5):677–82.
130. Stoohs RA, Facchini F, Guilleminault C. Insulin resistance and sleep-disordered breathing in healthy humans. Am J Respir Crit Care Med. 1996;154(1):170–4.
131. Punjabi NM, Shahar E, Redline S, et al. Sleep-disordered breathing, glucose intolerance, and insulin resistance: the Sleep Heart Health Study. Am J Epidemiol. 2004;160(6):521–30.
132. Reichmuth KJ, Austin D, Skatrud JB, et al. Association of sleep apnoea and type II diabetes: a population based study. Am J Respir Crit Care Med. 2005;172(12):1590–5.
133. Stamatakis K, Sanders MH, Caffo B, et al. Fasting glycemia in sleep disordered breathing: lowering the threshold on oxyhemoglobin desaturation. Sleep. 2008;31:1018–24.
134. Botros N, Concato J, Mohsenin V, et al. Obstructive sleep apnoea as a risk factor for type 2 diabetes. Am J Med. 2009;122:1122–7.
135. Grassi G, Seravalle G, Quarti-Trevano F, et al. Reinforcement of the adrenergic overdrive in the metabolic syndrome complicated by obstructive sleep apnoea. J Hypertens. 2010;28:1313–20.
136. Stamatakis KA, Punjabi NM. Effects of sleep fragmentation on glucose metabolism in normal subjects. Chest. 2010;137:95–101.
137. Naegele B, Thouvard V, Pepin JL, et al. Deficits of cognitive functions in patients with sleep apnea syndrome. Sleep. 1995;18(1):43–52.
138. Twigg GL, Papaioannou I, Jackson M, et al. Obstructive sleep apnea syndrome is associated with deficits in verbal but not visual memory. Am J Respir Crit Care Med. 2010;182:98–103.
139. Naegele B, Launois SH, Mazza S, et al. Which memory processes are affected in patients with obstructive sleep apnea? An evaluation of 3 types of memory. Sleep. 2006;29:533–44.
140. Quan SF, Wright R, Baldwin CM, et al. Obstructive sleep apnea-hypopnea and neurocognitive functioning in the Sleep Heart Health Study. Sleep Med. 2006;7:498–507.
141. Arnsten AF, Li BM. Neurobiology of executive functions: catecholamine influences on prefrontal cortical functions. Biol Psychiatry. 2005;57(11):1377–84.
142. Verstraeten E, Cluydts R. Executive control of attention in sleep apnea patients: theoretical concepts and methodological considerations. Sleep Med Rev. 2004;8(4):257–67.
143. Kales A, Caldwell AB, Cadieux RJ, Vela-Bueno A, Ruch LG, Mayes SD. Severe obstructive sleep apnea-II: associated psychopathology and psychosocial consequences. J Chron Dis. 1985;38(5):427–34.

144. Alchanatis M, Deligiorgis N, Zias N, Amfilochiou A, Gotsis E, Arakatsani A, et al. Frontal brain lobe impairment in obstructive sleep apnoea: a proton MR spectroscopy study. Eur Respir J. 2004;24(6):980–6.
145. Ayalon L, Ancoli-Israel S, Klemfuss Z, et al. Increased brain activation during verbal learning in obstructive sleep apnea. Neuroimage. 2006;31:1817–25.
146. Glasser M, Bailey N, McMillan A, Goff E, Morrell MJ. Sleep apnoea in older people. Breathe. 2011;7(3):249–56.
147. Mazza S, Pepin JL, Naegele B, et al. Driving ability in sleep apnoea patients before and after CPAP treatment: evaluation on a road safety platform. Eur Respir J. 2006;28:1020–8.
148. Young T, Peppard PE, Taheri S. Excess weight and sleep-disordered breathing. J Appl Physiol. 2005;99(4):1592–9.
149. Lévy P, Bonsignore MR, Eckel J. Sleep, sleep-disordered breathing and metabolic consequences. Eur Respir J. 2009;34:243–60.
150. Chobanian AV, Bakris GL, Black HR, et al. Seventh Report of the Joint National Committee on Prevention, Detection, Evaluation, and Treatment of High Blood Pressure. Hypertension. 2003;42:1206–52.
151. Angelico F, del Ben M, Augelletti T, et al. Obstructive sleep apnoea syndrome and the metabolic syndrome in an internal medicine setting. Eur J Int Med. 2010;21:191–5.
152. Sin DD, Fitzgerald F, Parker JD, et al. Risk Factors for central and obstructive sleep apnea in 450 men and women with congestive heart failure. Am J Respir Crit Care Med. 1999;160: 1101–6.
153. Vanderveken OM, Boudewijns A, Ni Q, et al. Cardiovascular implications in the treatment of obstructive sleep apnea. J Cardiovasc Transl Res. 2011;4(1):53–60.
154. Gami AS, Pressman G, Caples SM, et al. Association of atrial fibrillation and obstructive sleep apnea. Circulation. 2004;110:364–7.
155. Peker Y, Carlson J, Hedner J. Increased incidence of coronary artery disease in sleep apnoea: a long-term follow-up. Eur Respir J. 2006;28(3):596–602.
156. Grunstein R. Endocrine disorders. In: Kryger MH, Roth T, Dement W, editors. Principles and practice of sleep medicine, vol. 105. Philadelphia, PA: Elsevier Saunders; 2005. p. 1237–45.
157. Fritschi C, Quinn L. Fatigue in patients with diabetes: a review. J Psychosom Res. 2010; 69(1):33–41.
158. Chotinaiwattarakul W, O'Brien LM, Fan L, Chervin RD. Fatigue, tiredness, and lack of energy improve with treatment for OSA. J Clin Sleep Med. 2009;5(3):222–7.
159. Lewis G, Wessely S. The epidemiology of fatigue: more questions than answers. J Epidemiol Commun Health. 1998;46:2–97.
160. Trombetta IC, Somers VK, Maki-Nunes C, et al. Consequences of comorbid sleep apnea in the metabolic syndrome – implications for cardiovascular risk. Sleep. 2010;33(9):1193–9.
161. Parati G, Lombardi C, Hedner J, et al. Recommendations for the management of patients with obstructive sleep apnoea and hypertension. Eur Respir J. 2013;41:523–38.
162. Kushida CA, Littner MR, Morgenthaler T, et al. Practice parameters for the indications for polysomnography and related procedures: an update for 2005. Sleep. 2005;28(4):499–519.
163. Artz M, Young T, Finn L, et al. Sleepiness and sleep in patients with both systolic heart failure and obstructive sleep apnea. Arch Intern Med. 2006;166:1716–22.
164. Kanagala R, Murali NS, Friedman PA, Ammash NM, et al. Obstructive sleep apnea and the recurrence of atrial fibrillation. Circulation. 2003;107:2589–94.
165. Bansal A, Lee-Chiong T. Sleep and medical disorders. In: Butkov N, Lee-Chiong T, editors. Fundamentals of sleep technology, vol. 22. Philadelphia, PA: Lippincott Williams & Wilkins; 2007. p. 186–97.
166. Khawaja IT, Sayyed RT, Jaouni H. Obstructive sleep apnea: an unrecognized but prevalent condition. Compr Ther. 2000;26:294–7.
167. Bottini P, Tantucci C. Sleep apnea syndrome in endocrine diseases. Respiration. 2003;70: 320–7.
168. Weiss V, Sonka K, Pretl M, et al. Prevalence of sleep apnea syndrome in acromegaly population. J Endocrinol Invest. 2000;23:515–9.

169. Isono S, Sacki N, Tanaka A, et al. Collapsibility of passive pharynx in patients with acromegaly. Am J Respir Crit Care Med. 1999;160:64–8.
170. Bengtsson B, Brummer R, Eden S, et al. Body composition in acromegaly. Clin Endocrinol. 1989;30:121–30.
171. Shipley JE, Schteingart DE, Tandon R, et al. Sleep architecture and sleep apnea in patients with Cushing's syndrome. Sleep. 1992;15:514–8.
172. Yanovsky JA, Cutler JB. Glucocorticoid action and the clinical features of Cushing's syndrome. Endocrinol Metab Clin N Am. 1994;23:487–509.
173. Rosenow F, McCarthy V, Caruso AC. Sleep apnoea in endocrine disease. J Sleep Res. 1998; 7:3–11.
174. Harris MI, Flegal KM, Cowie CC, et al. Prevalence of diabetes, impaired fasting glucose, and impaired glucose tolerance in U.S. adults: the Third National Health and Nutrition Examination Survey, 1988–1994. Diabetes Care. 1998;21(4):518–24.
175. West SD, Nicoll DJ, Stradling JR. Prevalence of obstructive sleep apnea in men with type 2 diabetes. Thorax. 2006;61:945–50.
176. Babu AR, Herdegen J, Fogelfeld L, Shott S, Mazzone T. Type 2 diabetes, glycemic control, and continuous positive airway pressure in obstructive sleep apnea. Arch Intern Med. 2005;165(4):447–52.
177. Pallayova M, Donic V, Tomori Z. Beneficial effects of severe sleep apnea therapy on nocturnal glucose control in persons with type 2 diabetes mellitus. Diabetes Res Clin Pract. 2008; 81:e8–11.
178. Ficker JH, Dertinger SH, Siegfried W, et al. Obstructive sleep apnoea and diabetes mellitus: the role of cardiovascular autonomic neuropathy. Eur Respir J. 1998;11(1):14–9.
179. Park YW, Zhu S, Palaniappan L, Heshka S, Carnethon MR, Heymsfield SB. The metabolic syndrome: prevalence and associated risk factor findings in the US population from the Third National Health and Nutrition Examination Survey, 1988–1994. Arch Intern Med. 2003;163:427–36.
180. Reaven G. Role of insulin resistance in human disease. Banting lecture. Diabetes. 1997;37(12): 1595–607.
181. DeFronzo R, Ferrannini E. Insulin resistance: a multifaceted syndrome responsible for NIDDM, obesity, hypertension, dyslipidemia and atherosclerotic cardiovascular disease. Diabetes Care. 1991;14:173–94.
182. Kahn R, Buse J, Ferrannini E, et al. The metabolic syndrome: time for a critical appraisal. Diabetes Care. 2005;28:2289–304.
183. Dorkova Z, Petrasova D, Molcanyiova A, et al. Effects of CPAP on cardiovascular risk profile in patients with severe obstructive sleep apnea and metabolic syndrome. Chest. 2008;134: 686–92.
184. Agusti A, Hedner J, Marin JM, Barbé F, Cazzola M, Rennard S. Night-time symptoms: a forgotten dimension of COPD. Eur Respir Rev. 2011;20(121):183–94.
185. Klink ME, Dodge R, Quan SF. The relation of sleep complaints to respiratory symptoms in a general population. Chest. 1994;105(1):151–4.
186. Lee R, McNicholas WT. Obstructive sleep apnea in chronic obstructive pulmonary disease patients. Curr Opin Pulm Dis. 2011;17:79–83.
187. McNicholas WT, Verbraecken J, Marin JM. Sleep disorders in chronic obstructive pulmonary disease: the forgotten dimension. Eur Respir Rev. 2013;22(129):365–75.
188. Rodrigues CJO, Marson O, Tufic S, et al. Relationship among end-stage renal disease, hypertension, and sleep apnea in nondiabetic dialysis patients. Am J Hypertens. 2005;18:152–7.
189. Beecroft JM, Pierratos A, Hanly PJ. Clinical presentation of obstructive sleep apnea in patients with end-stage renal disease. J Clin Sleep Med. 2009;5:115–21.
190. Jean G, Piperno D, Francois B, et al. Sleep apnea incidence in maintenance hemodialysis patients: influence of dialysate buffer. Nephron. 1995;71:138–42.
191. Choi JB, Loredo JS, Norman D, et al. Does obstructive sleep apnea increase hematocrit? Sleep Breath. 2006;10:155–60.

192. Moore-Gillon JC, Treacher DF, Gaminara EJ, Pearson TC, Cameron IR. Intermittent hypoxia in patients with unexplained polycythaemia. Br Med J. 1986;293:588–90.
193. Carlson JT, Hedner J, Fagerberg B, Ejnell H, Magnusson B, Fyhrquist F. Secondary polycythaemia associated with nocturnal apnoea – a relationship not mediated by erythropoietin? J Int Med. 1992;231:381–7.
194. Krieger J, Sforza E, Delanoe C, Petiau C. Decrease in hematocrit with continuous positive airway pressure treatment in obstructive sleep apnoea patients. Eur Respir J. 1992;5: 228–33.
195. Young T, Blustein J, Finn L, Palta M. Sleep-disordered breathing and motor vehicle accidents in a population-based sample of employed adults. Sleep. 1997;20:608–13.
196. Tarasiuk A, Greenberg-Dotan S, Brin YS, Simon T, Tal A, Reuveni H. Determinants affecting health-care utilization in obstructive sleep apnea syndrome patients. Chest. 2005;128:1 310–4.
197. Sassani A, Findley LJ, Kryger M, Goldlust E, George C, Davidson TM. Reducing motor-vehicle collisions, costs, and fatalities by treating obstructive sleep apnea syndrome. Sleep. 2004;27:453–8.
198. Peker Y, Hedner J, Johansson A, Bende M. Reduced hospitalization with cardiovascular and pulmonary disease in obstructive sleep apnea patients on nasal CPAP treatment. Sleep. 1997;20:645–53.
199. Krieger J, Meslier N, Lebrun T, et al. Accidents in obstructive sleep apnea patients treated with nasal continuous positive airway pressure: a prospective study. The Working Group ANTADIR, Paris and CRESGE, Lille, France. Association Nationale de Traitement a Domicile des Insuffisants Respiratoires. Chest. 1997;112:1561–6.
200. Ayas NT, FitzGerald JM, Fleetham JA, et al. Cost-effectiveness of continuous positive airway pressure therapy for moderate to severe obstructive sleep apnea/hypopnea. Arch Intern Med. 2006;166:977–84.
201. Tousignant P, Cosio MG, Levy RD, et al. Quality adjusted life years added by treatment of obstructive sleep apnea. Sleep. 1994;17:52–60.
202. Alghanim N, Comondore VR, Fleetham J, Marra CA, Ayas NT. The economic impact of obstructive sleep apnea. Lung. 2008;186:7–12.
203. Prosser LA, Stinnett AA, Goldman PA, et al. Cost-effectiveness of cholesterol-lowering therapies according to selected patent characteristics. Ann Intern Med. 2000;132:769–79.
204. Albarrak M, Banno K, Sabbagh AA, et al. Utilization of healthcare resources in obstructive sleep apnea syndrome: a 5-year follow-up study in men using CPAP. Sleep. 2005;28: 1306–11.
205. Ulfberg J, Carter N, Talback M, Edling C. Excessive daytime sleepiness at work and subjective work performance in the general population and among heavy snorers and patients with obstructive sleep apnea. Chest. 1996;110:659–63.
206. Ayas NT, Marra C. Continuous positive airway pressure therapy for obstructive sleep apnea syndrome: do the dollars make sense? Sleep. 2005;28:1211–3.
207. Kapur VK, Alfonso-Cristancho R. Just a good deal or truly a steal? Medical cost savings and the impact on the cost-effectiveness of treating sleep apnea. Sleep. 2009;32:135–6.
208. Bahammam A, Delaive K, Ronad J, et al. Health care utilization in males with obstructive sleep apnea syndrome two years after diagnosis and treatment. Sleep. 1999;22:740–7.
209. Banno K, Manfreda J, Walld R, Delaive K, Kryger MH. Healthcare utilization in women with obstructive sleep apnea syndrome 2 years after diagnosis and treatment. Sleep. 2006;29: 1307–11.

Compliance of Various Forms of Obstructive Sleep Apnea Treatment

Madeline Ravesloot

Introduction

The therapeutic armamentarium for obstructive sleep apnea (OSA) comprises several treatment options. To provide effective treatment for OSA, careful consideration of the individual patient, available medical and surgical therapies, and inherent risks and complications of those interventions must be taken into account. Continuous positive airway pressure (CPAP) has the firmest evidence base in the treatment of OSA. A growing body of evidence is becoming available supporting the practice of other treatment modalities, especially mandibular advancement devices (MADs), weight loss, positional therapy (PT) and sleep surgery.

Treatment is generally approached in a stepwise manner and begins with behaviour modification, indicated for all patients with a modifiable risk factor [1]. This includes weight loss, alcohol and sedative abstinence and avoidance of worst sleeping position.

Continuous Positive Airway Pressure

Continuous positive airway pressure (CPAP) first introduced by Sullivan in 1981, is regarded as the gold standard in the treatment of moderate and severe cases and is the most efficacious treatment modality of OSA [2]. CPAP functions as a pneumatic splint to maintaining upper airway patency. CPAP is considered successful when the apnea-hypopnea index (AHI) is reduced to below 5 when CPAP is used. In a

M. Ravesloot (✉)
Department of Otorhinolaryngology, Sint Lucas Andreas Ziekenhuis,
Jan Tooropstraat 164, Amsterdam 1061 AE, The Netherlands
e-mail: m.ravesloot@slaz.nl

N. de Vries et al. (eds.), *Positional Therapy in Obstructive Sleep Apnea*,
DOI 10.1007/978-3-319-09626-1_3

meta-analysis of the Cochrane Collaboration, compared with control, CPAP was shown to be significantly effective in reducing the AHI as well as improving measurements of quality of life, cognitive function and objective and subjective measures of sleepiness [3]. Possible side effects can be related to the interface (skin abrasion from contact with the mask, claustrophobia, mask leak, irritated eyes), pressure (nasal congestion and rhinorrhea with dryness or irritation of the nasal and pharyngeal membranes, sneezing, gastric and bowel distension, recurrent ear and sinus infections) and negative social factors [4, 5].

Mandibular Advancement Devices

Mandibular advancement devices (MADs), also known as mandibular reposition appliances (MRA) or oral appliances (OA), have become increasingly popular as a treatment alternative [6]. By advancing the mandible and its attached soft tissue structures forward, they aim to increase upper airway size [7]. MADs have been found to be effective in reducing the AHI, especially in patients with mild to moderate OSA. Studies have shown that MADs are more effective when compared to "control devices" (which do not protrude the mandible), in reducing the AHI [6, 8–12]. When compared to CPAP, there was a significant effect in favor of CPAP compared with MADs [13–16].

Side effects have been reported with the use of MADs: excessive salivation or dryness of the mouth; gum irritation; discomfort of the temporomandibular joint, teeth or facial musculature; bite change; and temporomandibular disorders [6–8, 17–25]. Long-term treatment with a MAD can result in changes in dental morphology [24].

Sleep Surgery

Sleep surgery aims to increase the surface area of the upper airway, to bypass the pharyngeal airway or to remove a specific pathology [26, 27]. Surgical procedures developed to treat OSA can predominantly be classified according to site of intervention, mechanism of action and invasiveness [4].

Uvulopalatopharyngoplasty (UPPP) is the most commonly performed surgical procedure for OSA [28–31]. The procedure aims to increase the retropalatal lumen and reduce the collapsibility of the pharynx, by resection of the free edge of the uvula and soft palate, often in combination with a tonsillectomy [26, 27]. Unfortunately, UPPP is often misused as the first line of surgical therapy for OSA, without adequate assessment of obstruction site(s) and regardless of predictive factors such as obesity [32]. As a result, an isolated UPPP is often unsuccessful in treating OSA, especially in badly selected patients. Palatal surgery is indicated in patients who have airway collapse at the level of the velum. There are no widely accepted standardized methods or algorithms to identify suitable candidates.

In a literature review by Sher et al., published in 1996, an overall response rate of 40.7 % was reported (with response defined as a 50 % decrease in the respiratory disturbance index [RDI] and a postoperative RDI of 20, or as a 50 % decrease in the AI and a postoperative AI of 10) in patients with OSA treated with UPPP alone, regardless of site of obstruction. In patients with suspected hypopharyngeal obstruction, the response rate was a mere 5.3 %, whilst in patients with suspected palatal narrowing alone, the response rate increased to 52.3 % [33]. As in all surgery, meticulous patient selection is crucial. The type and extent of surgical intervention mainly depends on the severity of the disease and the site(s) of obstruction as well as patient's characteristics, sleep position dependence, comorbidity and the patient's preference [34]. Over the years, the scope of surgical treatment modalities has broadened significantly.

No surgery is without risks. Possible late complications, in order of descending frequency, of UPPP are pharyngeal dryness and hardening, postnasal secretion, dysphagia, incapability of initiating swallowing, prolonged angina, taste disorders, speech disorders, numbness of tongue, permanent velopharyngeal incompetence and nasopharyngeal stenosis. Furthermore, although more clarification is needed, studies suggest that the response to UPPP for OSA decreases progressively over the years after surgery [35–40].

Treatment modalities designed to prevent obstruction at the level of the hypopharynx vary from minimally invasive, such as radiofrequency ablation of the base of the tongue, to invasive genioglossal advancement (GA) or maxillomandibular advancement (MMA), for example. An evidence-based medicine review reported a success rate ranging from 20 % to 83 % achieved in patients undergoing tongue radiofrequency, 25–83 % in reports on midline glossectomy and 39–78 % on GA. Surgical success is defined as a reduction in AHI of 50 % or more and an AHI of less than 20 [41].

Compliance

CPAP and MAD treatment are regarded as successful if the AHI drops below 5 whilst the devices are used; an AHI below 5 is the bar for CPAP adjustment. It is however common knowledge that a majority of patients are not adherent to the treatment during 100 % of the total sleep time under everyday non-laboratory conditions [42]. Current arbitrary trends define compliance as 4 h per night as an average over all nights observed [43].

Treatment outcome based on individual compliance in conservative treatment can currently most reliably be reported in patients with CPAP. Built-in counters have become a standard feature in CPAP devices, and hours of use can easily be assessed by every physician. Until recently accurate assessment of compliance for other conservative interventions was limited to subjective self-report.

Despite the efficacy of CPAP, it is, however, a clinical reality that the use of CPAP is often cumbersome. Patients seem to either tolerate the device well or not at all—a bimodal distribution [44]. Studies have shown that 29–83 % of patients are non-adherent, when adherence is defined as at least 4 h of CPAP use per night. [45] More support and care is needed to improve compliance, especially on a long-term basis, such as addressing CPAP side effects.

Objective usage data for MAD are harder to collect than for CPAP, but self-reported treatment compliance is high [8, 11, 15, 17, 18]. Compliance rates vary greatly between studies varying between 4 and 82 % after 1 year of treatment [46]. Long-term compliance has been reported to decrease over time. Over a 2- to 5-year follow-up period, studies have reported a subjective therapeutic adherence ranging from 48 % to 90 % [47–50]. Discontinuation of treatment is due to side effects or lack of perceived benefit [51]. Self-reported adherence tends to overestimate actual use [4].

Reporting on the efficacy of OA in a 3-month prospective clinical trial, Vanderveken et al. took objective OA compliance into consideration through an embedded microsensor thermometer with on-chip integrated readout electronics [52]. The mean AHI was calculated based on the objective OA use and treatment period.

Compliance Positional Therapy

Ineffectiveness, backache, discomfort and no improvement in sleep quality or daytime alertness have been responsible for poor compliance and subsequent disappointing long-term results of PT of various tennis ball techniques.

Skinner et al. included 20 patients in a randomized cross-over comparing the efficacy of the thoracic anti-supine band (TASB) with nCPAP [51]. Subjects were randomly assigned to receive the TASB or nCPAP for the first month followed by a 1-week washout before commencing the alternative treatment. The self-reported compliance was significantly better with TASB than with nCPAP. Nineteen of 20 patients reported a 7-h nightly use with the TASB. In contrast only 9 of 20 subjects met the 4 h per night CPAP compliance criteria.

Next to the efficacy study of PT (vest with semi-rigid foam on dorsal part) by Wenzel et al., the group contacted the patients approximately 13.7 months later by telephone to assess PT compliance [53]. Only 4 of the 14 patients were still using PT (on average for 7.3 h and 6.4 nights); their ESS was reduced from 8.5–6.5. The remaining 10 patients had stopped using PT due to the following reasons: discomfort and tightness of the vest, frequent awakenings, restless sleep, increased sweating during the night and prevention of preferred sleeping position.

Oksenberg et al. assessed the use of PT (TBT) during a 6-month period in 78 consecutive POSA patients [54]. Of the 50 patients who returned the questionnaire, 38 % were still using PT; 24 % no longer used PT, as they claimed to have learned to avoid the supine position; and 38 % no longer used PT but had not learned to avoid the supine position.

Bignold et al. studied the compliance of 67 patients, who had been prescribed PT (TBT) 2.5 ± 1 year earlier, using a follow-up questionnaire [55]. 6 % were still using

PT; 13.4 % no longer used PT, as they claimed to have learned to avoid the supine position; and a staggering 80.6 % no longer used PT, but had not learned to avoid the supine position. Reasons to abort the PT included ineffectiveness, backache, discomfort and no improvement in sleep quality or daytime alertness.

Of the 9 patients randomized to PT (triangular pillow), in a study performed by Svatikova et al., 3 months post-stroke, the self-reported adherence was 3 (33 %) all nights, 1 (11 %) most nights, 2 (22 %) some nights and 3 (33 %) no nights [56].

In a second study performed by Bignold et al., patients were assigned with PT for 3 weeks (a position monitoring device and supine alarm device) [57]. The device was active for 1 of the 3 weeks. Patients used the device 85 % of nights over the full 3 weeks with an average of 6.8 h of use per night.

Recent developments have seen the introduction of a new generation of PT, which successfully prevents patients from adopting the supine position without negatively influencing sleep efficiency. In a recent study by van Maanen et al., studying the effect of the sleep position trainer (SPT) in patients with POSA, the median percentage of supine sleeping time decreased from 49.9 % [20.4–77.3 %] to 0.0 % [range: 0.0–48.7 %] ($p<0.001$) [58]. The median AHI decreased from 16.4 per hour [6.6–29.9] to 5.2 per hour [0.5–46.5] ($p<0.001$). 15 patients developed an overall AHI below 5 per hour. Sleep efficiency did not change significantly, the Epworth Sleepiness Scale decreased significantly, and Functional Outcomes of Sleep Questionnaire increased significantly. Compliance after 1 month was found to be 92.7 % [62.0–100.0 %].

At present, evidence of PT effectiveness is based on small-scale case series and a few randomized trials. Little is known about the long-term compliance of PT. It has been suggested that patients may learn to avoid the supine position following PT and therefore do not need to use PT on a regular basis [59]. Others may need PT either periodically to reinforce training or consistently.

Reporting on Compliance

The effectiveness of conservative treatment regarding the reduction of AHI depends both on its impact on airway obstruction and compliance. Current evidence demonstrates that clinical outcome is dependent on compliance to treatment in a dose-dependent manner.

In a double-blind, placebo-controlled cross-over trial by Sharma et al., 86 patients with OSA were randomly assigned to therapeutic CPAP or sham CPAP for a period of 3 months with a washout period of 1 month in between [60]. A statistically significant greater mean reduction in systolic and diastolic blood pressure (BP), glycated haemoglobin, triglycerides, LDL cholesterol and total cholesterol was observed in a subgroup of patients who used CPAP ≥ 5 h ($n=51$). Similar results were found in a prospective long-term follow-up study and a randomized controlled trial: a significant decrease in the 24-h mean arterial pressure (MAP) was achieved in patients who used CPAP >5.3 h per day ($n=27$), and a statistically significant decrease in systolic BP was observed in patients who use CPAP ≥ 5.6 h per night [61, 62]. Hours of CPAP use was an independent predictor of reduction in BP [61].

Campos-Rodriguez et al. reported in a retrospective cohort study that the 5-year cumulative survival rate was significantly higher in patients with sleep apnea and hypertension who used CPAP ≥ 6 h per night [63].

Weaver et al. reported a linear-dose relationship between hours of CPAP use and improvement in daytime sleepiness after 3 months of therapy in a recent follow-up cohort study of patients with severe OSA [64].

This current evidence demonstrates that clinical outcome is dependent on compliance to treatment in a dose-dependent manner.

As cardiovascular effects and long-term survival are relatively hard to assess, the AHI is mostly used as a surrogate outcome measure. The current evidence however demonstrates that compliance also needs to be taken into account when reporting treatment outcome in terms of AHI reduction.

Currently, when reporting on treatment effectiveness of conservative treatment, the reduction in AHI whilst using CPAP in laboratory situations is documented. An artificial compliance of 100 % is assumed.

Two current publications have suggested methods to include compliance into the calculation of the AHI under conservative treatment. Ravesloot and de Vries proposed mathematical formulas to assess mean AHI with regard to treatment compliance based on the hours of CPAP use as documented by the built-in counters of the CPAP devices [65]. They suggest that a mean AHI in CPAP therapy is more realistic than using arbitrary compliance rates which in fact hide insufficient reductions in AHI. Almost simultaneously, Stuck et al. published data on treatment effects of CPAP on the AHI in a cohort of patients with OSA. The mean AHI could also be calculated based on the treatment period and the hours of use of the device [66].

The following formula was described in both papers using the estimated total sleep time (TST), the hours of CPAP use in the treatment period as assessed with the devices' built-in counters (HOURSonCPAP), the AHI as assessed in the sleep lab before treatment (AHIoffCPAP) and whilst using CPAP (AHIonCPAP):

$$\text{Mean AHI for CPAP} = \frac{(\text{AHIonCPAP} \times \text{HOURSonCPAP}) + [\text{AHIoffCPAP} \times (\text{TST} - \text{HOURSonCPAP})]}{\text{TST}}$$

For example, if we take a patient with an AHI of 38 (*AHIoffCPAP*). Using the compliance criteria cut-off discussed, our patient sleeps using CPAP 7 nights per week (*NIGHTSonCPAP*). The AHI (*AHIoffCPAP*) is reduced to 2 (*AHIonCPAP*) during 4 h, again using the compliance cut-off criteria discussed (*HOURSonCPAP*). During the residual 4 h (*HOURSoffCPAP*), the AHI remains 38. Using the generalized formula above and the parameters for this patient, we can calculate the mean AHI during compliant use of CPAP:

$$\text{Mean AHI for CPAP} = \left(\frac{(4 \times 2) + (4 \times 38)}{8} \right) = 20.$$

The mean AHI is 20, so the AHI is reduced by 47.37 %.

This formula can be generalized to other PSG outcomes such as the apnea index or desaturation index. This mathematical formula is based on the assumption that the AHI will revert to baseline once the CPAP appliance is no longer used. CPAP is thought to play a role in reducing edema resulting from snoring-associated vibration and apnea-induced mechanical stress of the upper airway. It can be argued that the baseline AHI may be reduced by a fraction in chronic CPAP use and that after termination of CPAP during the night the AHI may not completely revert to baseline. The precise effect however remains to be elucidated. If future research allows quantification of the magnitude of this effect, the formula could easily be extended by a factor addressing this aspect.

Future Perspectives

Treatment outcome based on individual compliance in conservative treatment can currently most reliably be reported in patients with CPAP. Built-in counters have become a standard feature in CPAP devices, and hours of use can easily be assessed by every physician. Until recently accurate assessment of compliance for other conservative interventions was limited to subjective self-report.

Reporting on the efficacy of OA in a 3-month prospective clinical trial, Vanderveken et al. took objective OA compliance into consideration through an embedded microsensor thermometer with on-chip integrated readout electronics [52]. The mean AHI was calculated based on the objective OA use and treatment period. Their results support the hypothesis that higher compliance with OA therapy translates into a similar adjusted effectiveness as compared with CPAP [52, 67]. Despite not being a common practice as yet, compliance to OA devices can be measured objectively with the introduction of this new device [52].

In future studies comparing the effects of different devices (e.g. CPAP or OA) on the AHI with alternative treatment methods, especially those with 100 % adherence (e.g. surgery), adherence should to be taken into account with the formula mentioned above. In doing so, one could compare the effectiveness of OA, CPAP and surgery.

The following example may illustrate this approach: in a recent systematic review and meta-analysis reporting on the efficacy of maxillomandibular advancement (MMA) on the AHI in OSA patients, the mean AHI decreased from 63.9 to 9.5 per hour ($p < 0.001$) following surgery [12].

In the previously mentioned study by Stuck et al. addressing the effects of CPAP, the mean AHI decreased from 35.6 to 11.9 per hour when individual adherence was taken into account [12]. The mean AHI under CPAP was 2.4 per hour. Juxtaposed, these treatment modalities seem to be equally effective in reducing the AHI when adherence is taken into account, although the population in the MMA study was more severely affected. This approach may also be used to compare the effects of other current treatment strategies.

Following this train of thought, recent studies suggest that higher compliance with OA therapy translates into a similar adjusted effectiveness as compared with CPAP [11, 13].

References

1. Strohl KP. Overview of obstructive sleep apnoea in adults. In: Basner RC, editor. UpToDate 20S12.
2. Sullivan CE, Issa FG, Berthon-Jones M, Eves L. Reversal of obstructive sleep apnoea by continuous positive airway pressure applied through the nares. Lancet. 1981;1:862–5.
3. Giles TL, Lasserson TJ, Smith BH, White J, Wright J, Cates CJ. Continuous positive airways pressure for obstructive sleep apnoea in adults. Cochrane Database Syst Rev. 2006;CD001106.
4. McNicholas WT, Bonsignore MR, editors. Sleep apnoea. European Respiratory Society Monograph; 2010.
5. Gay P, Weaver T, Loube D, Iber C. Evaluation of positive airway pressure treatment for sleep related breathing disorders in adults. Sleep. 2006;29:381–401.
6. Lim J, Lasserson TJ, Fleetham J, Wright J. Oral appliances for obstructive sleep apnoea. Cochrane Database Syst Rev. 2006;CD004435.
7. Ferguson KA, Cartwright R, Rogers R, Schmidt-Nowara W. Oral appliances for snoring and obstructive sleep apnoea: a review. Sleep. 2006;29:244–62.
8. Mehta A, Qian J, Petocz P, Darendeliler MA, Cistulli PA. A randomized, controlled study of a mandibular advancement splint for obstructive sleep apnoea. Am J Respir Crit Care Med. 2001;163:1457–61.
9. Hans MG, Nelson S, Luks VG, Lorkovich P, Baek SJ. Comparison of two dental devices for treatment of obstructive sleep apnoea syndrome (OSAS). Am J Orthod Dentofacial Orthop. 1997;111:562–70.
10. Blanco J, Zamarron C, Abeleira Pazos MT, Lamela C, Suarez QD. Prospective evaluation of an oral appliance in the treatment of obstructive sleep apnoea syndrome. Sleep Breath. 2005;9:20–5.
11. Gotsopoulos H, Chen C, Qian J, Cistulli PA. Oral appliance therapy improves symptoms in obstructive sleep apnoea: a randomized, controlled trial. Am J Respir Crit Care Med. 2002;166:743–8.
12. Johnston CD, Gleadhill IC, Cinnamond MJ, Gabbey J, Burden DJ. Mandibular advancement appliances and obstructive sleep apnoea: a randomized clinical trial. Eur J Orthod. 2002;24:251–62.
13. Engleman HM, McDonald JP, Graham D, et al. Randomized crossover trial of two treatments for sleep apnoea/Hypopnoea syndrome: continuous positive airway pressure and mandibular repositioning splint. Am J Respir Crit Care Med. 2002;166:855–9.
14. Lam B, Sam K, Mok WY, et al. Randomised study of three non-surgical treatments in mild to moderate obstructive sleep apnoea. Thorax. 2007;62:354–9.
15. Randerath WJ, Heise M, Hinz R, Ruehle KH. An individually adjustable oral appliance vs continuous positive airway pressure in mild-to-moderate obstructive sleep apnoea syndrome. Chest. 2002;122:569–75.
16. Tan YK, L'Estrange PR, Luo YM, et al. Mandibular advancement splints and continuous positive airway pressure in patients with obstructive sleep apnoea: a randomized cross-over trial. Eur J Orthod. 2002;24:239–49.
17. Ferguson KA, Ono T, Lowe AA, al-Majed S, Love LL, Fleetham JA. A short-term controlled trial of an adjustable oral appliance for the treatment of mild to moderate obstructive sleep apnoea. Thorax. 1997;52:362–8.

18. Tegelberg A, Wilhelmsson B, Walker-Engstrom ML, et al. Effects and adverse events of a dental appliance for treatment of obstructive sleep apnoea. Swed Dent J. 1999;23:117–26.
19. Fritsch KM, Iseli A, Russi EW, Bloch KE. Side effects of mandibular advancement devices for sleep apnoea treatment. Am J Respir Crit Care Med. 2001;164:813–8.
20. Walker-Engstrom ML, Ringqvist I, Vestling O, Wilhelmsson B, Tegelberg A. A prospective randomized study comparing two different degrees of mandibular advancement with a dental appliance in treatment of severe obstructive sleep apnoea. Sleep Breath. 2003;7:119–30.
21. Rose E, Staats R, Virchow C, Jonas IE. A comparative study of two mandibular advancement appliances for the treatment of obstructive sleep apnoea. Eur J Orthod. 2002;24:191–8.
22. Bloch KE, Iseli A, Zhang JN, et al. A randomized, controlled crossover trial of two oral appliances for sleep apnoea treatment. Am J Respir Crit Care Med. 2000;162:246–51.
23. Hammond RJ, Gotsopoulos H, Shen G, Petocz P, Cistulli PA, Darendeliler MA. A follow-up study of dental and skeletal changes associated with mandibular advancement splint use in obstructive sleep apnoea. Am J Orthod Dentofacial Orthop. 2007;132:806–14.
24. Doff MH, Finnema KJ, Hoekema A, Wijkstra PJ, de Bont LG, Stegenga B. Long-term oral appliance therapy in obstructive sleep apnoea syndrome: a controlled study on dental side effects. Clin Oral Investig. 2013;17(2):475–82.
25. Doff MH, Veldhuis SK, Hoekema A, et al. Long-term oral appliance therapy in obstructive sleep apnoea syndrome: a controlled study on temporomandibular side effects. Clin Oral Investig. 2012;16:689–97.
26. Practice parameters for the treatment of obstructive sleep apnoea in adults: the efficacy of surgical modifications of the upper airway. Report of the American Sleep Disorders Association. Sleep 1996;19:152–5.
27. Sundaram S, Bridgman SA, Lim J, Lasserson TJ. Surgery for obstructive sleep apnoea. Cochrane Database Syst Rev. 2005;CD001004.
28. Ikematsu T. Study of snoring, 4th report: therapy. Japan Oto-Rhino-Laryngol. 1963;64: 434–5.
29. Fujita S, Conway W, Zorick F, Roth T. Surgical correction of anatomic abnormalities in obstructive sleep apnoea syndrome: uvulopalatopharyngoplasty. Otolaryngol Head Neck Surg. 1981;89:923–34.
30. Kezirian EJ, Maselli J, Vittinghoff E, Goldberg AN, Auerbach AD. Obstructive sleep apnoea surgery practice patterns in the United States: 2000 to 2006. Otolaryngol Head Neck Surg. 2010;143:441–7.
31. Kezirian EJ, Weaver EM, Yueh B, et al. Incidence of serious complications after uvulopalatopharyngoplasty. Laryngoscope. 2004;114:450–3.
32. Ishman SL, Wakefield TL, Collop NA. Sleep apnoea and sleep disorders. In: Flint PW, Haughey BH, Lund VJ, et al., editors. Cummings otolaryngology – head and neck surgery. 5th ed. Philadelphia, PA: Mosby; 2010.
33. Sher AE, Schechtman KB, Piccirillo JF. The efficacy of surgical modifications of the upper airway in adults with obstructive sleep apnoea syndrome. Sleep. 1996;19:156–77.
34. Ravesloot MJ, de Vries N. One hundred consecutive patients undergoing drug-induced sleep endoscopy: results and evaluation. Laryngoscope. 2011;121:2710–6.
35. Pirsig W, Verse T. Long-term results in the treatment of obstructive sleep apnoea. Eur Arch Otorhinolaryngol. 2000;257:570–7.
36. Larsson LH, Carlsson-Nordlander B, Svanborg E. Four-year follow-up after uvulopalatopharyngoplasty in 50 unselected patients with obstructive sleep apnoea syndrome. Laryngoscope. 1994;104:1362–8.
37. Lu SJ, Chang SY, Shiao GM. Comparison between short-term and long-term post-operative evaluation of sleep apnoea after uvulopalatopharyngoplasty. J Laryngol Otol. 1995;109: 308–12.
38. Janson C, Gislason T, Bengtsson H, et al. Long-term follow-up of patients with obstructive sleep apnoea treated with uvulopalatopharyngoplasty. Arch Otolaryngol Head Neck Surg. 1997;123:257–62.

39. Boot H, van Wegen R, Poublon RM, Bogaard JM, Schmitz PI, van der Meche FG. Long-term results of uvulopalatopharyngoplasty for obstructive sleep apnoea syndrome. Laryngoscope. 2000;110:469–75.
40. Hultcrantz E, Johansson K, Bengtson H. The effect of uvulopalatopharyngoplasty without tonsillectomy using local anaesthesia: a prospective long-term follow-up. J Laryngol Otol. 1999;113:542–7.
41. Kezirian EJ, Goldberg AN. Hypopharyngeal surgery in obstructive sleep apnoea: an evidence-based medicine review. Arch Otolaryngol Head Neck Surg. 2006;132:206–13.
42. Kryger MW. Diagnosis and management of sleep apnoea syndrome. Clin Cornerstone. 2000;2:39–47.
43. Young T, Hutton R, Finn L, Baddr S, Palta M. The gender basis in sleep apnoea diagnosis: are women missed because they have different symptoms? Arch Intern Med. 1996;156:2445–51.
44. Kribbs NB, Pack AI, Kline LR, et al. Objective measurement of patterns of nasal CPAP use by patients with obstructive sleep apnoea. Am Rev Respir Dis. 1993;147:887–95.
45. Weaver TE, Grunstein RR. Adherence to continuous positive airway pressure therapy: the challenge to effective treatment. Proc Am Thorac Soc. 2008;5:173–8.
46. Walker-Engström ML, Wilhelmsson B, Tegelberg A, Dimenäs E, Ringqvist I. Quality of life assessment of treatment with dental appliance or UPPP in patients with mild to moderate obstructive sleep apnoea. A prospective randomized 1-year follow-up study. J Sleep Res. 2000; 9:303–8.
47. Yoshida K. Effects of a mandibular advancement device for the treatment of sleep apnoea syndrome and snoring on respiratory function and sleep quality. Cranio. 2000;18:98–105.
48. Clark GT, Sohn JW, Hong CN. Treating obstructive sleep apnoea and snoring: assessment of an anterior mandibular positioning device. J Am Dent Assoc. 2000;131:765–71.
49. Pantin CC, Hillman DR, Tennant M. Dental side effects of an oral device to treat snoring and obstructive sleep apnoea. Sleep. 1999;22:237–40.
50. McGown AD, Makker HK, Battagel JM, L'Estrange PR, Grant HR, Spiro SG. Long-term use of mandibular advancement splints for snoring and obstructive sleep apnoea: a questionnaire survey. Eur Respir J. 2001;17:462–6.
51. Skinner MA, Kingshott RN, Filsell S, Taylor R. Efficacy of the 'tennis ball technique' versus nCPAP in the management of position-dependent obstructive sleep apnoea syndrome. Respirology. 2009;13:708–15.
52. Vanderveken OM, Dieltjens M, Wouters K, de Backer WA, van de Heyning PH, Braem MJ. Objective measurement of compliance during oral appliance therapy for sleep-disordered breathing. Thorax. 2013;68:91–6.
53. Wenzel S, Smith E, Leiacker R, Fischer Y. Efficacy and long-term compliance of the vest preventing the supine position in patients with obstructive sleep apnoea. Laryngorhinootologie. 2007;86:579–83.
54. Oksenberg A, Silverberg D, Offenbach D, Arons E. Positional therapy for obstructive sleep apnoea patients: a 6-month follow-up study. Laryngoscope. 2006;116:1995–2000.
55. Bignold JJ, Deans-Costi G, Goldsworthy MR, et al. Poor long-term patient compliance with the tennis ball technique for treating positional obstructive sleep apnoea. J Clin Sleep Med. 2009;5:428–30.
56. Svatikova A, Chervin RD, Wing JJ, Sanchez BN, Migda EM, Brown DL. Positional therapy in ischemic stroke patients with obstructive sleep apnoea. Sleep Med. 2011;12:262–6.
57. Bignold JJ, Mercer JD, Antic NA, McEvoy RD, Catcheside PG. Accurate Position monitoring and improved supine-dependent obstructive sleep apnoea with a new position recording and supine avoidance device. J Clin Sleep Med. 2011;7:376–83.
58. Oksenberg A, Silverberg DS, Arons E, Radwan H. Positional vs nonpositional obstructive sleep apnoea patients. Chest. 1997;112:629–39.
59. Cartwright RD, Lloyd S, Lilie J, Kravtiz H. Sleep position training as treatment for sleep apnoea syndrome: a preliminary study. Sleep. 1985;8:87–94.
60. Sharma SK, Agrawal S, Damodaran D, et al. CPAP for the metabolic syndrome in patients with obstructive sleep apnoea. N Engl J Med. 2011;365:2277–86.

61. Campos-Rodriguez F, Perez-Ronchel J, Grilo-Reina A, Lima-Alvarez J, Benitez MA, Almeida-Gonzalez C. Long-term effect of continuous positive airway pressure on BP in patients with hypertension and sleep apnoea. Chest. 2007;132:1847–52.
62. Barbé F, Durán-Cantolla J, Capote F, et al. Long-term effect of continuous positive airway pressure in hypertensive patients with sleep apnoea. Am J Respir Crit Care Med. 2010;181: 718–26.
63. Campos-Rodriguez F, Peña-Griñan N, Reyes-Nuñez N, et al. Mortality in obstructive sleep apnoea-Hypopnoea patients treated with positive airway pressure. Chest. 2005;128:624–33.
64. Weaver TE, Maislin G, Dinges DF, et al. Relationship between hours of CPAP use and achieving normal levels of sleepiness and daily function. Sleep. 2007;30:711–9.
65. Ravesloot MJL, de Vries N. Reliable Calculation of the efficacy of non-surgical and surgical treatment of obstructive sleep apnoea revisited. Sleep. 2011;34:105–10.
66. Stuck BA, Leitzbach S, Maurer JT. Effects of continuous positive airway pressure on apnoea-Hypopnoea index in obstructive sleep apnoea based on long-term compliance. Sleep Breath. 2012;16:467–71.
67. de Almeida FR. Complexity and efficacy of mandibular advancement splints: understanding their mode of action. J Clin Sleep Med. 2011;7:447–8.

Part II
Initial Work Up: Polysomnography

Prevalence of Positional Obstructive Sleep Apnea in Patients Undergoing Polysomnography and the Effect of Sleep Stage

Mahesh Shetty and M. Jeffery Mador

Introduction

Determining whether sleep apnea is positional or not has important therapeutic consequences as discussed elsewhere in this book. In this chapter, we will discuss the prevalence of positional sleep apnea in patients with sleep apnea, factors that make positional sleep apnea more likely in a patient with sleep apnea, and the effect of sleep stage on positional sleep apnea.

Prevalence

Obstructive sleep apnea (OSA) is a common disorder, estimated to occur in approximately 2 % and 4 % of middle-aged women and men, respectively (based on the presence of an abnormal sleep study plus self-reported sleepiness), in a landmark study published in 1993 [1]. The prevalence of sleep apnea in 2013 is likely greater than this based on the increase in obesity levels since then. A recent study examining changes in OSA prevalence using the same Wisconsin state cohort that was used in the original investigation show increases in prevalence rates from 14 % to 55 %

M. Shetty, M.D.
Division of Pulmonary, Critical Care and Sleep Medicine, University at Buffalo, Buffalo, NY, USA

M.J. Mador, M.D. (✉)
Division of Pulmonary, Critical Care and Sleep Medicine, University at Buffalo, Buffalo, NY, USA

Western New York Veteran Affairs Healthcare System, 3495 Bailey Ave, Buffalo, NY 14223, USA
e-mail: mador@buffalo.edu

N. de Vries et al. (eds.), *Positional Therapy in Obstructive Sleep Apnea*,
DOI 10.1007/978-3-319-09626-1_4

Table 1 Prevalence of positional sleep apnea

Definition	Author	Total sample size	Number of pos SA	Number of non-pos SA	Prevalence of pos SA (%)
Lenient definition	Richard [8]	120	67	53	55.8
	Sunwoo [9]	91	65	26	71.4
	Teerapraipruk [10]	144	96	48	66.7
	Gillman [4]	100	63	37	63
	Oksenberg [11]	574	321	253	55.9
Strict definition	Gillman [4]	100	23	77	23
	Mador [5]	258	69	189	26.7

Pos SA positional sleep apnea, *non-pos SA* non-positional sleep apnea

in 2007–2010 compared to those obtained in 1988–1994 [2]. Positional sleep apnea defined as a worsening of sleep apnea in the supine posture compared to the non-supine posture is extremely common. The exact prevalence depends on the definition used to diagnose positional sleep apnea.

The usual definition of positional sleep apnea is a supine apnea-hypopnea index (AHI) that is greater than twice the non-supine AHI as initially described by Cartwright in 1984 [3]. However, another perhaps more clinically useful definition is to define positional sleep apnea as the presence of sleep apnea only in the supine posture. With this definition, the AHI in the non-supine posture is less than 5 per hour *and* less than 50 % of the supine AHI, while the overall AHI and supine AHI both exceed 5 per hour [4, 5]. This definition is useful because in such patients elimination of supine sleep should result in resolution of sleep apnea. With the original definition while demonstrating a clear positional tendency, the clinical importance is less clear. A reduction in AHI from 60 per hour in the supine posture to 29 per hour in the non-supine posture meets the definition for positional sleep apnea. However, complete elimination of supine sleep would not successfully treat sleep apnea. Thus, positional therapy in this type of patient could only be used as an adjunct measure. Identification of this positional tendency would still be clinically useful if it predicted the response to therapy to different modalities. There have been recent studies that suggest that mandibular advancement devices are more effective in positional sleep apnea patients compared to non-positional sleep apnea patients [6, 7]. Thus, identification of a positional component is potentially a simple way of phenotyping patients with sleep apnea identifying patients more likely to respond to some sleep apnea treatment modalities. Using the original more lenient definition, studies have found that the prevalence varies from 56 % to 71.4 % [4, 8–11], mean 62.6 % ± 6.8 (SD) (Table 1). One of the studies examined the prevalence in a strictly Asian sample and found a prevalence of 67 % indicating that positional sleep apnea is common in non-Caucasian populations as well [10]. There have been some studies that have measured the prevalence data with the much stricter definition discussed above (ratio of the supine AHI and non-supine AHI greater than 2 along with a non-supine AHI less than 5 events per hour) [4, 5]. With this strict definition, the prevalence for positional sleep apnea was substantially less than with the original definition but still ranged from 23 % to 27 % (Table 1) [4, 5].

One of the abovementioned studies was a prospective cohort trial performed in Melbourne, Australia, on 100 consecutive OSA patients, and the prevalence was measured by both definitions [4]. When positional sleep apnea was defined using the lenient definition, the prevalence was 63 %, but when they used the stricter definition for positional sleep apnea, the prevalence decreased to 23 % [4]. In our study, the prevalence using the lenient definition was 58 % and decreased to 27 % with the stricter definition [5]. It is still noteworthy that even with the strict definition, positional sleep apnea is common (Table 1). Thus, methods that can successfully eliminate supine sleep and are tolerable have the potential to be an important treatment modality.

One methodologic point that needs to be considered is the effect that the polysomnographic procedure has on promoting supine sleep in the laboratory. During a sleep study, the patient is connected to a multitude of wires. The patient may try to sleep on his/her back in the sleep laboratory because they are concerned that other postures may promote lead dislodgement. In a prospective study in 12 positional sleep apnea patients, the patients were studied for 3 nights, once with standard PSG leads attached (PSG night) and the other 2 nights without any leads attached, but position was monitored with a position sensor [12]. The time spent supine was 56 % greater during the PSG night compared to the non-PSG nights [12]. This can artifactually magnify the severity of the patients' disease (when they have a positional component) compared to what would occur at home when supine sleep would be less.

There have also been significant differences in the AHI when tested in the right lateral compared to the left lateral position. A retrospective review performed in Turkey noted that the left lateral position had a higher AHI at 30.2 ± 32.6 per hour compared to the right lateral position at 23.6 ± 30.1 per hour that was statistically significant ($p < 0.001$) [13]. Another interesting study evaluated 105 sleep apnea patients in the sleep laboratory using a 9-position thoracic sensor. Positions identified were the left lateral (L), prone (P), prone left (PL), prone right (PR), right (R), supine (S), supine left (SL), supine right (SR), and upward position (UP) [14]. It was noted that the AHI gradually improved when the body position changed from the supine to prone position [14]. Thus, in this study, the AHI was worse in the supine posture, intermediate in the lateral posture, and best in the prone posture (Fig. 1). The AHI in the upright posture was similar to that observed in the prone position. The supine left or right was a position intermediate between the supine and lateral position and had an AHI that was similar to that observed in the lateral position. Similarly, the prone right and left was a position intermediate between the prone and lateral position and had an AHI similar to that observed in the prone position [14].

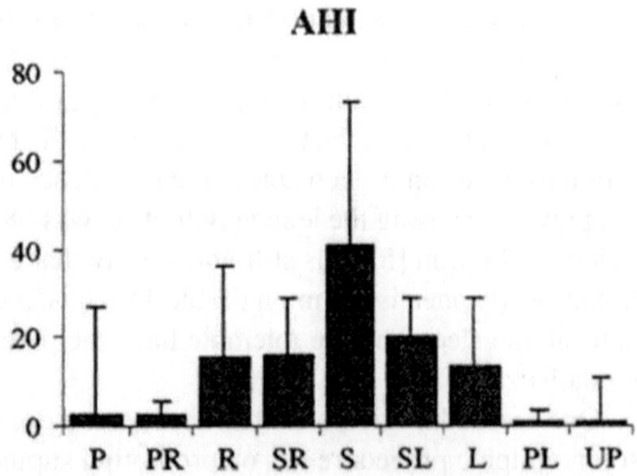

Fig. 1 AHI in different body positions. *L* left lateral, *P* prone, *PL* prone left, *PR* prone right, *R* right, *S* supine, *SL* supine left, *SR* supine right, and *UP* upward position. Figure adapted from Pneumologia, 2011. **60**(4): p. 216–21 [14] with permission

Factors That Predict Occurrence of Positional Sleep Apnea

Multiple factors have been evaluated in the last few decades that are strongly associated or directly affect the prevalence of positional sleep apnea.

Sleep Apnea Severity

As recommended by the American Academy of Sleep Medicine, sleep apnea severity is classified into three categories based on the AHI [15]. Mild sleep apnea has an AHI between 5 and 15 events per hour; moderate sleep apnea, an AHI between 15 and 30 events per hour; and severe sleep apnea, an AHI more than 30 events per hour [15].

There have been several studies performed to evaluate the prevalence of positional sleep apnea among the different severities of sleep-disordered breathing.

A study by Mador et al. evaluated patients at two different settings: at a veterans affairs medical center with a predominantly male population and a free-standing ambulatory sleep center with equal gender proportions. They noted that positional sleep apnea prevalence (defined using the strict definition for positional sleep apnea) decreased as the sleep apnea severity increased [5]. It was 49.5 % in mild sleep apnea, 19.4 % in moderate sleep apnea, and 6.5 % in severe sleep apnea [5]. Another study by the same group evaluated 80 sequential patients who were referred to the Veterans Affairs Medical Center in Western New York and enrolled 20 patients in each of the three sleep apnea severity categories and an additional 20 patients who did not meet the definition for sleep apnea [16]. The hazard ratio for events (apneas and hypopneas) was significant in patients during supine compared to non-supine sleep in the mild and moderate sleep apnea groups at 1.25 (95 % CI 1.02–1.52) and 1.24 (95 % CI 1.04–1.47), respectively [16], meaning that events were more likely to occur in the supine posture compared to the non-supine posture in patients with mild and moderate sleep apnea but not in the normal and severe sleep apnea groups [16].

A retrospective analysis by Oksenberg et al. evaluated 574 sleep apnea patients diagnosed by a respiratory distress index (RDI) greater than 10 per hour. They were further categorized into four different RDI categories (10–19.9, 20–29.9, 30–39.9, greater than 40 per hour). It was noted that the prevalence of positional sleep apnea (defined using the more lenient definition) remained high between 65.1 and 69.0 % in the mild, moderate, severe sleep apnea categories (RDI 10–19.9, 20–29.9, and 30–39.9 per hour), but showed a statistically significant reduction to 32.4 % in the most severe category (RDI greater than 40 per hour) [11]. Chung et al. evaluated 218 positional sleep apnea patients and randomly selected 109 of these patients to be matched with non-positional sleep apnea patients by age, gender, and body mass index (BMI) [17]. It was noted that both the matched and unmatched positional sleep apnea patients had less severe AHI values compared to the non-positional sleep apnea patients [17].

Although "positionality" gets weaker as the severity of sleep apnea worsens, it should be noted that in severe sleep apnea patients, the severity of each apneic event (apnea duration, the lowest oxygen desaturation, and duration of arousals) is still worse in the supine position compared to the non-supine position [18]. A retrospective review performed by Oksenberg et al. evaluated 638 patients undergoing two diagnostic polysomnograms (PSG)s at least 6 months apart [19]. Obstructive sleep apnea was seen in 566 patients [19]. They were then divided into four groups according to whether a positional component occurred during the two recorded PSGs: "non-positional sleep apnea (NPP) who remained NPP," "positional sleep apnea (PP) who remained PP," "PP who became NPP," and "NPP who became PP" [19]. The "NPP who remained NPP" group were found to have a higher AHI in their initial PSG compared to the other three groups. The group of patients that had "PP who became NPP" had a significant increase in the AHI compared to the other three groups [19]. Thus, worsening of the AHI reduces the prevalence of positional sleep apnea.

Ozeke et al. evaluated the AHI on the left side and compared it to the right side in patients with different severities of obstructive sleep apnea [13]. It was noted that on the left side, AHI was significantly higher compared to the right side in patients with moderate and severe OSA, but was not significantly different in patients with mild OSA [13].

Why is positional sleep apnea more common in patients with mild to moderate sleep apnea? Patients with positional sleep apnea might have a less collapsible upper airway that only collapses in the supine posture when gravity works against the patient. Patients with severe sleep apnea likely have a more collapsible airway that collapses in all postures, and since the AHI is already severely increased in the non-supine posture, it is difficult for that metric to substantially worsen in the supine posture. The prior study by Oksenberg et al. shows that as sleep apnea worsens, patients often will switch from a positional component to a non-positional component [19].

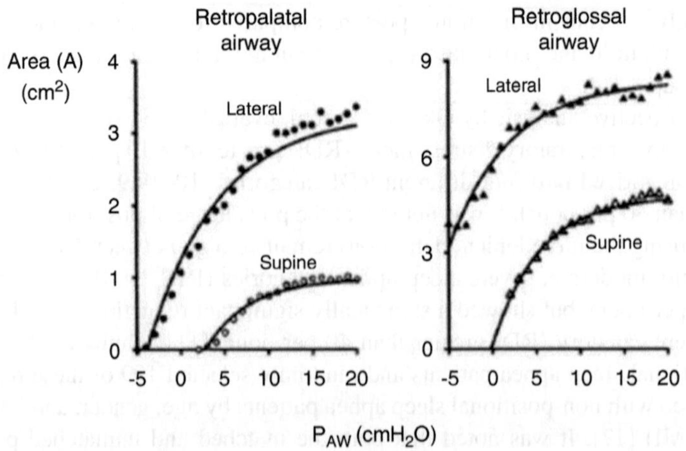

Fig. 2 Static pressure area plot in supine and lateral positions. P_{AW} airway pressure. Figure adapted from Anesthesiology, 2002. **97**(4): p. 780–5 [21] with permission

Anatomic/Morphological Factors

There are multiple studies performed to evaluate the anatomic factors that would determine the propensity of having positional sleep apnea.

A Belgium study evaluated the effect of changes in body position from prone to right side to supine by fast-computed tomography scanning in six awake position-dependent OSA patients and five position-nondependent OSA patients [20]. It was noted that the former (positional patients) had a larger minimum cross-sectional area than the latter and changes in body position affected the lateral but not the anteroposterior dimensions of the upper airway [20]. A study on 91 Korean patients with OSAS evaluated the level of obstruction based on video fluoroscopy [9]. The patients with soft palate obstruction had a higher chance of having positional sleep apnea compared to the patients with tongue base obstruction [9]. A Japanese study tried to evaluate the pathophysiology of positional sleep apnea [21]. They induced total muscle paralysis with general anesthesia in eight OSA patients in order to eliminate neuromuscular factors that could contribute to pharyngeal wall patency [21]. The cross-sectional area of the pharynx was measured endoscopically at different static airway pressures [21]. Then, a static pressure area plot between the positions was assessed to evaluate the influence of body position on the mechanical properties of the pharyngeal wall [21]. Static pressure area curves were higher in the lateral position compared to the supine position indicating a larger upper airway area at any given pressure in the lateral position (Fig. 2) [21]. In another small Japanese study, ten BMI-, age-, and AHI-matched positional and non-positional sleep apnea patients, respectively, underwent pharyngeal magnetic resonance imaging and cephalometric radiography during wakefulness [22]. They noted that positional sleep apnea patients have smaller volumes of the pharyngeal lateral wall soft tissues compared to non-positional sleep apnea patients [22]. They also have a larger maxilla-nasion-mandible angle and a smaller lower facial height than the latter [22]. They concluded that positional sleep apnea patients could have a wider airway laterally and a more backward position of the lower jaw compared to non-positional sleep apnea patients [22] which would lead to obstruction primarily in the supine posture. A Chinese study on 103 OSA patients revealed that the modified Mallampati (MMP) grade and the neck circumference were important morphological features that helped to predict which patients were likely to have positional sleep apnea [23]. Those with a thick neck or small airway by Mallampati score were less likely to have positional sleep apnea [23]. A Japanese study published in 2008 evaluated the upper airway morphology in positional sleep apnea compared to non-positional sleep apnea patients [24]. They noted that the horizontal distance between the tonsillar fauces was significantly greater in positional sleep apnea patients [24].

An Australian study that evaluated the critical pressure at which the pharynx collapses in 23 OSA patients noted a significant decrease in the passive pharyngeal collapsibility associated with change from supine to lateral position [25].

There is also a change of shape of the upper airway from the supine to non-supine posture. When anatomical optical coherence tomography was used to scan the upper airway in OSA patients, it was noted that the upper airway changed from a more transversely oriented elliptical shape when supine to a more circular shape in the non-supine position [26]. It was suggested that the increase in circularity has a lesser propensity for tube collapse and this may be responsible for the reduction in obstructive episodes in the non-supine position [26]. Another Chinese study noted that the distance from the velum tip to the pharyngeal wall was narrower in non-positional sleep apnea patients compared to positional sleep apnea patients [27]. Thus, changes in pharyngeal shape, size, and collapsibility all occur when patients shift from the lateral to supine posture promoting a worsening of sleep apnea in the supine posture. The less pronounced these changes are in the non-supine posture, the more likely the patient is to display a clinically significant worsening in the AHI when he/she moves to the supine posture.

Obesity

Obesity has always been strongly associated with sleep apnea. A longitudinal analysis of the Wisconsin cohort concluded that a 10 % increase in body weight could be associated with a six times risk of developing OSA in subjects who did not have sleep apnea on their original study [28]. With regard to positional sleep apnea, there have been many studies evaluating the effect of body weight on positional sleep apnea. The studies date back as early as 1985, when Cartwright et al. evaluated 24 male patients with sleep apnea [3]. Fourteen out of the 24 were classified as having positional sleep apnea, 12 of whom were nonobese (defined as less than 25 % above their ideal weight), while 7 out of the 10 non-positional sleep apnea patients met the obesity criterion (more than 25 % above their ideal weight) [3]. In a retrospective study performed on 574 sleep apnea patients subjects were divided into five different categories depending on the BMI (20–24.9; 25–29.9; 30–34.9; 35–39.9; and greater than 40) [11]. There was a significant decrease in the prevalence of positional sleep apnea as the BMI increased [11]. The authors also found that when the total group was divided into obese (BMI greater than 30) and nonobese (BMI less than or equal to 30) groups, the prevalence of positional sleep apnea was 42.2 % and 68 %, respectively. Three of the four severely obese patients, who had non-positional sleep apnea, successfully lost weight and converted to positional sleep apnea [11]. In another study of 218 positional sleep apnea patients and 123 non-positional sleep apnea patients, the BMI correlated with the AHI severity only in non-positional sleep apnea patients [17]. A study that evaluated 120 sleep apnea patients observed a higher BMI in non-positional sleep apnea patients compared to the positional sleep apnea patients, although the difference did not reach statistical significance [8]. A Japanese study classified 257 sleep apnea patients into a normal weight group (BMI under 24.0), mild obese group (BMI 24.0–26.4), and obese group (BMI 26.4 and heavier), which is different from the classification of obesity in the United States [29]. They noted that the prevalence of positional sleep apnea proportionally decreased as the BMI increased from 90.9 % in the normal weight group to 74.0 % in the mild obese group and to 57.4 % in the obese group [29]. Another Japanese study that evaluated the effect of BMI on positional sleep apnea concluded that improvements due to changes in posture became increasingly smaller with increases in the BMI [30].

A retrospective review of 2,077 OSA patients concluded that non-positional sleep apnea patients had a higher BMI compared to positional sleep apnea patients [31].

These authors also noted in another study that weight gain could convert patients with positional sleep apnea to non-positional sleep apnea, while weight loss could convert patients with non-positional sleep apnea to positional sleep apnea [19].

Thus, BMI has an inverse relationship with positional sleep apnea [11]. An increase in weight makes positional sleep apnea less likely. One mechanism that could explain this phenomenon is the changes noted in upper airway size and shape with weight gain due to deposition of adipose tissue in the upper airway that could convert positional sleep apnea to non-positional sleep apnea.

Age

In one study, the prevalence of positional sleep apnea decreased to 48.6 % in patients 60 years and older compared to 59.2 % in patients who were younger than 60 years [11]. A subsequent larger study performed by the same author revealed no significant age difference between the positional sleep apnea and the non-positional sleep apnea patients [31]. Another study noted a statistically significant difference in the ages between positional sleep apnea and non-positional sleep apnea patients, 47.1 years and 53.9 years, respectively [8].

Age may play a small role in identifying positional sleep apnea patients although results are conflicting. The positional effect seems to decrease with increase in age, and thus younger patients have a higher probability of having positional sleep apnea.

Effect of Sleep Stage on Positional Sleep Apnea

The effect of sleep stages on OSA has been well studied and documented in the past with worsening of respiratory events during rapid eye movement (REM) sleep compared to non-rapid eye movement (NREM) sleep. Muscle atonia is more prominent during REM sleep, and this is felt to be the major reason why sleep apnea worsens during this sleep stage. There is a significant amount of literature that has evaluated the effects of various sleep stages on positional sleep apnea, especially the effect of REM sleep compared to NREM sleep. A study of 263 subjects noted that sleep architecture was better preserved in positional sleep apnea patients than in non-positional sleep apnea patients with a lower arousal index of 26.0 ± 17.4 per hour and 45.4 ± 30.5 per hour, respectively, and higher slow wave sleep 15.2 ± 10.1 % and 10.2 ± 9.5 %, respectively [10].

A study published in Germany on 16 male OSA patients evaluated the pharyngeal critical pressure and the resistance of the upstream segment during light sleep, slow wave sleep, and REM sleep in the supine and non-supine position [32]. It was noted that during light sleep, the pharyngeal critical pressure decreased from 0.6 ± 0.8 cm H_2O (supine) to -2.2 ± 3.6 cm H_20 (non-supine) ($p < 0.01$) [32]. A more negative critical closing pressure means that the airway is less collapsible in that state. During slow wave sleep stage, the pharyngeal critical pressure decreased from 0.3 ± 1.4 cm H_2O (supine) to -1.7 ± 2.6 cm H_20 (non-supine) ($p < 0.05$), and during REM sleep the pharyngeal critical pressure decreased from 1.2 ± 1.5 cm H_2O (supine) to -2.0 ± 2.2 cm H_2O (non-supine) ($p < 0.05$) [32]. The resistance of the upstream segment had no dependence on body position or sleep stages except in the non-supine position during REM sleep [32].

A carefully performed study evaluated 253 PSGs performed over 3 months. Since the study was from Australia, subjects were classified as having OSA by an AHI ≥ 15 events per hour [33]. In this study, the AHI and to a lesser extent the arousal index progressively decreased from stage 1 NREM sleep to slow wave sleep (Fig. 3). The AHI during REM sleep was intermediate between that observed in stage 1 and stage 2 NREM sleep. The AHI in the lateral position was less than that observed in the supine posture during all NREM sleep stages and also during REM sleep. In both patients with sleep apnea and those who would be characterized in the United States or Europe as having either mild sleep apnea (AHI 5–15 per hour) or no sleep apnea (AHI less than 5 per hour), respiratory events in the lateral position were 50–60 % of that observed in the supine position and arousal events 60–80 % of the supine values.

Studies in the past have examined the phenomena of REM-related OSA that has been defined as an AHI during REM sleep that is more than twofold higher than that

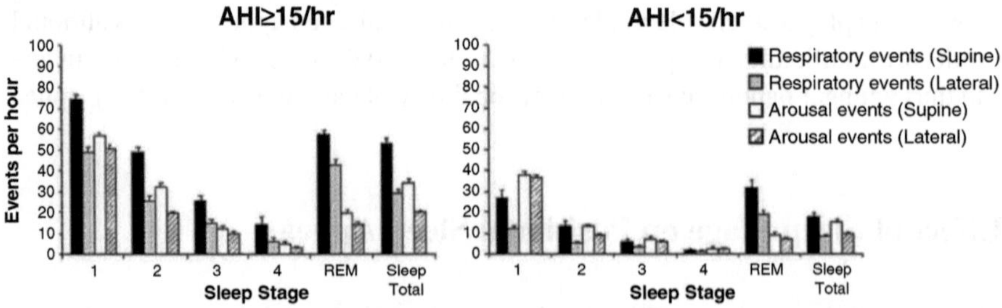

Fig. 3 Respiratory and arousal event frequencies in various sleep stages in supine and lateral positions. Figure adapted from J Clin Sleep Med, 2009. **5**(6): p. 519–24 [33] with permission

observed during NREM sleep with a total AHI greater than 5 per hour [34]. In a study by Eiseman et al., REM-related OSA was observed in about 50 % of patients, and positional sleep apnea (lenient definition) was noted in about 60 % of the patients [34]. The median amount of REM sleep was 16 % of total sleep time, while the median amount of supine sleep was 65 % of total sleep time [34]. It was thus noted that body position had a greater impact on the overall AHI than did the REM sleep AHI [34] simply because the subjects spent more time supine than they spent in REM sleep. Since normally patients spend 15–25 % of total sleep time in REM sleep, there are greater limits to how much REM sleep apnea can influence the overall severity of sleep apnea compared with positional sleep apnea [35].

A prospective analysis by Mador et al. evaluated 80 sequential PSGs performed at the Veterans Affairs Hospital in Buffalo and classified them into four groups: no OSA, mild OSA, moderate OSA, and severe OSA [16]. The hazard ratio for respiratory events in REM sleep compared with NREM sleep was significantly increased for the no OSA, mild, and moderate OSA groups but not the severe group. The hazard ratio for respiratory events in the supine compared with the non-supine position was significant for the mild and moderate OSA groups but not the normal or severe groups [16]. There was no statistically significant interaction effect between the various sleep stages and the supine and non-supine positions [16]. Thus, in this particular study, patients were not additively worse when in the supine posture during REM sleep compared to when they were in the supine posture during NREM sleep. The odds ratio of sleeping in the supine position for REM sleep versus NREM sleep was 0.47 (95 % CI 0.27–0.82) for moderate OSA and 0.54 (95 % CI 0.3–0.95) for severe OSA [16]. Thus, in this study, patients with moderate or severe sleep apnea avoided or at least had less REM sleep in the supine posture which may have in part explained the lack of additive effect of REM and supine sleep.

In an older smaller study [36], it was noted that 9 out of 22 patients who had "positional dependency" during NREM sleep lacked the feature during REM sleep [36]. Another small study [37] noted that the apnea duration was longer in REM sleep compared to NREM sleep even after adjusting for body position [37]. Although the AHI was greater in the supine position compared to the non-supine position, this difference was only noted in NREM sleep [37]. A subsequent study noted that the sleep apnea severity was worse in REM sleep in supine position, followed by NREM sleep in supine position, followed by REM sleep in non-supine position, and lastly by NREM sleep in non-supine position [38].

Some studies have shown that the AHI is worse during REM stage in supine sleep compared to supine NREM sleep or REM non-supine sleep while others have not. However, when one study carefully looked for an interaction between sleep stage and body position, it was not found. Some studies have also shown that positional sleep apnea is more prominent during NREM compared to REM sleep.

However, the largest studies have found a positional effect during both NREM and REM sleep. The finding that patients with moderate and severe OSA had a lesser tendency to sleep in the supine position during REM sleep compared to NREM sleep stage could be the bodies' way of responding to worsening of respiratory events and hypoxemia [16]. In patients with severe neurologic disease who demonstrate significant nocturnal hypoventilation, the amount of REM sleep decreases, and in the most severe cases, no REM sleep is observed at all.

References

1. Young T, et al. The occurrence of sleep-disordered breathing among middle-aged adults. N Engl J Med. 1993;328(17):1230–5.
2. Peppard PE, et al. Increased prevalence of sleep-disordered breathing in adults. Am J Epidemiol. 2013;177(9):1006–14.
3. Cartwright RD. Effect of sleep position on sleep apnea severity. Sleep. 1984;7(2):110–4.
4. Gillman A, et al. Comparison of supine-only and REM-only obstructive sleep apnoea. Sleep Med. 2012;13(7):875–8.
5. Mador MJ, et al. Prevalence of positional sleep apnea in patients undergoing polysomnography. Chest. 2005;128(4):2130–7.
6. Lee CH, et al. The effect of positional dependency on outcomes of treatment with a mandibular advancement device. Arch Otolaryngol Head Neck Surg. 2012;138(5):479–83.
7. Chung JW, et al. Treatment outcomes of mandibular advancement devices in positional and nonpositional OSA patients. Oral Surg Oral Med Oral Pathol Oral Radiol Endod. 2010;109(5):724–31.
8. Richard W, et al. The role of sleep position in obstructive sleep apnea syndrome. Eur Arch Otorhinolaryngol. 2006;263(10):946–50.
9. Sunwoo WS, et al. Association between positional dependency and obstruction site in obstructive sleep apnea syndrome. Clin Exp Otorhinolaryngol. 2012;5(4):218–21.
10. Teerapraipruk B, et al. Clinical and polysomnographic data of positional sleep apnea and its predictors. Sleep Breath. 2012;16(4):1167–72.
11. Oksenberg A, et al. Positional vs nonpositional obstructive sleep apnea patients: anthropomorphic, nocturnal polysomnographic, and multiple sleep latency test data. Chest. 1997;112(3): 629–39.
12. Metersky ML, Castriotta RJ. The effect of polysomnography on sleep position: possible implications on the diagnosis of positional obstructive sleep apnea. Respiration. 1996; 63(5):283–7.
13. Ozeke O, et al. Influence of the right- versus left-sided sleeping position on the apnea-hypopnea index in patients with sleep apnea. Sleep Breath. 2012;16(3):617–20.
14. Tiotiu A, et al. Body position and breathing abnormalities during sleep: a systematic study. Pneumologia. 2011;60(4):216–21.

15. Sleep-related breathing disorders in adults: recommendations for syndrome definition and measurement techniques in clinical research. The Report of an American Academy of Sleep Medicine Task Force. Sleep 1999;22(5):667–89.
16. Mador MJ, et al. Are the adverse effects of body position in patients with obstructive sleep apnea dependent on sleep stage? Sleep Breath. 2010;14(1):13–7.
17. Chung JW, et al. Patients with positional versus nonpositional obstructive sleep apnea: a retrospective study of risk factors associated with apnea-hypopnea severity. Oral Surg Oral Med Oral Pathol Oral Radiol Endod. 2010;110(5):605–10.
18. Oksenberg A, et al. Association of body position with severity of apneic events in patients with severe nonpositional obstructive sleep apnea. Chest. 2000;118(4):1018–24.
19. Oksenberg A, et al. Obstructive sleep apnoea in adults: body postures and weight changes interactions. J Sleep Res. 2012;21(4):402–9.
20. Pevernagie DA, et al. Effects of body position on the upper airway of patients with obstructive sleep apnea. Am J Respir Crit Care Med. 1995;152(1):179–85.
21. Isono S, Tanaka A, Nishino T. Lateral position decreases collapsibility of the passive pharynx in patients with obstructive sleep apnea. Anesthesiology. 2002;97(4):780–5.
22. Saigusa H, et al. Three-dimensional morphological analyses of positional dependence in patients with obstructive sleep apnea syndrome. Anesthesiology. 2009;110(4):885–90.
23. Weihu C, et al. Relationship of body position, upper airway morphology, and severity of obstructive sleep apnea/hypopnea syndrome among Chinese patients. Acta Otolaryngol. 2011; 131(2):173–80.
24. Soga T, et al. Upper airway morphology in patients with obstructive sleep apnea syndrome: effects of lateral positioning. Auris Nasus Larynx. 2009;36(3):305–9.
25. Ong JS, et al. Variability of human upper airway collapsibility during sleep and the influence of body posture and sleep stage. J Sleep Res. 2011;20(4):533–7.
26. Walsh JH, et al. Effect of body posture on pharyngeal shape and size in adults with and without obstructive sleep apnea. Sleep. 2008;31(11):1543–9.
27. Chang ET, Shiao GM. Craniofacial abnormalities in Chinese patients with obstructive and positional sleep apnea. Sleep Med. 2008;9(4):403–10.
28. Peppard PE, et al. Longitudinal study of moderate weight change and sleep-disordered breathing. JAMA. 2000;284(23):3015–21.
29. Itasaka Y, et al. The influence of sleep position and obesity on sleep apnea. Psychiatry Clin Neurosci. 2000;54(3):340–1.
30. Akita Y, et al. Posture of patients with sleep apnea during sleep. Acta Otolaryngol Suppl. 2003;550:41–5.
31. Oksenberg A, et al. The significance of body posture on breathing abnormalities during sleep: data analysis of 2077 obstructive sleep apnea patients. Harefuah. 2009;148(5):304–9. 350, 351.
32. Penzel T, et al. Effect of sleep position and sleep stage on the collapsibility of the upper airways in patients with sleep apnea. Sleep. 2001;24(1):90–5.
33. Ratnavadivel R, et al. Marked reduction in obstructive sleep apnea severity in slow wave sleep. J Clin Sleep Med. 2009;5(6):519–24.
34. Eiseman NA, et al. The impact of body posture and sleep stages on sleep apnea severity in adults. J Clin Sleep Med. 2012;8(6):655–6A.
35. Kryger MH, Roth T, Dement WC. Principles and practice of sleep medicine. 5th ed. Philadelphia, PA: Saunders/Elsevier; 2011.
36. Pevernagie DA, Shepard Jr JW. Relations between sleep stage, posture and effective nasal CPAP levels in OSA. Sleep. 1992;15(2):162–7.
37. George CF, Millar TW, Kryger MH. Sleep apnea and body position during sleep. Sleep. 1988;11(1):90–9.
38. Oksenberg A, et al. REM-related obstructive sleep apnea: the effect of body position. J Clin Sleep Med. 2010;6(4):343–8.

The Contribution of Head Position to the Apnea/Hypopnea Index in Patients with Position-Dependent Obstructive Sleep Apnea

Ellen R. van Kesteren and Anthony A.J. Hilgevoord

Introduction

It is generally known that body position affects apnea/hypopnea occurrence during sleep in patients with OSA. A substantial proportion of OSA patients have the highest apnea/hypopnea index (AHI) when lying in supine position compared to other sleep positions. Thus, in these patients, turning sideways results in a substantial decrease of respiratory events. In literature, this group is classified as having a position-dependent OSA [1–7].

The gold standard for diagnosing OSA is an overnight polysomnography. To identify position-dependent OSA, a polysomnograph measurement system is required which offers the possibility to record body position. Several commercially available recording systems have an integrated position sensor. These portable devices are strapped to the chest of the patient. Alternatively, recording systems are used with separate position sensors connected to the recorder by a wire. These sensors are usually placed anteriorly in the midline of the trunk on the elastic belts which are used to record respiratory movements. In some centers, the chest belt is used for this, in others the abdominal belt.

The clustering of respiratory events in the supine position, with significantly higher AHI over these episodes, is usually directly apparent from the hypnogram (Fig. 1a).

However, quite often one encounters hypnograms with a clear clustering of apnea/hypopnea events without this straightforward relationship to supine or another body position. Often, a cluster of apnea/hypopnea events may start or cease abruptly without seeing a change of body position or sleep stage (Fig. 1b).

E.R. van Kesteren, B.Sc. (✉) • A.A.J. Hilgevoord, M.D., Ph.D.
Department of Neurology and Clinical Neurophysiology, St. Lucas Andreas Hospital, Jan Tooropstraat 164, Amsterdam 1061 AE, The Netherlands
e-mail: e.vankesteren@slaz.nl

N. de Vries et al. (eds.), *Positional Therapy in Obstructive Sleep Apnea*,
DOI 10.1007/978-3-319-09626-1_5

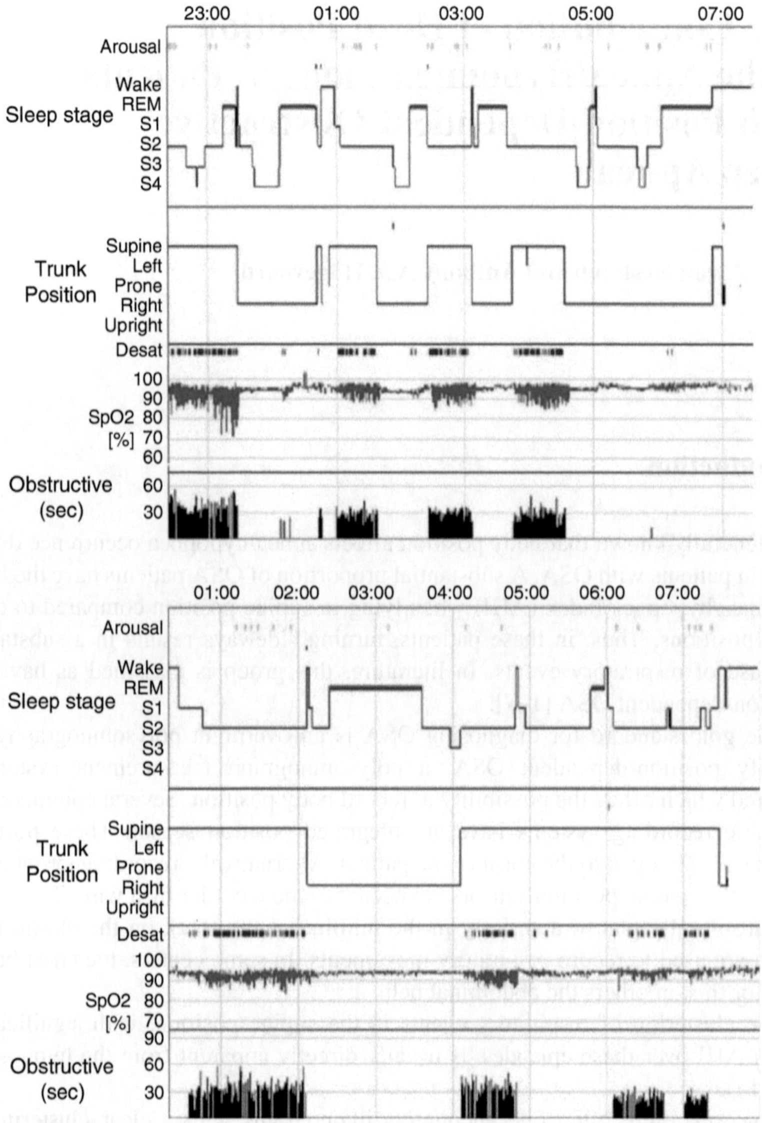

Fig. 1 Overnight polysomnograms of two separate OSA patients. (**a**) Trunk supine position-dependent OSA: the apneas are primarily related to the position of the trunk. (**b**) Clusters of apnea are related to the position of the trunk, but also periods without any apnea in this position are seen

This observation was the basis for some additional investigations in our sleep clinic. In this we looked at several aspects of current practice of measurement of body position.

Ultimately, this led to a study in 300 subjects in whom we recorded both the position of the trunk and of the head. The results of this study will be discussed to demonstrate the importance of head position, separately of trunk position, in patients with position-dependent OSA [1].

How to Measure Body Position During Polysomnography of Suspected OSA Patients?

In literature, no clear research-based guidelines are found on the technical aspects of recording body position. There are no reports on how to attach the position sensors to the body of the patient to achieve the most reliable position detection and recording. One might think that the frequently observed discrepancy between apnea/hypopnea clustering and body position is due to artifacts from the position-sensor data or is caused by sensor displacement during the night.

We set out to investigate this matter more into detail. Firstly we looked at the position sensor. The position sensor we use is an electromechanical one, mainly based on the displacement of a small mercury droplet within the sensor in different orientations due to gravity. The sensor generates five discrete output voltage levels corresponding to five different sleep positions; left, right, supine, prone and upright, with a threshold angle of ±10° from the 45° position boundary. The position sensor should reliably reflect the orientation of the sensor relative to the direction of gravity. This was assured by regularly checking and calibrating the sensors. Also position output was checked by turning over the patient when the sensors were attached. Of additional importance is that sensor characteristics remain stable throughout the night. Potential confounders are slow drifts in the output of devices based on acceleration sensors. The electromechanical type we used should not be prone to this problem. The recorded voltage levels are digitized by the polysomnographic device and stored in a raw data file on the computer as a sequence of numbers. Numerical analysis of these data files demonstrated a good reproducibility and did not show significant overnight drifts or possibly confounding spurious sensor output signals.

The second step of our investigation focused on the fixation of the position sensor on the trunk. In our center, we use a polysomnography system with a separate position sensor connected by wire to the recording device. To exclude sensor displacement, the position sensor was taped directly to the chest of the patient at the lower part of the sternum. At this location, under normal circumstances, the body surface is fairly horizontal when the patient is lying supine. Also, the lower part of the sternum has the least possible amount of subcutaneous tissue, which minimizes possible movement of the sensor relative to the rigid underlying structures of the trunk (Fig. 2). To assure a reliable readout, the surface of the bed was kept horizontal overnight.

All patients were also checked at the end of the overnight recording session to exclude position sensor dislocation. This procedural refinement did show a more consistent recording of trunk position. Also in a number of patients, it was verified that there was a good correspondence between position sensor indicated position and that visually observed by overnight video surveillance. With these procedural refinements, we are quite confident that the position recording faithfully reflects the position of the trunk of the patients under investigation.

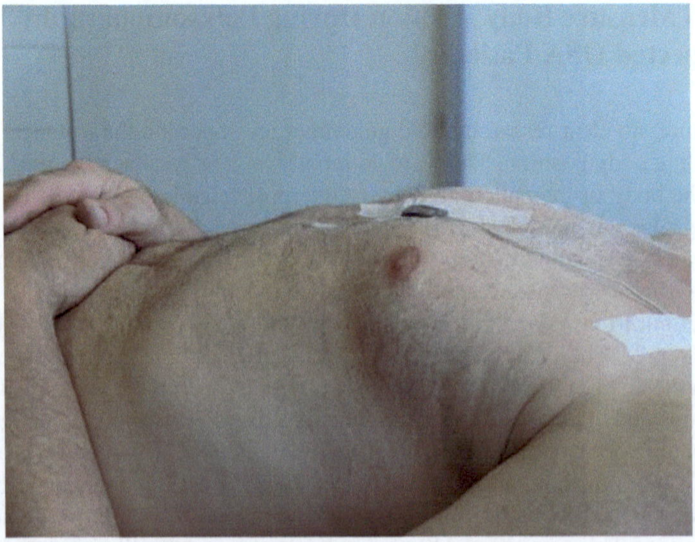

Fig. 2 Location of the trunk position sensor

However, despite our efforts at procedural optimizations, we still regularly encountered hypnograms with clusters of apnea/hypopnea, without any clear relation with the recorded body position or sleep stage.

One could hypothesize that the position of the trunk is not the only important factor for having a position-dependent OSA. The position of the head could additionally affect the appearance of respiratory events in some OSA patient. We investigated this more specifically.

How to Measure Head Position?

In literature also, no studies are found on the most reliable recording methods of head position in patients suspected of OSA. The diagnosis of position-dependent OSA is commonly related to the position of the trunk only. This is also because the vast majority of polygraph systems can record only one position parameter. To investigate head position in addition to the trunk position, we performed polysomnogram recordings with dual position sensors. The position sensor on the trunk was attached to the sternum as described previously. An identical sensor was taped directly to the skin in the middle of the forehead, just above the eyebrows (Fig. 3). This location is approximately horizontal when the head lies in supine position.

To make sure this position readout gives the correct values, patients were asked to sleep with a single pillow (Fig. 4). It was assured that this setup could reliably detect visually observed lateral rotation of the head during sleep, with or without rotation of the trunk. A limitation is that our type of sensor does not allow a

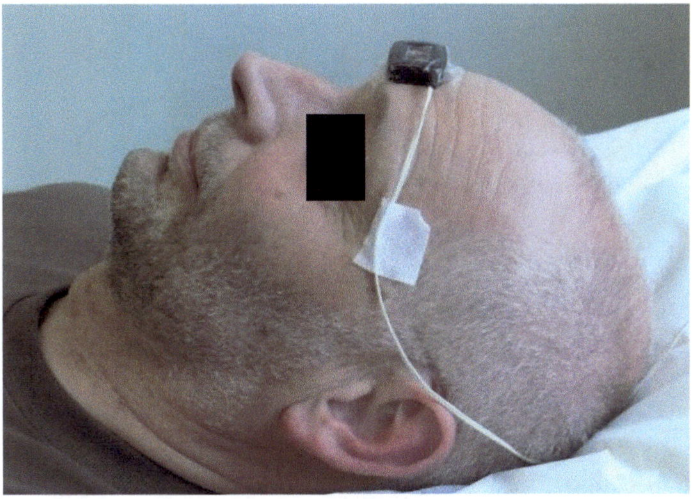

Fig. 3 Location of the head position sensor

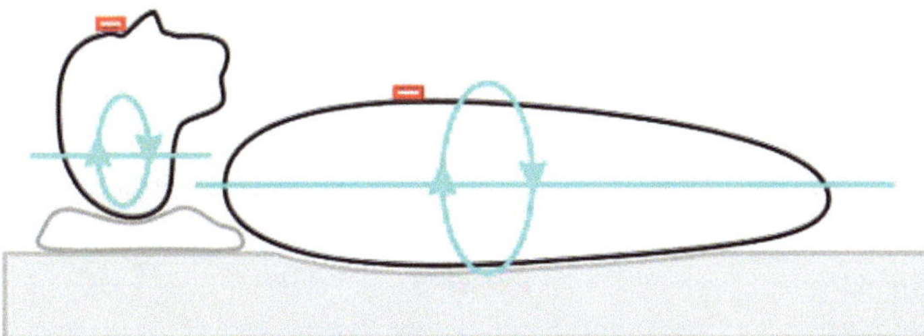

Fig. 4 Schematic representation of our dual-rotation recording setup

continuous recording of the exact angle of lateral rotation. It only detects rotation of more than 45° to the left or right.

The electromechanical sensor on the forehead could potentially also record flexion and extension. However, because of the detection thresholds, only major flexion and extension movements may be detected. Such large flexion-extension movements are not likely to occur during sleep lying supine with the head supported by a single pillow. Recording of flexion-extension movements would require a more elaborate setup. Also, because the trunk-neck-head complex does not have a single flexion-extension rotation axis. In the most simplified form, one might use a model with two rotation axes (Fig. 5). The figure illustrates that a "neutral" head position may occur in very different postures of the neck.

Ideally, one would also record lateroflexion of the neck and the orientation of the mandible relative to the skull.

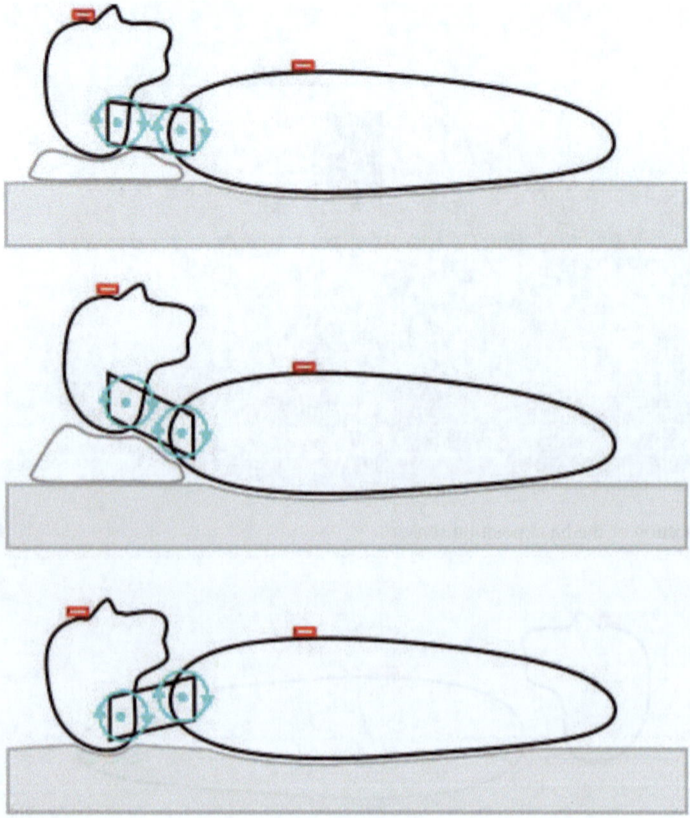

Fig. 5 Schematic representation of freedom of movement in flexion-extension

How to Combine Head and Trunk Position Analysis?

As we were limited in our technical means, the focus of our investigation was aimed primarily at lateral rotation of the head, and not at flexion-extension. The standard software we used for generating the hypnograms from the recorder data does not allow analysis of multiple position data channels at the same time. However, the recording device did allow simultaneous recording of the output of an additional position sensor at a separate recording channel. The data from each recording channel was transferred to a separate digital computer data file. During analysis, we could choose which position data file to use. Thus, two overnight polysomnograms were constructed: one employed the data from the trunk position sensor and the other employed the data from the head position sensor. All other hypnographic data channels and parameters remained the same.

The setup described allowed us to assess two hypnograms using either head position data or trunk position data but not the interaction between the two.

To achieve this, we synthesized a new position data file from the head and trunk data which reflected all possible combinations of head and trunk position. This was subsequently again entered into the standard analysis process.

Study Setup

To explore the effect of trunk and head position on the AHI, we conducted a study on 300 consecutive adult subjects (>18 years). The group consisted of 227 men (with a mean age of 50 years and an average BMI of 28.7) and 73 women (with a mean age of 49 years and an average BMI of 32.2). Subjects were referred to our department because of clinically suspected OSA and underwent overnight polysomnography. From overnight polysomnograms, the AHI in different positions was determined, and the effect of the trunk and head position on the AHI was investigated. All subjects gave informed consent for participation in this study. Respiratory events were scored according to the AASM 2007 criteria [8]. Sleep stages were scored by using the standard criteria of Rechtschaffen and Kales [9]. Automated hypnogram analysis results were manually reviewed by an experienced sleep investigator.

Firstly, the patients with an AHI > 5 were identified as having OSA.

Secondly, OSA patients who spent >5 and <95 % of the total sleeping time in supine position, based on the trunk position sensor readout, were further analyzed for position dependence. Position dependence was defined as an overnight AHI in supine position (determined for both the trunk position sensor and the head position sensor) at least twice as high as AHI in non-supine positions [1, 2, 4]. Since we used two position sensors, this led to four possible classifications: both trunk and head supine dependent, only trunk supine dependent, only head supine dependent, and not supine dependent.

Thirdly, to evaluate the importance of the head position relative to the trunk position, we further analyzed all subjects with trunk supine position dependence. If the overnight AHI in head supine position proves to be higher than in trunk supine position, this would support our initial hypothesis that in some patients the clustering of respiratory events is related more to head position than to trunk position.

If the overnight AHI in head supine position exceeded the AHI in trunk supine position by ≥5, the patient was classified as having head position-aggravated trunk supine position dependence. This group was evaluated further on the quantitative aspects of the interaction between the position of the head and trunk.

Therefore, finally, we combined the data from both position sensors to determine the AHI over four possible situations: (1) trunk supine + head supine; (2) trunk supine + head not supine; (3) trunk not supine + head supine; and (4) trunk not supine + head not supine.

Results

The results of the study are summarized in the flowchart shown in Fig. 6. Three hundred subjects were included in the study. Based on an overnight AHI>5, of these 300 subjects 241 were diagnosed with OSA. Forty-two of these 241 subjects had to be excluded from the study: 20 because of technical problems due to sensor displacement or due to artifacts and another 22 because of spending too much (>95 %, $n=10$) or too little (<5 %, $n=12$) of the total sleep time in supine position.

The data from the remaining 199 patients were further analyzed for trunk and head position dependence. In 82 of these subjects (41.2 %), the overnight AHI did not meet the criteria of position dependence. Hundred and four patients were classified as trunk supine dependent (the overnight AHI in supine position determined from the trunk position sensor was at least twice as high as AHI in non-supine positions [1, 2, 4]). Hundred and two of these 104 subjects were trunk as well as head supine dependent. Thirteen subjects were only head supine dependent, but not trunk supine dependent.

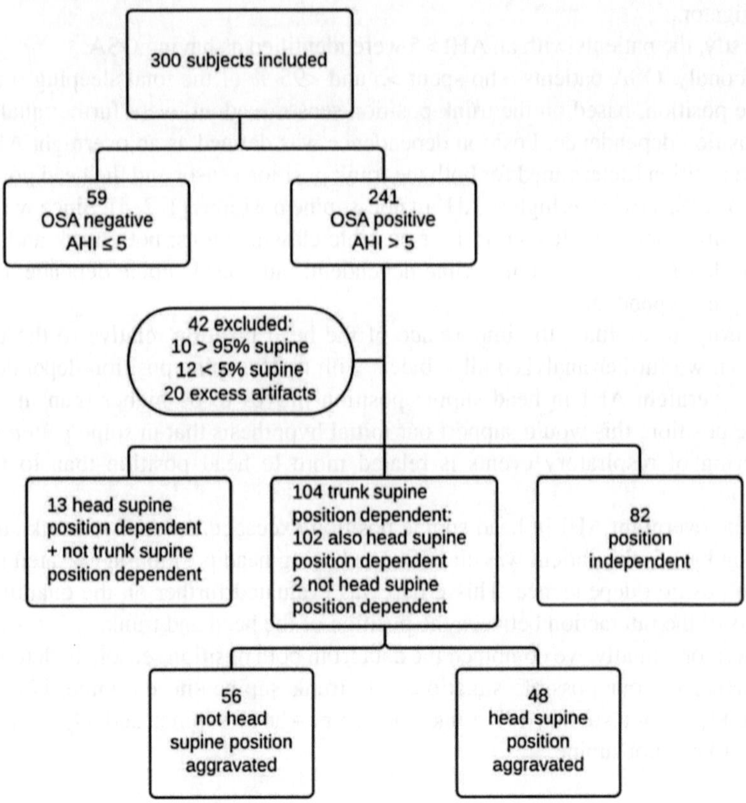

Fig. 6 Flowchart of the 300 subjects included in the study

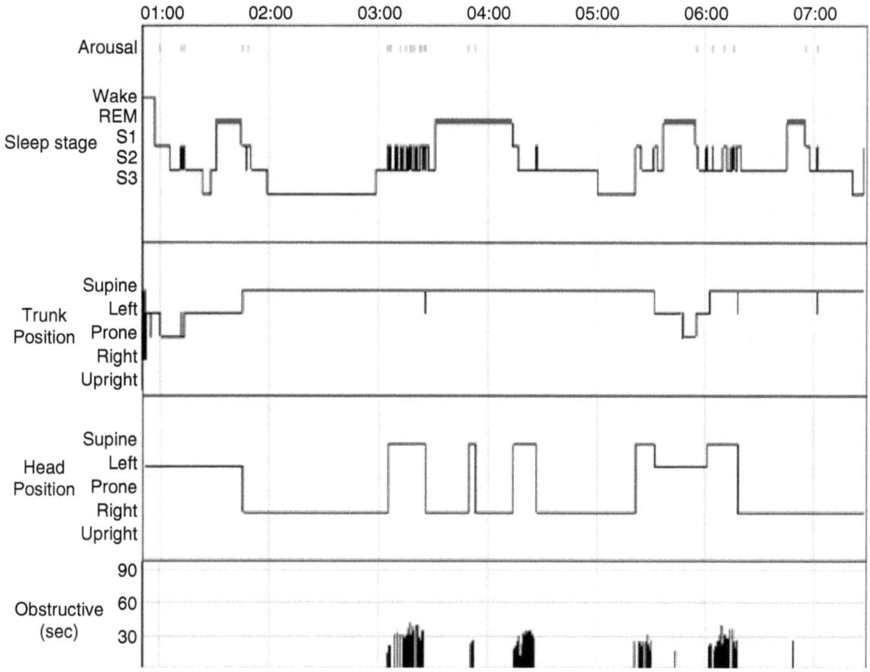

Fig. 7 Overnight polysomnogram in a single subject. Two position channels are displayed: the head position and the trunk position. Apneas are primarily related to the position of the head

In 48 of the 104 trunk supine-dependent subjects (46.2 %), the overnight AHI in supine position was considerably higher when based on the head position sensor than when based on the trunk position sensor. These subjects were classified as having a head position-aggravated trunk supine position-dependent OSA.

Figure 7 shows the polysomnogram of one single subject. A clear clustering of apnea is seen specifically related to the supine position of the head. This subject slept a major part of total sleep time in trunk supine position, and only a small part of this time with the head also in supine position. When the head was turned sideways, the respiratory events disappeared. The AHI in trunk supine position (21.4 per hour, sleeping in trunk supine position 79.9 % of the total sleeping time) was almost the same as the AHI calculated over the total sleep time (23.6 per hour). Based on the criteria for position dependence, this patient does not have a position-dependent OSA. However, since the AHI in head supine position was very high compared to the AHI in trunk supine position (76.8, during 16.6 % of the total sleeping time), this subject is classified as having a head supine position-dependent OSA and not a trunk supine position-dependent OSA. In our study, this was seen in 13 subjects.

Table 1 summarizes the demographic and polysomnographic characteristics of the 199 subjects diagnosed with OSA and further analyzed for trunk and head position dependence. The table shows that more men than women were included in

Table 1 Demographic and polysomnographic characteristics of OSA-positive patients (average ± standard deviation)

	Male	Female	Total
Characteristics			
Patients (*n*)	161	38	199
Age (years)	47.7 (10.5)	49.4 (13.6)	48.0 (11.1)
BMI (kg/m²)	28.7 (4.6)	32.4 (9.4)	29.4 (6.0)
AHI (events/h)			
Total	28.6 (21.3)	23.4 (18.8)	27.6 (20.9)
Trunk supine	40.1 (24.0)	25.6 (19.8)	37.3 (23.9)
Head supine	44.9 (26.9)	33.3 (26.5)	42.7 (27.1)
AHI head supine minus AHI trunk supine	4.8 (16.8)	7.7 (13.7)	5.3 (16.2)
Time percentage			
% time in trunk supine position	44.2 (20.7)	53.3 (22.9)	45.9 (21.4)
% time in head supine position	31.6 (20.4)	31.1 (24.2)	31.5 (21.1)

BMI body mass index, *AHI* apnea-hypopnea index

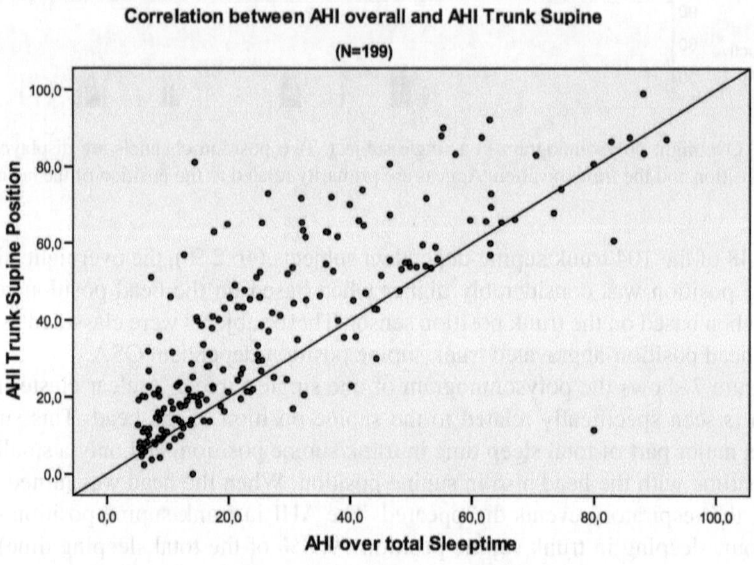

Fig. 8 Correlation of the AHI determined over the total sleep time and the AHI determined over the time spent in trunk supine position. The *line* indicates the unity line

the study, which is similar to the difference between men and women in a general OSA population.

Figure 8 is a graph of the entire OSA-positive study population ($n = 199$). It shows the correlation of the AHI determined over the total sleep time with the AHI during trunk supine position. Notice that a lot of points are lying above the unity line ($x = y$), meaning many OSA patients have a higher AHI in trunk supine position. These are

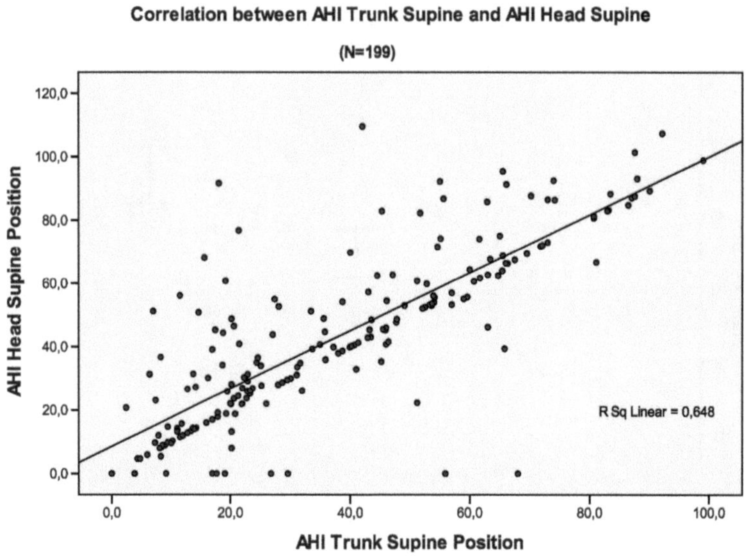

Fig. 9 Correlation of the AHI determined over the time spent in trunk supine position and the time spent in head supine position. The *line* indicates the linear regression line

classified as having trunk supine position dependence. This is also seen in literature on position-dependent OSA.

Figure 9 shows the correlation between the overnight supine AHI based on the trunk and head position sensor in the entire OSA group ($n=199$). Most points lie on the unity line ($x=y$), indicating that the AHI in trunk supine position and head supine position are the same (the unity line is not drawn, but is clearly visible by the large number of points lying on the $x=y$ line). This is reflected in the correlation coefficient ($r^2=0.65$). Still, there is still a large number of outliers above the unity line. This causes that the linear regression line lies parallel with, but above, the unity line. A number of points are seen where the head supine position AHI is zero. This mainly reflects subjects who always had their heads turned sideways while sleeping on their back.

Figure 10 shows the mean AHI values determined over the three different time periods in the entire OSA group ($n=199$). The average AHI determined over the total sleep time was 28 (SD 21, median 21). The average AHI over the time period spent in supine position based on the trunk position sensor was 37 (SD 24, median 32). Based on the head position sensor, this was 43 (SD 27, median 41). These differences were all significant. Clearly is seen that AHI values are highest over the time period in which the head is in supine position.

The data presented thus far show that head supine overnight AHI values are higher than trunk supine overnight AHI values, but give no insight into the interaction between the position of the head and trunk. That was the subject of the next step in our analysis.

Figure 11 first shows the relation between the time spent in trunk supine and in head supine positions. The graph demonstrates that for a large proportion of

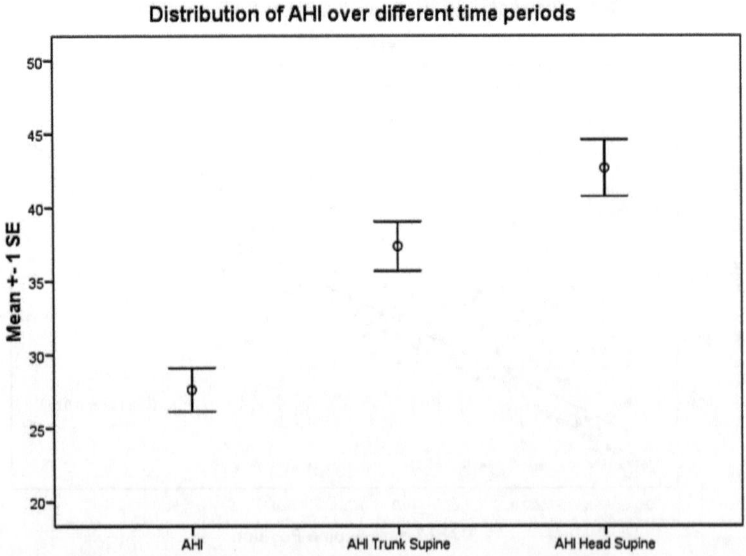

Fig. 10 Mean AHI values determined over the total sleep time, the time spent in trunk supine position, and the time spent in head supine position (in the entire OSA group: $n = 199$)

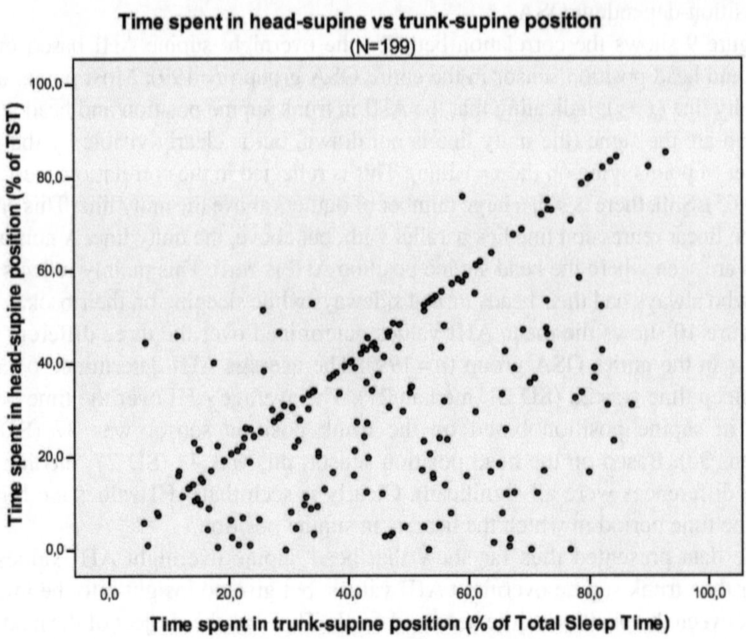

Fig. 11 Correlation of the time spent in head supine position and trunk supine position in the OSA-positive group ($n = 199$)

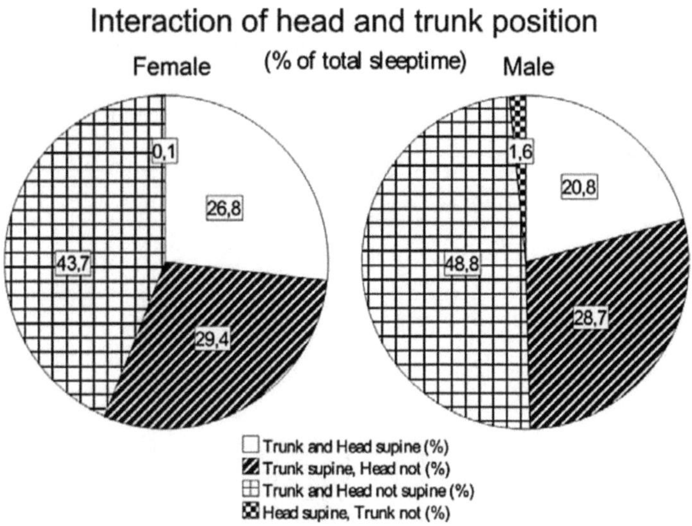

Fig. 12 Relative time spent in trunk supine position and head supine position in the head position-aggravated trunk supine position-dependent group ($n=47$)

subjects, this is the same (the points lie on the unity line, $x=y$). This suggests that the position of the head and the trunk is highly correlated. However, there is also a significant proportion of subjects in whom the time spent in head supine position is considerably shorter than the time spent in trunk supine position. This indicates that these subjects have their head rotated laterally during at least part of the time spent in trunk supine position. In a minority of patients, we even see that the time spent in head supine position remains zero, even when sleeping on the back for a large percentage of the time. This suggests that these subjects always sleep with their head laterally rotated while sleeping on their back.

The remaining part of our investigation dealt with the interaction of the position of the head and trunk. Therefore, we combined the information from the two position sensors. This is a possibility not offered in the standard sleep recorder hard- and software. For this reanalysis, we only reevaluated the hypnograms of the subjects with a head-aggravated trunk supine position dependence ($n=47$). During analysis, we found that these results were different for men and women, and therefore these are presented separately.

Figure 12 shows the relative time spent in the different positions of the head and trunk for men and women in the head position-aggravated trunk supine position-dependent group ($n=47$). Subjects in this group spent approximately half of the total sleep time in trunk supine position. Also seen is that more than half of this trunk supine position time, the head is not in supine position, thus laterally rotated.

The remaining question was whether apnea incidence indeed decreased when the head was turned laterally in head position-aggravated trunk supine position-dependent patients. The answer was yes, as is demonstrated in Fig. 13. The AHI is

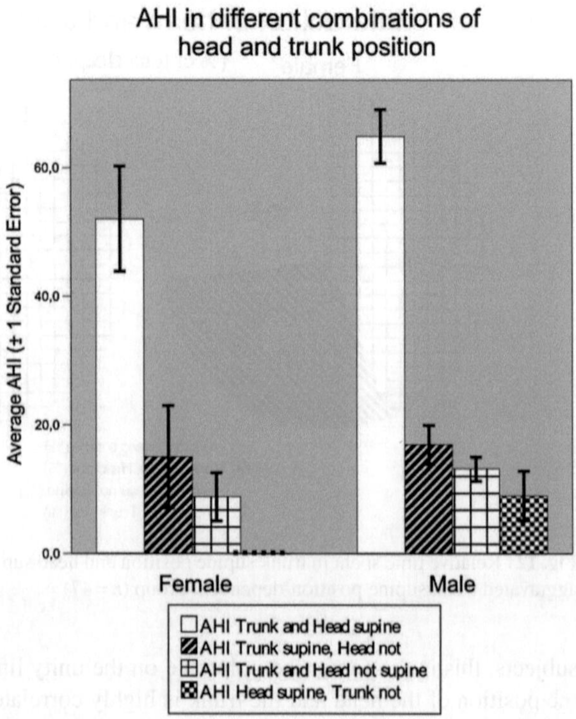

Fig. 13 Average AHI over the time spent in the different combinations of head and trunk position in the head position-aggravated trunk supine position-dependent group ($n=47$)

clearly the highest in the combination of head supine and trunk supine, which means that the head and trunk are both in supine position. The AHI clearly decreases when the head is rotated laterally while lying supine. Sideways rotation of the head had a larger effect for men than for women.

Conclusion

In this study, we first demonstrated that approximately half of our OSA patients show a clear position dependence, a factor comparable to that previously reported in literature. A novel finding is that in approximately a quarter of all OSA patients the head position is an important additional factor next to the position of the trunk. In these patients, the AHI calculated over the time when the head lies supine is higher than the AHI determined over the time when the trunk is in supine position. This finding may have consequences for the manner we diagnose and treat OSA patients in the future [10, 11].

The mechanisms behind the head position dependence of the AHI were not the primary subject of our study. Also flexion-extension movements of the neck were not specifically taken into account.

Investigators, in our group and others, have recently addressed these subjects in more detail.

As stated, most standard software does not allow inclusion of multiple position sensors in the analysis. We had to use some custom computer programming to get around these limitations. This may not be within the reach of every center. Therefore, we hope that the producers of commercially available recorders will add these features in the near future.

References

1. van Kesteren ER, van Maanen J, Hilgevoord AAJ, Laman DM, de Vries N. Quantitative effects of trunk and head position on the apnea hypopnea index in obstructive sleep apnea. Sleep. 2011;34(8):1075–81.
2. Richard W, Kox D, den Herder C, Laman M, van Tinteren H, de Vries N. The role of sleep position in obstructive sleep apnea syndrome. Eur Arch Otorhinolaryngol. 2006;263:946–50.
3. Oksenberg A, Silverberg DS, Arons E, Radwan H. Positional vs non-positional obstructive sleep apnea patients: anthropomorphic, nocturnal polysomnographic, and multiple sleep latency test data. Chest. 1997;112:629–39.
4. Cartwright RD, Diaz F, Lloyd S. The effects of sleep posture and sleep stage on apnea frequency. Sleep. 1991;14:351–3.
5. George CF, Millar TW, Kryger MH. Sleep apnea and body position during sleep. Sleep. 1988;11:90–9.
6. Kavey NB, Blitzer A, Gidro-Frank S, Korstanje K. Sleeping position and sleep apnea syndrome. Am J Otolaryngol. 1985;6:373–7.
7. Cartwright RD. Effect of sleep position on sleep apnea severity. Sleep. 1984;7:110–4.
8. American Academy of Sleep Medicine. The international classification of sleep disorders: diagnostic and coding manual. 2nd ed. Westchester, IL: American Academy of Sleep Medicine; 2005.
9. Rechtschaffen A, Kales A. A manual of standardized terminology: techniques and scoring systems for sleep stages of human subjects. Brain Information Service/Brain Research Institute, UCLA, Los Angeles. 1968;1–15.
10. Bignold JJ, Deans-Costi G, Goldsworthy MR, et al. Poor long-term patient compliance with the tennis ball technique for treating positional obstructive sleep apnea. J Clin Sleep Med. 2009;5:428–30.
11. Oksenberg A, Silverberg D, Offenbach D, Arons E. Positional therapy for obstructive sleep apnea patients: a 6-month follow-up study. Laryngoscope. 2006;116:1995–2000.

Influence of Sleep Position on the Transition of Mild to Moderate and Severe OSA

Linda B.L. Benoist, Sharon Morong, and Nico de Vries

Introduction

Various chapters have shown that positional OSA patients are younger and have a lower BMI, neck circumference, and AHI compared to non-positional OSA patients. In this chapter, several theories about the influences of sleep position on the transition of mild to moderate and severe OSA will be discussed.

POSA

It has been well proven that many patients suffering from OSA have a different rate of apneic events in the lateral position, when compared with the supine position [1]. Position-dependent OSA (POSA) is defined as an AHI which is at least twice as high in supine sleeping position compared to the AHI during sleep in other positions [2–5]. Overall, 56 % of patients with OSA are diagnosed with POSA [4–6].

This chapter is a modified version of the articles "Evaluation of position dependency in non-apneic snorers" 2014 and "The effect of weight loss on OSA severity and position dependence in the bariatric population." The final publications are available at link.springer.com.

L.B.L. Benoist, M.D. (✉)
Ear Nose and Throat, Sint Lucas Andreas Ziekenhuis,
Jan Tooropstraat 164, Amsterdam 1061 AE, The Netherlands
e-mail: l.benoist@slaz.nl

S. Morong, M.D., M.Sc., F.R.C.S.C.
Department of Otolaryngology, Sint Lucas Andreas Ziekenhuis, Amsterdam, The Netherlands

N. de Vries, M.D., Ph.D.
Department of Otolaryngology, Sint Lucas Andreas Ziekenhuis, Amsterdam, The Netherlands

Department of Otolaryngology, University Hospital Antwerp, Antwerp, Belgium

N. de Vries et al. (eds.), *Positional Therapy in Obstructive Sleep Apnea*,
DOI 10.1007/978-3-319-09626-1_6

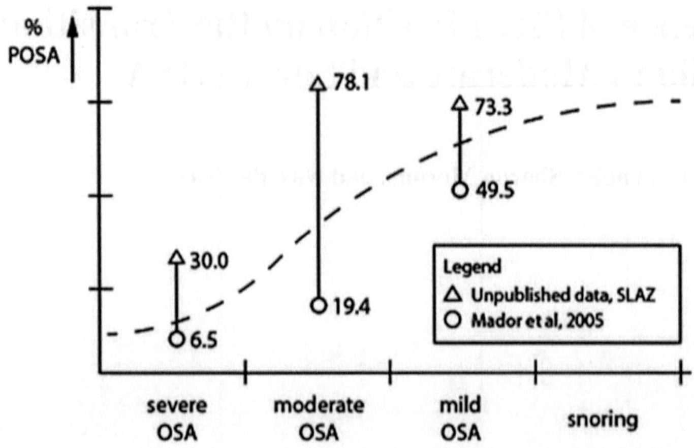

Fig. 1 POSA percentages with results from Mador et al. [7] and unpublished data Sint Lucas Andreas Ziekenhuis (SLAZ)

One study reported that the effect of sleep position in patients with OSA is inversely related to the severity of the disease; in other words, the lower a patient's apnea-hypopnea index (AHI), the more often they were found to be position dependent [7]. Mador et al.'s study population consisted of 144 patients. They found that while almost 50 % of patients with mild OSA (AHI of 5–15) were position dependent, only 19.4 % patients with moderate OSA (AHI of 15–30) were position dependent and even less (6.5 %) patients with severe OSA (AHI > 30) were position dependent. Our study group has found that in a sample size of 248 patients, 73.3 % of the patients were diagnosed with mild POSA, 78.1 % with moderate POSA, and only 30.0 % with severe POSA (unpublished data). Cartwright's definition for POSA was used for the above findings [1]. From these results, an inverse relationship was found between an increasing AHI and the predominance of position dependence. Figure 1 shows the results of these findings in one graph, including a trend line which reflects our hypothesis that position dependency is increased in non-apneic snorers. One possible theory for the development and subsequent worsening of OSA is the transition from having an elevated AHI in the supine position only (mild OSA) to having an elevated AHI in all body positions (severe OSA). This would partly explain why patients with severe OSA are hardly ever position dependent and also suggest that the prevalence of patients with no OSA who snore may be currently underestimated.

Various Theories

Different studies support the statement that patients with POSA are more likely to have a lower BMI, neck circumference, and AHI than their non-positional counterparts. The mechanism underlying this, however, is still unclear. Saigusa et al.

performed awake pharyngeal magnetic resonance imaging and cephalometric radiography on 10 positional and 10 non-positional Japanese patients that were matched for BMI, AHI, and age. The authors found both craniofacial and soft tissue volume differences in positional patients compared to those who were non-positional. Positional patients had more backward positioning of the lower jaw with smaller lower facial height and craniofacial volume. They were also noted to have a smaller volume of lateral pharyngeal wall soft tissue [8].

Teerapraipruk et al. also concur that craniofacial structural changes may play an important role in POSA given that in their population of Asian patients, the average BMI noted in both positional and non-positional patients was lower than the average BMI noted in the Western population [9]. It is possible that a subgroup of patients initially develops OSA that is positional, but when left untreated or undiagnosed, they increase in weight as a consequence of their disease and further develop an OSA that is more severe and non-positional in nature.

Spiegel et al. performed a randomized 2-period, 2-condition crossover clinical study in 12 healthy young men where subjects underwent 2 days of sleep restriction and 2 days of sleep extension. It was found that sleep restriction was associated with increased levels of ghrelin, a hunger-stimulating hormone, and decreased levels of the hunger-suppressing hormone leptin. As a result, increases in hunger and appetite were noted in this sleep-deprived population [10]. It can be postulated that patients with OSA who suffer from fragmented sleep may experience the metabolic changes described above with an increase in weight and subsequently become obese. Patients may also have decreased energy secondary to sleep deprivation, rendering physical activity more difficult and less desirable, which compounds the issue of weight gain and obesity.

Sunnergren et al. believe that the underlying etiology may be neurological [11]. The airway remains open during sleep due to reflexes that dilate the upper airway musculature. These reflexes would be most active in the supine position to counteract gravity and muscular hypotonia. A literature review by Svanborg et al. reports on various studies looking at neurological and electrophysiological findings in the upper airway of non-apneic snorers and patients with OSA [12]. Snoring occurs as a result of vibration of the upper airway soft tissues. Studies have reported that long-term soft tissue vibration can cause local nerve lesions and injury [13, 14]. Svanborg et al. then theorized that repeated snoring over time may cause neuronal lesions with compromise to the dilator reflexes of the upper airway [15]. A study was performed using concentric needle electromyography (EMG) in the palatopharyngeus muscle of 12 OSA patients and 15 non-apneic snorers and 5 controls. Ten out of 12 OSA patients had local motor neuropathy, while only 3 out of 15 non-apneic snorers and none of the controls had neuropathy. They used this finding to hypothesize that progression from non-apneic snoring to OSA may be due to neurogenic injury [15]. Sunnergren et al. have further theorized that the severity of upper airway neuropathy may not only determine progression of non-apneic snoring to OSA but also place POSA as an intermediary between snoring and OSA. The more severe the neuropathy, the more likely that a patient would have problems dilating their upper airway in all sleeping positions and not just supine [11].

Conclusion

The arguments above generate a provocative theory that severe non-positional OSA can in fact be reversed to a mild positional OSA or even positional non-apneic snoring with weight loss. Patients may initially have had non-apneic snoring which subsequently progressed to a mild OSA that was positional in nature. When left untreated, metabolic and neuronal imbalances may have occurred that led to increased weight and obesity and resulted in a transition from mild to moderate sleep apnea noted only in the supine position (POSA) to a more severe sleep apnea noted in all sleeping positions.

References

1. Cartwright RD. Effect of sleep position on sleep apnea severity. Sleep. 1984;7(2):110–4.
2. Cartwright RD, Diaz F, Lloyd S. The effects of sleep posture and sleep stage on apnea frequency. Sleep. 1991;14(4):351–3.
3. Oksenberg A, Silverberg DS. The effect of body posture on sleep-related breathing disorders: facts and therapeutic implications. Sleep Med Rev. 1998;2(3):139–62.
4. Oksenberg A, Silverberg DS, Arons E, Radwan H. Positional vs nonpositional obstructive sleep apnea patients: anthropomorphic, nocturnal polysomnographic, and multiple sleep latency test data. Chest. 1997;112(3):629–39.
5. Richard W, Kox D, den Herder C, Laman M, van Tinteren H, de Vries N. The role of sleep position in obstructive sleep apnea syndrome. Eur Arch Otorhinolaryngol. 2006;263(10): 946–50.
6. Ravesloot MJL, van Maanen JP, Dun L, de Vries N. The undervalued potential of positional therapy in position-dependent snoring and obstructive sleep apnea-a review of the literature. Sleep Breath. 2013;17(1):39–49.
7. Mador MJ, Kufel TJ, Magalang UJ, Rajesh SK, Watwe V, Grant BJ. Prevalence of positional sleep apnea in patients undergoing polysomnography. Chest. 2005;128(4):2130–7.
8. Saigusa H, Suzuki M, Higurashi N, Kodera K. Three-dimensional morphological analyses of positional dependence in patients with obstructive sleep apnea syndrome. Anesthesiology. 2009;110(4):885–90.
9. Teerapraipruk B, Chirakalwasan N, Simon R, et al. Clinical and polysomnographic data of positional sleep apnea and its predictors. Sleep Breath. 2012;16(4):1167–72.
10. Spiegel K, Tasali E, Penev P, Van CE. Brief communication: sleep curtailment in healthy young men is associated with decreased leptin levels, elevated ghrelin levels, and increased hunger and appetite. Ann Intern Med. 2004;141(11):846–50.
11. Sunnergren O, Brostrom A, Svanborg E. Positional sensitivity as a confounder in diagnosis of severity of obstructive sleep apnea. Sleep Breath. 2013;17(1):173–9.
12. Svanborg E. Impact of obstructive apnea syndrome on upper airway respiratory muscles. Respir Physiol Neurobiol. 2005;147(2–3):263–72.
13. Brismar T, Ekenvall L. Nerve conduction in the hands of vibration exposed workers. Electroencephalogr Clin Neurophysiol. 1992;85(3):173–6.
14. Takeuchi T, Futatsuka M, Imanishi H, Yamada S. Pathological changes observed in the finger biopsy of patients with vibration-induced white finger. Scand J Work Environ Health. 1986;12(4 Spec No):280–3.
15. Svanborg E. Upper airway nerve lesions in obstructive sleep apnea. Am J Respir Crit Care Med. 2001;164(2):187–9.

Clinical Characteristics of Positional Obstructive Sleep Apnea Among Asians

Naricha Chirakalwasan

Prior investigations have shown that when matched patients for age, gender, and body mass index, Asians were observed to have more severe OSA based on polysomnographic data [1]. The study comparing Asian and Caucasian OSA patients matching for age, gender, skeletal pattern, body mass index, and respiratory disturbance index revealed that the Chinese group, when compared with the Caucasian group, were found to have smaller maxillas and mandibles, more severe mandibular retrognathism, proclined lower incisors, increased total and upper facial heights, and steeper and shorter anterior cranial bases. Interestingly, the Chinese group was found to have a larger superior-posterior airway space, a larger nasopharynx and oropharynx cross-sectional area, and smaller tongue height [2]. A previous study which compared Far Eastern OSA with white men found that after matched for age, respiratory disturbance index (RDI), and the lowest oxygen desaturation, Asian OSA patients were observed to have more prominent SNA [angle measurement from sella (S) to nasion (N) to subspinate (A)], SNB [angle measurement from sella (S) to nasion (N) to supramental (B)], wider PAS (posterior airway space), and shorter MP-H (mandibular plane to hyoid bone) distance. However, they were noted to have a shorter anterior cranial base (NS) and narrower cranial base flexure (NSBa) than white men with OSA. The authors concluded that the nasopharyngeal and retropalatal regions may have a greater impact in the airway of Asian subjects because of the decreased cranial base dimensions, as opposed to the hypopharyngeal region, which may have a greater effect in the white subjects as reflected in the lower hyoid position [3] (Fig. 1). This notion is confirmed by a study using a videoendoscopic evaluation of the upper airway in Southeast Asian adults with OSA. They observed

N. Chirakalwasan, M.D. (✉)
Division of Pulmonary and Critical Care Medicine, Department of Medicine, Faculty of Medicine, Chulalongkorn University, Bangkok, Thailand

Excellence Center for Sleep Disorders, King Chulalongkorn Memorial Hospital, Thai Red Cross Society, 1873 King Rama IV Road, Bangkok 10330, Thailand
e-mail: narichac@hotmail.com

N. de Vries et al. (eds.), *Positional Therapy in Obstructive Sleep Apnea*,
DOI 10.1007/978-3-319-09626-1_7

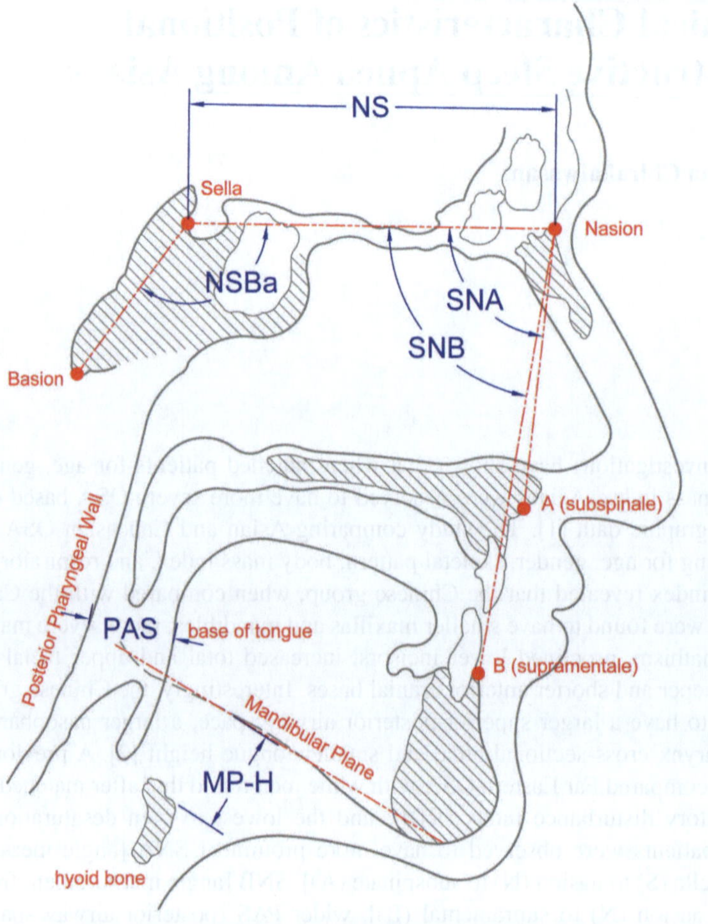

Fig. 1 SNA, angle measurement from sella (S) to nasion (N) to point A (subspinale); SNB, angle measurement from sella (S) to nasion (N) to point B (supramentale); MP-H, distance from mandibular plane (MP) to hyoid bone (H); PAS (posterior airway space), the distance between base of the tongue and the posterior pharyngeal wall; NSBa (cranial base flexure), angle formed by the intersection between lines drawn from nasion (N) to sella (S) to basion (Ba); NS (anterior cranial base), distance from nasion (N) to sella (S)

that the retropalatal region has more severe obstruction compared with retroglossal region in either erect or supine position [4]. A study comparing the differences in craniofacial structures and obesity between an Australian OSA and a Hong Kong OSA group found that at the same level of AHI, the Chinese OSA group was observed to be less obese with lower BMI and smaller neck circumference; however, they were observed to have more restricted cephalometric measurement [5]. It is believed that central obesity, which is generally more prevalent in Asians, may have predisposed them to develop OSA at a lower BMI compared to Caucasians [6–8]. Even though the clinical characteristics of Asian OSA patients appeared to be different, the prevalence of OSA was observed to be comparable to the other population. If OSA is defined as RDI ≥ 5, the prevalence of OSA was observed to be 8.8–27 % and 3.7–16 % in males and females, respectively. If OSA is defined as RDI ≥ 5 plus excessive daytime sleepiness, the prevalence of OSA was observed to be 4.1–7.5 % and 1.9–3.2 % in males and females, respectively [9–14].

Contrarily, positional OSA, which is a form of OSA noted predominantly during supine sleep, was reported with higher prevalence among Asians. The first data on positional OSA by Cartwright et al. using criteria for positional OSA as 50 % or more in apneic index between back and side sleep positions reported a prevalence of 58.3 % (14 in 24 subjects) [15]. Pevernagie et al. demonstrated overall positional OSA prevalence of 58.2 % using positional OSA criteria of apnea-hypopnea index (AHI)-O (off back)/AHI-B (back) ≤0.5 (similar to Cartwright criteria) [16]. Oksenberg et al. subsequently reported a prevalence of 55.9 % (321 in 574 subjects) for positional OSA using criteria for positional OSA as a ratio of supine RDI to the lateral RDI ≥2 and required sleep time more than 30 min in either supine or lateral position [17]. Mador et al. published a paper using a more rigid positional OSA criteria which was >50 % reduction in the AHI between the supine and non-supine position and the AHI in the non-supine position <5 with data of at least 15 minutes of both the supine and non-supine position [18]. They reported an overall prevalence of 27.4 % (68 in 248 subjects). For each severity of OSA, positional OSA prevalence was reported as 49.5 %, 19.4 %, and 6.5 % in mild, moderate, and severe OSA, respectively. Richard et al. reported overall positional OSA prevalence of 55.8 % using positional OSA criteria as at least two times higher AHI in supine position than the average AHI in the other positions (similar to Cartwright criteria) [19]. All these combined reports represent an overall prevalence of positional OSA in the Western population of approximately 27.4–58.3 %.

However, positional OSA among Asians was reported with higher prevalence ranging between 49 and 74.5 % [20–27] (Table 1). The prevalence of positional OSA was observed to be less as the severity of OSA increases [26, 27]. For clinical characteristics, most of the studies did not show differences in terms of age; however, two studies reported that the positional OSA group was older [23, 26]. Half of the studies with available information on BMI reported that positional OSA group was found to have lower BMI [23, 26, 27]. Two out of three studies with available information on neck circumference reported positional OSA to have smaller neck size [25, 27]. Excessive daytime sleepiness determined by Epworth Sleepiness Scale (ESS) was observed to be no different between the two groups. However, one study reported the positional OSA group to be less sleepy compared to the non-positional OSA group [23] (Table 2). For polysomnographic characteristics, all studies reported the AHI or RDI to be lower in the positional OSA group. Mean and nadir oxygen saturations were observed to be higher in positional OSA group [25, 26]. Only two papers on positional OSA in Asians described the details on sleep architecture. Both papers did not find a difference in sleep efficiency between the two groups. One study found less N1 and increase in REM sleep with no difference in NREM3 in the positional OSA group, compared to the non-positional OSA group [23]. Another study found the positional OSA group to have an increase in N3 with

Table 1 Prevalence of positional OSA

Author/year	Country	Ethnicity	Population/*N*	Positional OSA criteria	Prevalence of positional OSA	Prevalence of positional OSA (subgroup analysis)
Itasaka Y et al. [20]	Japan	Japanese	OSA patients/257	≥50 % reduction in AHI in lateral position	69.3 % (178 in 257 subjects)	90.9 % in normal weight group (BMI < 24), 74 % in mild obese group (BMI 24–26.4), 57.4 % in obese group (BMI > 26.4)
Nakano H et al. [21]	Japan	Japanese	Habitual snoring diagnosed with OSA/51	Lateral AHI/supine AHI < 0.5; ≥10 min of recorded lateral sleep	49 % (25 in 51 subjects)	No data
Chang ET et al. [22]	Taiwan	Chinese	OSA, central sleep apnea or mixture of obstructive and central sleep apnea excluded/75	Total AHI ≥ 5, <50 % reduction in the AHI between supine and non-supine postures, AHI < 5 in the non-supine posture	57.3 % (43 in 75 subjects)	No data
Tanaka F et al. [23]	Japan	Japanese	OSA patients/462	Supine AHI ≥2 times of lateral AHI	74.5 % (344 in 462 subjects)	No data
Lee CH et al. [24]	Korea	Korean	OSA patients undergoing uvulopalatopharyngoplasty (UPPP)/74	Supine AHI >2 times of lateral AHI; ≥5 % of sleep time in both supine and lateral position	70.3 % (52 in 74 patients)	No data
Teerapraipruk B et al. [25]	Thailand	Thai	OSA patients/144	Supine RDI/non-supine RDI ≥ 2, total RDI ≥ 5, supine and non-supine sleep time ≥30 min	66.7 % (96 in 144 patients)	No data
Sunwoo WS et al. [26]	Korea	Korean	OSA patients undergoing sleep videofluoroscopy	Supine AHI >2 times of lateral AHI, ≥5 % of sleep time in supine and lateral position	71.4 % (65 in 91 patients)	91.3 % in mild OSA group, 82.6 % in moderate OSA group, 55.6 % in severe OSA group
Hu B et al. [27]	China	Chinese	OSA patients undergoing nasal surgery/79	Supine AHI/non-supine AHI ≥ 2, supine and non-supine sleep time ≥30 min	53.2 % (42 in 79 patients)	70.4 % in mild OSA group, 61.5 % in moderate OSA group, 26.9 % in severe OSA group

Table 2 Baseline clinical characteristics (positional OSA/non-positional OSA)

Author/year	Age (years)	Sex (%M)	BMI	Neck size (cm)	ESS
Itasaka Y et al. [20]	No data	No data	No data	No data	No data
Nakano H et al. [21]	No data	No data	No data	No data	No data
Chang ET et al. [22]	54.8 ± 11.1/ 53.0 ± 14.6; p = ns	No data	26.9 ± 3.5/ 28.1 ± 4.5; p = ns	39.6 ± 3.7/ 39.9 ± 5.9; p = ns	9.1 ± 5.2/ 6.8 ± 4.6; p = ns
Tanaka F et al. [23]	49.5 ± 13.3/ 46.5 ± 11.7; $p = 0.0287$	91.6/87.3; p = no data	26.0 ± 3.5/ 29.6 ± 5.2; $p \leq 0.0001$	No data	10.6 ± 5.0/ 11.8 ± 5.5; $p = 0.0238$
Lee CH et al. [24]	47/47.2; p = ns	No data	26/26.5; p = ns	No data	No data
Teerapraipruk B et al. [25]	53.2 ± 11.5/ 50.8 ± 11.9; $p = 0.27$	76/81.3; $p = 0.53$	26.3 ± 4.8/ 27.9 ± 5.4; $p = 0.074$	14.9 ± 1.5/ 15.7 ± 1.4; $p = 0.001$ (in.)	9.6 ± 4.8/ 10.5 ± 5.3; $p = 0.335$
Sunwoo WS et al. [26]	49.5 ± 11.9/ 43.8 ± 10.4; $p = 0.035$	83.1/88.5; $p = 0.520$	26.1 ± 3.2/ 28.1 ± 3.5; $p = 0.009$	No data	10.0 ± 3.7/ 12.0 ± 4.3; $p = 0.059$
Hu B et al. [27]	41.8 ± 11.8/ 43.2 ± 8; p = ns	78.6/81.1; p = ns	26.6 ± 2.6/ 29.8 ± 3.3; $p < 0.01$	42.4 ± 1.6/ 43.7 ± 1.5; $p < 0.01$	No data

Data displayed in mean ± SD or the median
ns nonsignificance

no difference in N1 or REM sleep [25]. Two studies reported information on sleep position duration [23, 26]. One out of these two papers reported that the patients with positional OSA spent less time in supine position when compared to the non-positional OSA patients [23] (Table 3). Tanaka et al. [23] reported that the lateral AHI but not the supine AHI significantly correlated with excessive daytime sleepiness using ESS ($r = 0.102$; $p < 0.05$). For cephalometric measure, Chang et al. found the MP-H to be correlated with ESS [22]. Predictors for positional OSA were studied by Teerapraipruk et al. [25]. Low snoring frequency (less than 20 % of total sleep time) was a significant predictor for positional OSA (odd ratio of 3.27; $p = 0.011$). Low mean oxygen saturation <95 % was found to be a negative predictor (odd ratio of 0.31; $p = 0.009$). Low RDI (<15) was a significant predictor for normalization of RDI to less than 5 in non-supine position (odd ratio of 8.77; $p < 0.001$). Furthermore, Nakano et al. also reported an interesting finding that positional dependency of snoring was observed in terms of snoring intensity but not in terms of % of snoring time [21]. Position change in snoring was significantly correlated with AHI, especially in supine position.

Anatomical characteristics of positional OSA among Asians have been previously reported in literature. Chang et al. published a paper on clinical and cephalometric characteristics of positional OSA compared to non-OSA and non-positional OSA [22]. They reported that positional OSA when compared to non-positional OSA was observed to have longer PAS measurement (9.8 ± 3.1 mm and 8.1 ± 2.6 mm,

Table 3 Polysomnographic characteristics (positional OSA/non-positional OSA)

Author/year	RDI or AHI	Sleep efficiency (%)	Mean oxygen saturation (%)	Nadir oxygen saturation (%)	%N1 or N1 (min)	%N3 or N3 (min)	%REM or REM (min)	%Supine sleep time or supine sleep time (min)	%Lateral sleep time
Itasaka Y et al. [20]	No data	No data	No data	No data	No data	No data	No data	No data	No data
Nakano H et al. [21]	No data	No data	No data	No data	No data	No data	No data	No data	No data
Chang ET et al. [22]	36.4 ± 23.4/ 48.1 ± 25.4; $p<0.001$ (AHI)	No data	No data	No data	No data	No data	No data	No data	No data
Tanaka F et al. [23]	22.4 (11.6–35.7)/ 63.2 (39.5–80.9); $p<0.0001$ (RDI)	81.9 (71.6–88.4)/ 80.4 (71.8–86.0); $p=0.2943$	No data	No data	115.9 ± 57.7/ 160.5 ± 73.5; $p<0.0001$ (min)	0.5 (0.0–7.7)/ 0.5 (0.0–3.3); $p=0.2095$ (min)	58.7 ± 24.1/ 49.0 ± 10.1; $p=0.0002$ (min)	200.4 ± 96.9/ 222.4 ± 97.6; $p=0.0344$ (min)	156.1 ± 84.2/ 126.5 ± 77.8; $p=0.0008$ (min)
Lee CH et al. [24]	30.9/50; $p<0.001$ (AHI)	No data	No data	No data	No data	No data	No data	No data	No data
Teerapraipruk B et al. [25]	23.8 ± 14.2/ 43.0 ± 23.9; $p<0.001$ (RDI)	89.5 ± 10.7/ 90.2 ± 7.6; $p=0.715$	95.1 ± 1.5/ 93.3 ± 2.7; $p<0.001$	81.2 ± 8.2/ 77.9 ± 9.3; $p=0.032$	13.2 ± 10.2/ 15.6 ± 14.4; $p=0.252$ (%)	15.2 ± 10.1/ 10.2 ± 9.5; $p=0.005$ (%)	16.0 ± 7.0/ 14.0 ± 6.9; $p=0.109$ (%)	No data	No data
Sunwoo WS et al. [26]	25.4 ± 14.7/ 51.4 ± 23.8; $p<0.001$ (AHI)	No data	No data	85.8 ± 5.6/ 76.7 ± 11.6; $p=0.033$	No data	No data	No data	61.8 ± 21.9/ 55.7 ± 21.9; $p=0.268$ (%)	No data
Hu B et al. [27]	No data	No data	No data	No data	No data	No data	No data	No data	No data

Data displayed in mean ± SD or the median with interquartile ranges given in parentheses

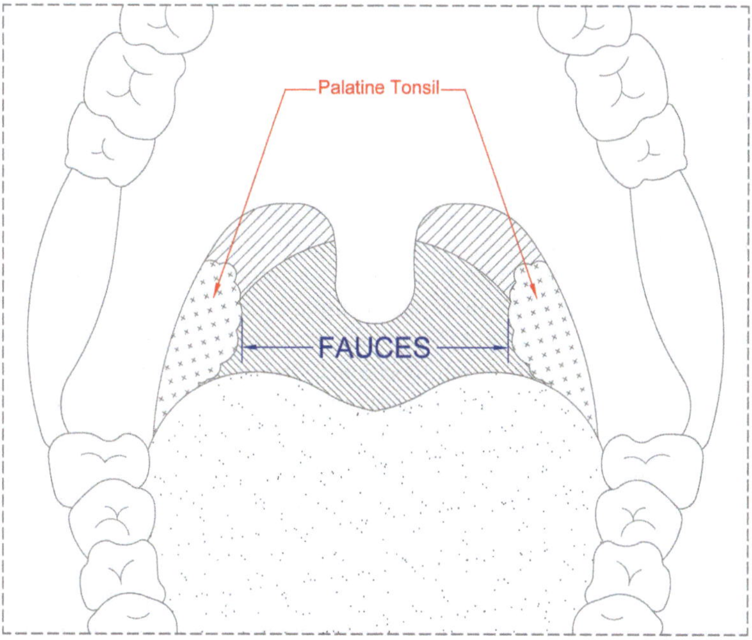

Fig. 2 The width of the fauces. Grade 1: the palatopharyngeal arch intersects at the tongue's edge. Grade 2: the palatopharyngeal arch intersects at ≥25 % of the whole width of the tongue. Grade 3: the palatopharyngeal arch intersects at ≥50 % of the whole width of the tongue. Grade 4: the palatopharyngeal arch intersects at ≥75 % of the whole width of the tongue

respectively). Saigura et al. revealed that patients with positional OSA when compared to non-positional OSA patients were noted to have a larger angle of the maxilla–nasion–mandible (the angle between A-N and N-B in Fig. 1) and smaller lower facial height (LFH) from cephalometric parameters and smaller volume of the pharyngeal lateral wall soft tissues from three-dimensional MRI reconstruction [28]. Soga et al. demonstrated that patients with positional OSA when compared with non-positional OSA patients were noted to have a lower grade of fauces width (50 % grade 2 compared to 8 % grade 2 in non-positional sleep apnea group) when a designated otolaryngologist performed an oral examination with the patient sitting in the upright position [29] (Fig. 2). Different risk factors for developing OSA in various ethnicities may have implications for OSA treatment. Asian OSA patients may be more beneficial from treatment options aiming to reposition the craniofacial structure such as maxillomandibular advancement surgery (MMA) or mandibular advancement device (MAD) [30]. A tongue-retaining device (TRD) which prevents a flaccid tongue from retrolapsing during supine sleep was also previously shown to be selectively effective in the group with positional OSA [31] as well as those patients with positional OSA who were unable to avoid supine sleep [32]. However, data for the effectiveness of palatal surgery for positional OSA treatment is controversial. A prior study performed in Korea utilizing sleep videofluoroscopy (SVF) demonstrated that patients with soft palate obstruction (SP type) were observed to have more positional OSA than the patients with tongue base obstruction (TB). The authors concluded that positional OSA may have higher success rates with palatal surgery alone [26]. A follow-up study from Korea by Kwon et al. also revealed similar findings. They demonstrated that in the responsive UPPP group—which was defined by reduction in postoperative AHI to less than 20 % and reduction of more than 50 % compared to the preoperative value—significant reduction in AHI was observed in supine AHI (40.5 ± 4.3 to 10.6 ± 9.3; $p < 0.001$). However, reduction in non-supine AHI did not reach statistically significant difference (13.5 ± 25 to 2.5 ± 4; $p = 0.25$) [33]. Another study also from Korea demonstrated a contradicting result; UPPP was more successful when events occurred in lateral position specifically in patients with non-positional OSA. They indicated that the improvement in lateral sleep-specific AHI may convert non-positional OSA to positional OSA [24]. The same group also concluded in another study that due to high positional dependency observed among Asians, effectiveness of surgical outcome should be interpreted with caution. They suggested using postoperative position-corrected AHI (P-AHI). P-AHI can be calculated from simple equation [(postoperative supine AHI × preoperative supine sleep time %) + (postoperative lateral AHI × preoperative lateral sleep time %)/100]. This P-AHI may be a more precise method of determining the success of OSA surgical treatment outcome [34]. Lastly, positional therapy, which can reposition the mandible by means of preventing the mandible from moving posteriorly, should obviously be theoretically beneficial among OSA. A previous study demonstrated a combination of lateral position (LP), cervical vertebrae support with head tilting (CVSHT), and scapula support (SS) to be effective treatment in Asian positional OSA patients. They demonstrated that in order to achieve at least 80 % reduction of AHI, LP and SS should be >30° and/or 20 mm, respectively [35]. Even prone position also was previously shown to be effective in ameliorating AHI in a case report from Japan which demonstrated that most dilated upper airway was observed in prone position according to an MRI study [36]. Recent meta-analysis of randomized trials comparing effectiveness of positional therapy versus continuous positive airway pressure (CPAP) demonstrated the superior efficacy of CPAP over positional therapy [37]. However, all three trials which were included in this meta-analysis were conducted in non-Asians. Further future randomized controlled studies on the effectiveness of positional therapy specifically performed among Asians are strongly encouraged.

Acknowledgment I would like to thank my beloved husband, Pannasan Sombuntham, for his contribution in providing two beautiful illustrations for this chapter. He has always been my true support in every aspect of my life. I love you so much.

References

1. Ong KC, Clerk AA. Comparison of the severity of sleep-disordered breathing in Asian and Caucasian patients seen at a sleep disorders center. Respir Med. 1998;92(6):843–8.
2. Liu Y, Lowe AA, Zeng X, Fu M, Fleethamc JA. Cephalometric comparisons between Chinese and Caucasian patients with obstructive sleep apnea. Am J Orthod Dentofacial Orthop. 2000;117:479–85.

3. Li KK, Kushida C, Powell NB, Riley RW, Guilleminault C. Obstructive sleep apnea syndrome: a comparison between Far-East Asian and white men. Laryngoscope. 2000;110:1689–93.
4. Abdullah B, Rajet KA, Abd Hamid SS, Mohammad WM. A videoendoscopic evaluation of the upper airway in South East Asian adults with obstructive sleep apnea. Sleep Breath. 2011;15(4):747–54.
5. Lee RWW, Vasudavan S, Hui DS, Prvan T, Petocz P, Darendeliler MA, et al. Differences in craniofacial structures and obesity in Caucasian and Chinese patients with obstructive sleep apnea. Sleep. 2010;33(8):1075–80.
6. James WP. The epidemiology of obesity: the size of the problem. J Intern Med. 2008;263: 336–52.
7. Kagawa M, Binns CB, Hills AP. Body composition and anthropometry in Japanese and Australian Caucasian males and Japanese females. Asia Pac J Clin Nutr. 2007;16 Suppl 1:31–6.
8. Rush EC, Freitas I, Plank LD. Body size, body composition and fat distribution: comparative analysis of European, Maori, Pacific Island and Asian Indian adults. Br J Nutr. 2009;102: 632–41.
9. Ip MS, Lam B, Lauder IJ, Tsang KW, Chung KF, Mok YW, Lam WK. A community study of sleep-disordered breathing in middle-aged Chinese men in Hong Kong. Chest. 2001;119(1): 62–9.
10. Ip MS, Lam B, Tang LC, Lauder IJ, Ip TY, Lam WK. A community study of sleep-disordered breathing in middle-aged Chinese women in Hong Kong: prevalence and gender differences. Chest. 2004;125(1):127–34.
11. Udwadia ZF, Doshi AV, Lonkar SG, Singh CI. Prevalence of sleep-disordered breathing and sleep apnea in middle-aged urban Indian men. Am J Respir Crit Care Med. 2004;169(2): 168–73.
12. Kim J, In K, Kim J, You S, Kang K, Shim J, et al. Prevalence of sleep-disordered breathing in middle-aged Korean men and women. Am J Respir Crit Care Med. 2004;170(10):1108–13.
13. Sharma SK, Kumpawa S, Banga A, Goel A. Prevalence and risk factors of obstructive sleep apnea syndrome in a population of Delhi, India. Chest. 2006;130:149–56.
14. Neruntarat C, Chantapant S. Prevalence of sleep apnea in HRH Princess Maha Chakri Srinthorn Medical Center, Thailand. Sleep Breath. 2011;15(4):641–8.
15. Cartwright RD. Effect of sleep position on sleep apnea severity. Sleep. 1984;7(2):110–4.
16. Pevernagie DA, Shepard Jr JW. Relations between sleep stage, posture and effective nasal CPAP levels in OSA. Sleep. 1992;15(2):162–7.
17. Oksenberg A, Silverberg DS, Arons E, Radwan H. Positional vs non positional obstructive sleep apnea patients: anthropomorphic, nocturnal polysomnographic, and multiple sleep latency test data. Chest. 1997;112(3):629–39.
18. Mador MJ, Kufel TJ, Magalang UJ, Rajesh SK, Watwe V, Grant BJ. Prevalence of positional sleep apnea in patients undergoing polysomnography. Chest. 2005;128:2130–7.
19. Richard W, Kox D, den Herder C, Laman M, van Tinteren H, de Vries N. The role of sleep position in obstructive sleep apnea syndrome. Eur Arch Otorhinolaryngol. 2006;263(10): 946–50.
20. Itasaka Y, Miyazaki S, Ishikawa K, Togawa K. The influence of sleep position and obesity on sleep apnea. Psychiatry Clin Neurosci. 2000;54(3):340–1.
21. Nakano H, Ikeda T, Hayashi M, et al. Effects of body position on snoring in apneic and non-apneic snorers. Sleep. 2003;2:169–72.
22. Chang ET, Shiao GM. Craniofacial abnormalities in Chinese patients with obstructive and positional sleep apnea. Sleep Med. 2008;9(4):403–10.
23. Tanaka F, Nakano H, Sudo N, Kubo C. Relationship between the body position-specific apnea-hypopnea index and subjective sleepiness. Respiration. 2009;78(2):185–90.
24. Lee CH, Kim SW, Han K, Shin JM, Hong SL, Lee JE, et al. Effect of uvulopalatopharyngoplasty on positional dependency in obstructive sleep apnea. Arch Otolaryngol Head Neck Surg. 2011;137(7):675–9.

25. Teerapraipruk B, Chirakalwasan N, Simon R, Hirunwiwatkul P, Jaimchariyatam N, Desudchit T, et al. Clinical and polysomnographic data of positional sleep apnea and its predictors. Sleep Breath. 2012;16(4):1167–72.
26. Sunwoo WS, Hong SL, Kim SW, Park SJ, Han DH, Kim JW, et al. Association between positional dependency and obstruction site in obstructive sleep apnea syndrome. Clin Exp Otorhinolaryngol. 2012;5(4):218–21.
27. Hu B, Han D, Li Y, Ye J, Zang H, Wang T. Polysomnographic effect of nasal surgery on positional and non-positional obstructive sleep apnea/hypopnea patients. Acta Otolaryngol. 2013;133(8):858–65.
28. Saigusa H, Suzuki M, Higurashi N, Kodera K. Three-dimensional morphological analyses of positional dependence in patients with obstructive sleep apnea syndrome. Anesthesiology. 2009;110(4):885–90.
29. Soga T, Nakata S, Yasuma F, Noda A, Sugiura T, Yatsuya H. Upper airway morphology in patients with obstructive sleep apnea syndrome: effects of lateral positioning. Auris Nasus Larynx. 2009;36(3):305–9.
30. Lee CH, Jung HJ, Lee WH, Rhee CS, Yoon IY, Yun PY, et al. The effect of positional dependency on outcomes of treatment with a mandibular advancement device. Arch Otolaryngol Head Neck Surg. 2012;138(5):479–83.
31. Cartwright R. Predicting response to the tongue retaining device for sleep apnea syndrome. Arch Otolaryngol. 1985;111:385–8.
32. Cartwright R, Ristanovic R, Diaz F, Caldarelli D, Alder G. A comparative study of treatments for positional sleep apnea. Sleep. 1991;14:546–52.
33. Kwon M, Jang YJ, Lee BJ, Chung YS. The effect of uvula-preserving palatopharyngoplasty in obstructive sleep apnea on globus sense and positional dependency. Clin Exp Otorhinolaryngol. 2010;3(3):141–6.
34. Lee CH, Shin HW, Han DH, Mo JH, Yoon IY, Chung S, et al. The implication of sleep position in the evaluation of surgical outcomes in obstructive sleep apnea. Otolaryngol Head Neck Surg. 2009;140(4):531–5.
35. Lee JB, Park YH, Hong JH, Lee SH, Jung KH, Kim JH, et al. Determining optimal sleep position in patients with positional sleep-disordered breathing using response surface analysis. J Sleep Res. 2009;18(1):26–35.
36. Matsuzawa Y, Hayashi S, Yamaguchi S, Yoshikawa S, Okada K, Fujimoto K, et al. Effect of prone position on apnea severity in obstructive sleep apnea. Intern Med. 1995;34(12):1190–3.
37. Ha SC, Hirai HW, Tsoi KK. Comparison of positional therapy versus continuous positive airway pressure in patients with positional obstructive sleep apnea: a meta-analysis of randomized trials. Sleep Med Rev. 2014;18(1):19–24.

Positional Therapy: Left Lateral Decubitus Position Versus Right Lateral Decubitus Position

Zhang Huankang, Huang Jingjing, Hou Xiaolin, J. Peter Van Maanen, and Xiao Kuanlin

Introduction

Visceral organs in the thoracic cavity, i.e., the right and left lungs, the heart, the esophagus, and the trachea, are not symmetrically distributed in the thorax. It has been reported that right-side sleepers had better sleep quality and less nightmares compared to left-side sleepers [1]. Furthermore, patients with congestive heart failure avoid the left lateral decubitus position spontaneously during sleep [2]. In congestive heart failure patients, sympathetic nervous modulation was most attenuated in the right lateral decubitus sleep position [3, 4].

Obstructive sleep apnea (OSA) is associated with increased cardiovascular and cerebrovascular morbidity and mortality rates [5–7]. Sleeping position has a major influence on sleep-related breathing disorders [8, 9]. The deleterious effect of the supine posture and the helpful effect of the lateral position on sleep-related breathing abnormalities have been reported consistently [10–12]. Ozeke et al. [13, 14] found that right lateral decubitus sleep position decreased the frequency of obstructive respiratory events in patients with moderate and severe disease. They speculate that the presence of underlying OSA, which is frequently encountered in

Z. Huankang, M.S. • H. Jingjing, M.S. • X. Kuanlin, M.D. (✉)
Department of Otorhinolaryngology-Head and Neck Surgery, Fudan University, Eye, Ear, Nose and Throat Hospital, 83 Fenyang Rd, Shanghai 200031, China
e-mail: xiaokuanlin@hotmail.com

H. Xiaolin, M.S.
Department of Otorhinolaryngology-Head and Neck Surgery, Xinhua Hospital, Shanghai Jiaotong University, Shanghai, China

J.P. Van Maanen, M.D.
Department of Otolaryngology, Sint Lucas Andreas Ziekenhuis, Amsterdam, The Netherlands

N. de Vries et al. (eds.), *Positional Therapy in Obstructive Sleep Apnea*,
DOI 10.1007/978-3-319-09626-1_8

patients with heart failure, may be one of the mechanisms explaining the demonstrated preference of patients with heart failure for the right lateral decubitus sleep position. However, evidence for whether or not the numbers of respiratory events are different between left and right lateral decubitus position is lacking. The purpose of the present study was to observe the effects of supine and left and right lateral decubitus positions on the rapid eye movement (REM) sleep, apnea-hypopnea index (AHI), and minimum arterial oxygen saturation (SaO_2) in adult OSA patients.

Materials and Methods

We retrospectively reviewed all subjects with suspected OSA who underwent consecutive overnight diagnostic polysomnographies (PSGs) between June 2009 and June 2012 in the Sleep Center of the Affiliated Eye, Ear, Nose, and Throat Hospital of Fudan University, Shanghai, China. Sleep data were scored manually and automatically according to standard criteria [15]. Body position was monitored continuously by a body position sensor, which was taped onto the skin overlying the sternum. After calibration, the patient was instructed to rotate in the bed to confirm that every position would be recorded correctly.

Adult subjects age ≥ 18 with an AHI ≥ 5 were included in the study. To control for intrasubject differences caused by sleep architecture, only subjects who spent more than 20 % of total sleep time in supine and left and right positions were included for further analysis.

Left positional OSA was defined as a total AHI ≥ 5 with a supine AHI that is at least two times higher than their left AHI, and right positional OSA was defined as a total AHI ≥ 5 with a supine AHI that is at least two times higher than their right AHI. To further study the theoretical efficacy of postural intervention in OSA patients, subgroup analysis of the following parameters was performed: sex, age, BMI, and the severity of OSA. Subjects were divided on the basis of their age into three groups (18–39 years, 40–59 years, and above 60 years). BMI was divided into three categories: normal body weight (18.5–23.9 kg/m^2), overweight (24.0–27.9 kg/m^2), and obesity (≥28 kg/m^2). According to Bei-Fan et al. [16], AHI was defined by the standard criteria [17]. The severity of sleep apnea was classified using the total AHI: mild sleep apnea was defined as a total AHI of 5–14.9 per hour, moderate sleep apnea as a total AHI of 15–29.9 per hour, and severe sleep apnea as a total AHI ≥ 30 per hour.

All results were expressed as mean ± standard deviation. SPSS (Statistical Package for Social Sciences) 17.0 program for Windows was used for statistical analysis of the results in our study. T-test and ANOVA were used to compare continuous results. Statistical significance was set at $P < 0.05$.

Results

Influence of Body Posture on Percentage of REM Sleep, AHI, and Minimum SaO_2

Out of a total of 2,221 studied subjects, 327 cases were included for further analysis. A male preponderance was found (314 patients or 96.0 %). The age distribution is shown in Fig. 1. 45 (13.8 %) cases suffered from mild, 70 (21.4 %) from moderate, and 212 (64.8 %) from severe OSA (Fig. 2).

The percentages of total sleep time spent in supine and left and right lateral decubitus positions showed no differences (33.5 % ± 6.7 %, 32.8 % ± 8.2 %, and 33.2 % ± 8.6 %, respectively; $P = 0.483$, Table 1). No significant difference could be found in the percentages of REM sleep in supine and left and right lateral decubitus positions (6.1 % ± 4.2 %, 6.5 % ± 4.2 %, and 6.4 % ± 4.2 %, respectively; $P = 0.424$, Table 1). Supine AHI was 60.5 ± 24.3 per hour, which was higher compared to 36.4 ± 28.4 per hour in the left lateral decubitus position ($P < 0.001$) and 35.3 ± 28.1 per hour in the right lateral decubitus position ($P < 0.001$, Table 1 and Fig. 3). In the supine position, the minimum SaO_2 was 76.5 % ± 10.8 %, which was lower compared to 80.0 % ± 10.2 % in the left lateral decubitus position ($P < 0.001$) and 80.0 % ± 10.1 % in the right lateral decubitus position ($P < 0.001$, Table 1 and Fig. 4). No significant difference could be found between left and right AHI ($P = 0.607$), and between left and right minimum SaO_2 ($P = 0.798$).

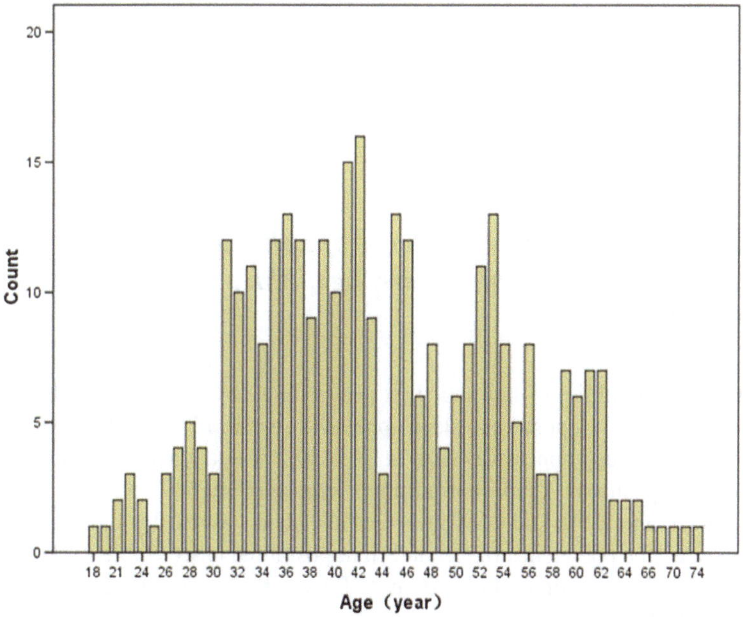

Fig. 1 Age distribution of 327 patients

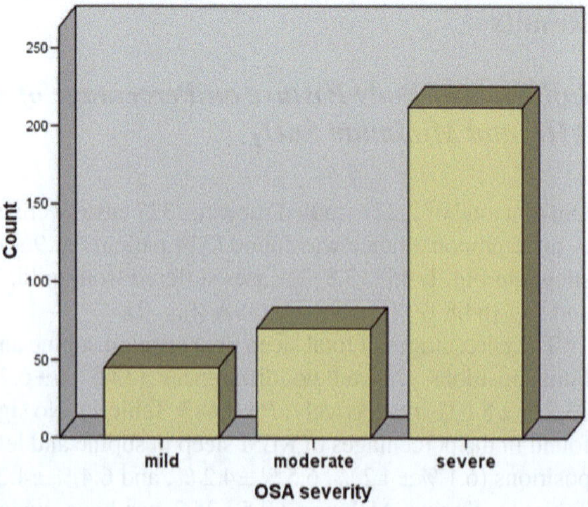

Fig. 2 Distribution of OSA severity: 45 (13.8 %) cases were mild OSA, 70 (21.4 %) cases were moderate OSA, and 212 (64.8 %) cases were severe OSA

Table 1 Comparison of supine and left and right lateral decubitus positions

	Supine	Left lateral decubitus	Right lateral decubitus	*P*-value
Sleep time (% TST)	33.5±6.7	32.8±8.2	33.2±8.6	0.483
REM (% TST)	6.1±4.2	6.5±4.2	6.4±4.2	0.424
AHI (per hour)	60.5±24.3	36.4±28.4	35.3±28.1	<0.001
Min SaO_2 (%)	76.5±10.8	80.0±10.2	80.0±10.1	<0.001

Values are given as mean±SD

REM rapid eye movement, *TST* total sleep time, *AHI* apnea-hypopnea index, *Min* SaO_2 minimum arterial oxygen saturation

Factors Influencing the Prevalence of Left and Right Positional OSA: Effect of Gender, Age, BMI, and OSA Severity

Based on the definition of left and right positional OSA mentioned earlier, out of 327 OSA patients, left positional sleep apnea was seen in 155 (47.4 %) patients, and right positional sleep apnea was seen in 161 (49.2 %) patients. The prevalence of left and right positional OSA showed no difference ($P=0.639$). Subgroup analysis using gender, age, BMI, and OSA severity showed no statistically significant difference between the prevalence of left and right positional OSA (Table 2). Prevalence of left and right positional OSA was not affected by gender or age. However, as BMI and AHI increased, prevalence of left and right positional OSA decreased (Table 2).

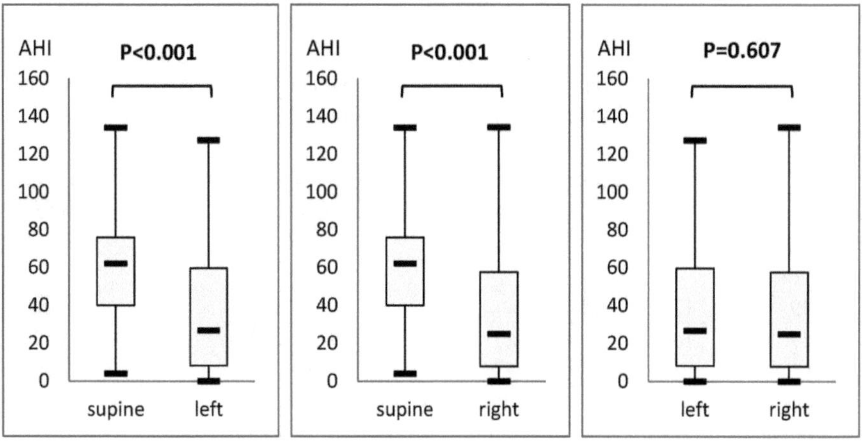

Fig. 3 Supine AHI was 60.5 ± 24.3 per hour, which was higher compared to 36.4 ± 28.4 per hour in left position ($P < 0.001$) and 35.3 ± 28.1 per hour in right position ($P < 0.001$). No statistically significant differences could be found between left and right AHI ($P = 0.607$)

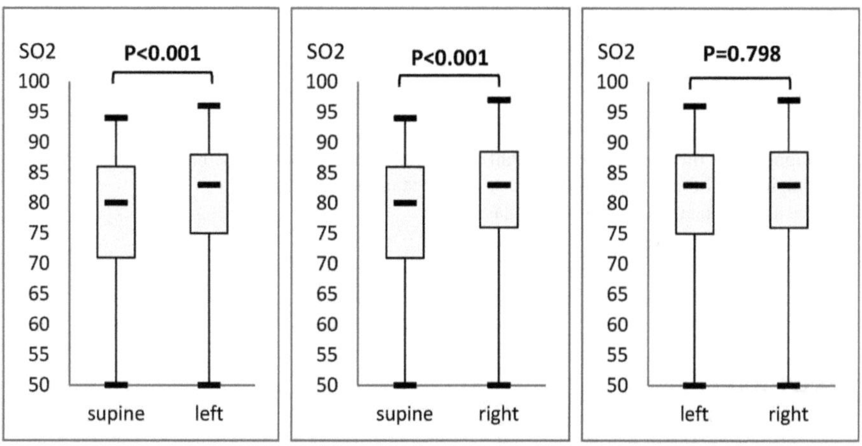

Fig. 4 Minimum SaO_2 in supine position was 76.5 ± 10.8 %, which was lower compared to 80.0 ± 10.2 % in left position ($P < 0.001$) and 80.0 ± 10.1 % in right position ($P < 0.001$). No statistically significant differences could be found between left and right minimum SaO_2 ($P = 0.798$)

Table 2 Factors influencing the prevalence of left and right positional OSA: effect of gender, age, BMI, and OSA severity

Factors	No.	Supine AHI/left AHI>2	Supine AHI/right AHI>2	*P*-value
Total	327	155 (47.4 %)	161 (49.2 %)	0.639
Gender				
Male	314	148 (47.1 %)	155 (49.4 %)	0.576
Female	13	7 (53.8 %)	6 (46.2 %)	0.695
P-value		0.635	0.821	
Age (years)				
18–39	128	65 (50.8 %)	67 (52.3 %)	0.802
40–59	168	77 (45.8 %)	81 (48. 2 %)	0.662
≥60	31	13 (41.9 %)	13 (41.9 %)	1.000
P-value		0.570	0.542	
BMI (kg/m^2)				
Normal	49	30 (61.2 %)*	30 (61.2 %)*	1.000
Overweight	161	85 (52.8 %)*	88 (54.7 %)*	0.737
Obesity	117	40 (34.2 %)	43 (36.8 %)	0.682
P-value		0.001	0.002	
Total AHI (per hour)				
Mild	45	37 (82.2 %)**	35 (77.8 %)**	0.598
Moderate	70	56 (80.0 %)**	60 (85.7 %)**	0.370
Severe	212	62 (29.2 %)	66 (31.1 %)	0.672
P-value		<0.001	<0.001	

Left positional sleep apnea was defined as a total AHI ≥ 5 with a supine AHI that is at least two times higher than their left AHI, and right positional sleep apnea was defined as a total AHI ≥ 5 with a supine AHI that is at least two times higher than their right AHI
AHI apnea-hypopnea index, *BMI* body mass index
*$P<0.05$ vs. obesity subjects
**$P<0.001$ vs. severe OSA subjects

Discussion

In this study, left and right lateral decubitus positions were compared with regard to their influence on the percentage of REM sleep, AHI, and minimum SaO_2. As we currently know, sleeping state influences many aspects of respiration. People in REM sleep are most vulnerable for having sleep-disordered breathing, and many OSA patients have higher AHI and lower SaO_2 in REM sleep than in non-REM sleep [18, 19]. To eliminate interindividual differences caused by sleep architecture, subjects should spend enough time in the supine and left and right lateral decubitus positions during PSG examinations. To provide this validity, adult OSA patients who spent more than 20 % of total sleep time in each of the three study sleeping positions were enrolled in the analysis. This inclusion criterion was so strict that, among 2,221 subjects, only 327 patients met the eligibility criteria. This is a population with a lot of severe OSA (212 in 327) and male (314 in 327) patients.

A staggering percentage of severe OSA patients and male preponderance are not uncommon in the sleep centers of China. A multicenter investigation in China showed that, among 2,297 consecutive patients (aged 18–85 years; 1,981 males and 316 females), 257 patients had AHI $\leq$5, 402 patients had AHI>5 and $\leq$15, 460 patients had AHI>15 and $\leq$30, and 1,178 patients had AHI>30 [20]. This is due to poor-quality health care and lack of health consciousness in China. A large quantity of Chinese patients won't go to hospital and take PSGs unless their OSA complaints are serious.

Using the inclusion criteria, subjects spent an almost equal percentage of sleep time in supine and left and right lateral decubitus positions ($P=0.483$). Percentages of REM sleep time in supine and left and right lateral decubitus positions showed no significant difference ($P=0.424$), although AHI was higher and minimum SaO_2 was lower in the supine position (Table 1). This could mean that percentage of REM sleep time is associated with sleep time and is unaffected by sleep position, AHI, and minimum SaO_2 in OSA patients. Nakano et al. [21] showed that percentage of REM sleep time in a non-apneic snorer group (AHI<15) and an apneic group (AHI>15) showed no differences (14.6 % ± 7.9 % of TST vs. 14.0 % ± 5.6 % of TST, $P>0.05$), indicating that percent of REM sleep time is unaffected by AHI. However, Nakano et al. [21] also reported that apneic patients tended to have more REM sleep in the lateral than in the supine position. This means that percentage of REM sleep time was affected by sleep position in apneic patients and is not in line with our present findings. A possible explanation for this discrepancy is that Nakano et al. didn't balance the lateral time and supine time during PSG examination when analyzing REM sleep time in lateral and supine position.

OSA patients have higher AHI scores in supine position which are often associated with the greatest decrease in SaO_2 [18]. Studying AHI and minimum SaO_2, the theoretical interventional efficacy of left and right lateral decubitus positions showed no statistically significant differences. These results differ from Ozeke et al. [13], who reported that the left lateral decubitus positional AHI score was significantly higher than that of right lateral decubitus position (30.2 ± 32.6 per hour vs. 23.6 ± 30.1 per hour; $P<0.001$). We don't know if this difference is related to ethnical differences. We assume that the upper airway structure is symmetrical. When the lower jaw and soft palate move downward from gravitational forces, the width of the upper airway must be the same in left and right lateral decubitus positions. Furthermore, our study is based on a much larger sample than Ozeke et al. Therefore, our results may lead to more reliable statistical inferences.

When positional OSA was defined as a supine AHI that is at least two times higher than their non-supine AHI, the percentage of positional OSA patients varies in different reports from 9 % to 60 % [9, 22–24]. This variation is probably due to the different types of OSA patients studied. In our study, left positional sleep apnea was seen in 47.4 % patients, and right positional sleep apnea was seen in 49.2 % patients.

In subgroup analysis, we found that both left and right positional OSA are common in nonobese and non-severe OSA patients. This was similar to findings in other studies that showed positional OSA patients to be thinner and have less severe OSA than non-positional patients [9].

For some patients, when the percentage of supine time would be reduced to 0 (and the AHI in the supine position would not be of influence any longer), the AHI values of left and right lateral decubitus positions are ≥30. This indicates that if this group of patients would be prescribed some kind of ideal positional therapy, their lowest possible AHI after treatment still is ≥30. So the clinical consequence of positional therapy for this group of patients could be of limited value. However, as a free, and in the future possibly convenient, treatment for OSA, positional therapy (e.g., using the tennis ball technique) is available to patients who can't afford other treatments (e.g., surgery, continuous positive airway pressure, oral appliances, etc.). This is especially true for patients in developing countries.

Conclusion

Percentage of REM sleep seems to be unaffected by sleep position in OSA patients. Left and right lateral decubitus positions had a same influence on AHI and minimum SaO_2. The prevalence of left and right positional OSA is similar. Positional therapy could be an effective treatment for OSA, especially for the nonobese and non-severe OSA patients.

References

1. Agargun MY, Boysan M, Hanoglu L. Sleeping position, dream emotions, and subjective sleep quality. Sleep Hypnosis. 2004;6:8–13.
2. Leung RS, Bowman ME, Parker JD, Newton GE, Bradley TD. Avoidance of the left lateral decubitus position during sleep in patients with heart failure: relationship to cardiac size and function. J Am Coll Cardiol. 2003;41(2):227–30.
3. Fujita M, Miyamoto S, Sekiguchi H, Eiho S, Sasayama S. Effects of posture on sympathetic nervous modulation in patients with chronic heart failure. Lancet. 2000;356(9244):1822–3.
4. Miyamoto S, Fujita M, Sekiguchi H, et al. Effects of posture on cardiac autonomic nervous activity in patients with congestive heart failure. J Am Coll Cardiol. 2001;37(7):1788–93.
5. Partinen M, Guilleminault C. Daytime sleepiness and vascular morbidity at seven-year follow-up in obstructive sleep apnea patients. Chest. 1990;97(1):27–32.
6. Hung J, Whitford EG, Parsons RW, Hillman DR. Association of sleep apnoea with myocardial infarction in men. Lancet. 1990;336(8710):261–4.
7. Koskenvuo M, Kaprio J, Telakivi T, Partinen M, Heikkila K, Sarna S. Snoring as a risk factor for ischaemic heart disease and stroke in men. Br Med J (Clin Res Ed). 1987;294(6563): 16–9.
8. Oksenberg A, Silverberg DS. The effect of body posture on sleep-related breathing disorders: facts and therapeutic implications. Sleep Med Rev. 1998;2(3):139–62.
9. Oksenberg A, Silverberg DS, Arons E, Radwan H. Positional vs nonpositional obstructive sleep apnea patients: anthropomorphic, nocturnal polysomnographic, and multiple sleep latency test data. Chest. 1997;112(3):629–39.
10. Oksenberg A, Khamaysi I, Silverberg DS, Tarasiuk A. Association of body position with severity of apneic events in patients with severe nonpositional obstructive sleep apnea. Chest. 2000;118(4):1018–24.

11. Richard W, Kox D, den Herder C, Laman M, van Tinteren H, de Vries N. The role of sleep position in obstructive sleep apnea syndrome. Eur Arch Otorhinolaryngol. 2006;263(10): 946–50.
12. Oksenberg A, Silverberg DS. Avoiding the supine posture during sleep for patients with mild obstructive sleep apnea. Am J Respir Crit Care Med. 2009;180(1):101. 101–2.
13. Ozeke O, Erturk O, Gungor M, et al. Influence of the right- versus left-sided sleeping position on the apnea-hypopnea index in patients with sleep apnea. Sleep Breath. 2012;16(3):617–20.
14. Ozeke O, Ertan C, Demir AD. Sleep apnea, heart failure, and sleep position. Sleep Breath. 2012;16(4):933–5.
15. Hori T, Sugita Y, Koga E, et al. Proposed supplements and amendments to 'A Manual of Standardized Terminology, Techniques and Scoring System for Sleep Stages of Human Subjects', the Rechtschaffen & Kales (1968) standard. Psychiatry Clin Neurosci. 2001;55(3): 305–10.
16. Bei-Fan Z. Predictive values of body mass index and waist circumference for risk factors of certain related diseases in Chinese adults: study on optimal cut-off points of body mass index and waist circumference in Chinese adults. Asia Pac J Clin Nutr. 2002;118:S685–93.
17. Sleep-related breathing disorders in adults: recommendations for syndrome definition and measurement techniques in clinical research. The Report of an American Academy of Sleep Medicine Task Force. Sleep 1999;22(5):667–89.
18. Series F, Cormier Y, La Forge J. Influence of apnea type and sleep stage on nocturnal post-apneic desaturation. Am Rev Respir Dis. 1990;141(6):1522–6.
19. Okabe S, Hida W, Kikuchi Y, Taguchi O, Takishima T, Shirato K. Upper airway muscle activity during REM and non-REM sleep of patients with obstructive apnea. Chest. 1994;106(3): 767–73.
20. He QY, Feng J, Zhang XL, et al. Relationship of daytime blood pressure and severity of obstructive sleep apnea among Chinese: a multi-center investigation in China. Chin Med J (Engl). 2010;123(1):18–22.
21. Nakano H, Ikeda T, Hayashi M, Ohshima E, Onizuka A. Effects of body position on snoring in apneic and nonapneic snorers. Sleep. 2003;26(2):169–72.
22. Cartwright RD. Effect of sleep position on sleep apnea severity. Sleep. 1984;7(2):110–4.
23. George CF, Millar TW, Kryger MH. Sleep apnea and body position during sleep. Sleep. 1988;11(1):90–9.
24. Braver HM, Block AJ. Effect of nasal spray, positional therapy, and the combination thereof in the asymptomatic snorer. Sleep. 1994;17(6):516–21.

Part III
Initial Work Up: Drug Induced Sleep Endoscopy

Drug-Induced Sleep Endoscopy and Sleep Position

Ioannis Koutsourelakis, Faiza Safiruddin, and Nico de Vries

Introduction

A major goal of surgical evaluation of snoring and obstructive sleep apnea (OSA) is the determination of the site(s) of obstruction so that the surgeon can tailor the operative procedure to the specific condition of each patient. Multiple evaluation techniques have been developed to examine an individual's pattern of upper airway obstruction, each with important strengths and weaknesses. These techniques are commonly performed during wakefulness and include largely static observations rather than dynamic assessments (e.g., Müller maneuver, lateral radiographic cephalometry, computed tomography scanning, and magnetic resonance imaging). Due to the difficulty in establishing the site of obstruction in the conscious patient who carries a diagnosis of OSA, the diagnosis and treatment of OSA is a complex and multidimensional issue. Croft and Pringle first proposed sleep endoscopy in 1991 [1]. Using midazolam as a sedating agent, they demonstrated the utility of passing a fiberoptic endoscope through a sleeping patient's nasal cavity to assess pharyngeal structures for evidence of obstruction. They were able to induce the preexisting snoring in 95 % of their patients [1].

We have previously renamed the technique as drug-induced sleep endoscopy (DISE) in order to reflect the three key features of this method of assessment: (1) the

I. Koutsourelakis, M.D., Ph.D. (✉) • F. Safiruddin, M.D.
Department of Otolaryngology, Saint Lucas Andreas Ziekenhuis, Jan Tooropstraat 164, Amsterdam 1061 AE, The Netherlands
e-mail: ikoutsourelakis@gmail.com

N. de Vries, M.D., Ph.D.
Department of Otolaryngology, Sint Lucas Andreas Ziekenhuis, Jan Tooropstraat 164, Amsterdam 1061 AE, The Netherlands

Department of Otolaryngology, University Hospital Antwerp, Antwerp, Belgium

N. de Vries et al. (eds.), *Positional Therapy in Obstructive Sleep Apnea*,
DOI 10.1007/978-3-319-09626-1_9

use of various pharmacologic agents to achieve sedation, (2) the goal of reproducing upper airway behavior similar to that which occurs during natural sleep, and (3) endoscopic upper airway evaluation. Other terms used in the literature include sleep endoscopy, sleep nasendoscopy, somnoendoscopy, somnoscopy, sedated endoscopy, and propofol sleep endoscopy [2].

The importance of DISE has been highlighted very recently by two studies which showed an association between DISE findings and surgical outcome. Indeed, Soares et al. pointed out that the presence of severe lateral pharyngeal wall and/or supraglottic collapse on preoperative DISE is associated with OSA surgical failure [3]. The authors added that the identification of this failure-prone collapse pattern may be useful in preoperative patient counseling as well as in directing an individualized and customized approach to the treatment of OSA. Furthermore, Koutsourelakis et al. documented that the presence of circumferential collapse at the velum and of complete collapse at the tongue base were independently associated with failure of OSA surgery [4].

Indications and Contraindications of Drug-Induced Sleep Endoscopy

DISE is indicated when surgery or therapy with mandibular repositioning devices are being considered as treatment options by the patient and the physician [5, 6]. Consequently, DISE is not necessary if continuous positive airway pressure, weight loss, or positional therapy is being considered, as visualization of the level of obstruction is not mandatory for these treatment modalities. A high American Society of Anesthesiologists score (ASA 3) and propofol or midazolam allergies (albeit rare) are considered contraindications. Because of a higher procedure-associated risk and lesser effects on treatment decisions, markedly severe OSA (such as an apnea-hypopnea index (AHI) > 70 events/h) and severe obesity are relative contraindications [5].

Prior to DISE, polysomnography must be performed. The results of these examinations are mandatory and at the basis of performing of DISE.

Technique

Patients should have basic cardiorespiratory monitoring (pulse oximetry, blood pressure, electrocardiogram), and it must be possible to administer oxygen if needed. A computerized target-controlled infusion system for propofol can be helpful as well as a bispectral index score system for monitoring the depth of sedation, respectively; neither are compulsory [7].

Table 1 Pharmacological properties of midazolam and propofol

Midazolam	Propofol
Benzodiazepine derivative	2-6 Disopropylphenol
Large therapeutic range	Small therapeutic range
Active etabolites (accumulation)	No accumulation
Functional half life 45 min	Functional half life 4–6 min
Elimination half life 150 min	Elimination half life 55 min
Central muscle relaxation	Central breathing depression
Paradoxal reaction in 1 %	Hypopharyngeal reflex depression

Patients should remain nil per os before the DISE, to prevent regurgitation and aspiration. To reduce salivation, atropine or other anticholinergic agents can be administered 30 min before starting the procedure.

A topical anesthetic, with or without a decongestant, should be administered to 1 or both nostrils at least 20 min before starting the procedure, being careful not to overanesthetize the pharynx, as the risk of aspiration and coughing increases.

The patient should lie in a supine position on an operating table or in a bed. The position should attempt to mimic sleeping habits at home (e.g., one or two pillows, with or without dentures). To gain added value, the body position should be easily changeable, should one want to visualize potential consequences of another position. It is practical to be able to view the film of the flexible endoscopy on a screen and record it. With the help of a microphone, acoustic and visual signals can be recorded simultaneously. The lights should be dimmed and the room quiet to minimize awaking stimuli.

The sedative agents commonly used for DISE are propofol and/or midazolam; however, in some units both the drugs are used. If midazolam is used, a flumazenil injection should be readily available in case reversal of the benzodiazepine effect should be necessary [8].

With the presence of an anesthetist in an operating theater or in a clinic setting, propofol (1.5 mg/kg or continuous infusion) can be administered. Propofol, an ultra-short-acting hypnotic, enables greater control of the depth of sedation, albeit limited by a smaller therapeutic/diagnostic range. The pharmacologic properties of both drugs are shown in Table 1. Depending on the organization of the examination, a combined procedure may be useful: commence by administrating midazolam intravenously (3–4 mg) followed by propofol (30–50 mg or continuous infusion), titrated individually.

Subjects with an AHI below 30, or to be more accurate patients with a supine AHI below 30 and with good health (ASA I or II), can undergo midazolam-induced sleep endoscopy in the clinic. Midazolam is administered by the ear, nose, and throat surgeon (the presence of an anesthetist is not obligatory) or by an anesthetist. Sleep is induced by giving midazolam intravenously, slowly titrated up to 0.07 mg/kg per patient, followed by a saline flush. If insufficient, a bolus of 1–2.5 mg is given (a maximum of 7.5 mg per patient). Patients who are extremely nervous or who habitually use antidepressants or sedatives may need an extra bolus.

Previous studies reported that propofol did not change the respiratory pattern nor significantly influence the AHI, but did interfere with the sleep architecture, specifically, reduction in rapid eye movement (REM) sleep in patients undergoing propofol-induced sleep endoscopy [9]. Respiratory and sleep parameters did not change significantly during diazepam-induced sleep endoscopy in comparison with natural sleep either, except for a small increase in the apnea index and a minor change in the duration of the longest apnea and REM sleep [10].

Anesthetic depth is of key importance. The ideal concentration of the respective sedative is variable according to an individual's susceptibility to the sedative effect of the drug. Slow stepwise induction is key to avoid oversedation, resulting in a loss of consciousness. The latter is related to a decrease of upper airway muscle tone and an increase in pharyngeal critical closing pressure.

Once the patient has reached a satisfactory level of sedation, a flexible endoscope (e.g., 3.5 mm) lubricated and coated with anticondense is introduced into the nasal cavity.

The nasal passage, nasopharynx, velum, tongue base, epiglottis, and larynx are observed. The levels of snoring and/or obstruction are assessed.

During the DISE, maneuvers such as a chin lift (a manual closure of the mouth) or a jaw thrust (or Esmarch maneuver) should be performed, with reassessment of the airway after each maneuver. A jaw thrust is a gentle advancement of the mandible by up to 5 mm, mimicking the effect of a mandibular repositioning device. It is thought that, using DISE, one can predict the likelihood that an appliance would be effective by examining the changes in the airway. Although the effects during sedation may not be identical to those of natural sleep, the distance of protrusion can be measured and can inform decisions about the necessary degree of mandibular repositioning with an appliance.

In patients with an insufficient effect of a mandibular repositioning device, DISE can be performed without the device both in and out, to assess obstruction site(s) and surgical alternatives.

VOTE Classification

There is a wide range of systems which describe the complex interactions of upper airway structures during DISE. Some exclude the epiglottis; others try to group multiple structures together in various combinations. However, there is no universally used DISE scoring system—hence one is needed.

We therefore recently proposed the VOTE classification system for reporting DISE findings, with a focus on the primary structures that contribute to upper airway obstruction, either alone or in combination: the velum, oropharyngeal lateral walls (including the tonsils), tongue, and epiglottis [11].

The VOTE classification may be an oversimplification that overlooks some interactions, but we believe it is a foundation for further study of pharyngeal obstruction in OSA and for assessment of the response of upper airway structures

STRUCTURE	DEGREE OF OBSTRUCTION[a]	CONFIGURATION[c]		
		A-P	LATERAL	CONCENTRIC
Velum				
Oropharynx[b]				
Tongue Base				
Epiglottis				

Fig. 1 The VOTE classification. For each structure, there should be a classification as to the degree of obstruction and configuration of obstruction. *Open boxes* reflect the potential configuration that can be visualized related to a specific structure. *Shaded boxes* reflect the fact that a specific structure–configuration cannot be seen (e.g., oropharynx lateral walls in an anteroposterior direction). *A-P* anteroposterior. [a]Degree of obstruction has one number for each structure: 0, no obstruction (no vibration); 1, partial obstruction (vibration); 2, complete obstruction (collapse); X, not visualized. [b]Oropharynx obstruction can be distinguished as related solely to the tonsils or including the lateral walls, with or without a tonsillar component. [c]Configuration noted for structures with degree of obstruction greater than 0

to directed interventions. Our experience suggests that a focus on structures could help answer two central questions: treatment selection and the association between DISE findings and treatment outcomes—for surgery, mandibular repositioning devices, or combined therapy. The VOTE classification represents a common language to describe the patterns of obstruction during DISE and may ultimately determine treatment interventions (Fig. 1).

The most common and well-known sites of obstruction and vibration are located in the soft palate and the lateral pharyngeal walls, including tonsils and the base of tongue. Obstruction at epiglottic level occurs less often but has clinical significance. Previous large series of DISE in patients with OSA reported a majority of multilevel obstruction, a retropalatinal as well as retrolingual obstruction in a large percentage of cases. In general, a unilevel obstruction is more common in patients with mild OSA, while in severe OSA, a multilevel obstruction is more likely, being the "culprit" for the severity of the OSA.

The subsequent surgical treatment with different, site-specific procedures will not be discussed here. For many years, surgical evaluation techniques have focused on categorizing patients first according to the Fujita classification system that encompasses the two primary regions of pharyngeal upper airway obstruction: the palatal/velopharyngeal and hypopharyngeal/retrolingual regions. However, there are two major limitations of a region-based classification. First, there is substantial anatomical overlap between these regions, including the extension of the lateral pharyngeal walls throughout the length of the pharynx and the physical overlap of the tongue and soft palate. Second, a region-based approach may not determine surgical treatment adequately. For example, in patients with hypopharyngeal/retrolingual obstruction, the oropharyngeal lateral walls, tongue, and epiglottis can each play a more prominent role.

One of the biggest advantages of DISE is the individual analysis, which allows patient-specific and site-specific therapies according to location and degree of obstruction. Maurer et al. have found that in difficult cases, the therapeutic plans are changed after DISE in up to 75 %. Although we have the impression that surgical success rates in patients selected by DISE are better than average, this has to be confirmed in more studies.

The Structures of the VOTE Acronym

Our experience with over 7,500 DISE examinations suggests that a selected group of structures contribute to upper airway narrowing and/or obstruction in sleep-disordered breathing, individually or in combination. The VOTE classification (Fig. 1) evaluates these structures and the degree of airway narrowing.

Velum

Velopharyngeal obstruction occurs at the level of the soft palate, uvula, or lateral pharyngeal wall tissue at the level of the velopharynx. Because these three structures are not entirely distinct entities—both anatomically and on DISE—we have grouped them together. Airway closure related to the velum can occur with collapse in an anteroposterior or concentric configuration, but rarely in a lateral configuration.

Oropharyngeal Lateral Walls Including the Tonsils

The oropharyngeal lateral walls include two structures: the tonsils and the lateral pharyngeal wall tissues that include musculature and the adjacent parapharyngeal fat pads. Both structures collapse in a lateral configuration, although this may occur in combination with collapse of other structures, with a resulting concentric pattern. In the presence of lateral wall collapse, it can be difficult (but certainly not impossible) to determine whether the tonsils or lateral walls are playing a significant role, reflecting potential subtypes; importantly, the distinction can have important implications for treatment selection and outcomes. While the VOTE classification is largely based on DISE findings alone, the examination of tonsil size and lateral pharyngeal wall tissues during routine oral cavity examination are also important. Obstruction related to the oropharynx can only occur with collapse in a lateral configuration.

Tongue Base

Tongue base obstruction is a common DISE finding, and it results in anteroposterior narrowing of the upper airway. In natural sleep, there is a reduction in muscle tone of the tongue, especially during non-REM and REM sleep that is more pronounced in OSA patients compared to healthy individuals. Airway closure related to the base of tongue occurs with collapse in an anteroposterior direction.

Epiglottis

Epiglottic collapse occurs in one of two configurations, anteroposterior or lateral, but not concentric. Anteroposterior collapse can result with folding of the epiglottis with what appears to be decreased structural rigidity of the epiglottis or with an apparent posterior displacement of the entire epiglottis against the posterior pharyngeal wall, with normal epiglottic structural integrity. The second pattern, a lateral folding or involution, is consistent with a central vertically oriented crease of decreased rigidity of the epiglottis. The epiglottis may be under-recognized as a factor in patients with sleep-disordered breathing, and a substantial proportion of patients with OSA do demonstrate a significant epiglottic contribution to airway obstruction during DISE. DISE may provide a unique assessment of the epiglottis, as its apparent role has not been demonstrated as clearly demonstrated with other evaluation techniques (Fuyita, Mallampati/Friedman).

Other Structures

Although less common, airway obstruction in sleep-disordered breathing can be related to other structures. In rare cases, collapse above the VOTE level, for example, by massive nasal polyps, adenoid hypertrophy, or nasopharyngeal neoplasms, or below the VOTE level, for example, vocal cord level, in postradiation edema, or vocal cord paralysis, can be visualized. This is usually detected by awake examination already. If indicated, they are noted separately. We do not mean to minimize their potential role but believe the VOTE classification reflects patterns seen in the large majority of patients.

Degree of Airway Narrowing

The VOTE classification involves a qualitative assessment of the degree of airway narrowing, divided into the following:

1. None (typically with no vibration of the involved structure and less than 50 % airway narrowing compared to dimensions during nonapneic state)

2. Partial (vibration, 50–75 % narrowing, reduced airflow)
3. Complete (obstruction, greater than 75 % narrowing, and no airflow)

We recognize that differentiating between the three categories is not always clear, although the evaluation of degree of obstruction has been demonstrated as having moderate reliability. At level 1 in the upper airway, a partial collapse (vibration, snoring) might be present, while at the other level a complete collapse might be detected.

Complications

There are no severe side effects or emergency situations described with DISE in the literature. In more than 7,500 combined endoscopies, endotracheal intubation, tracheostomy, or the use of flumazenil was never necessary. Depending on the execution and performance, artificial ventilation with the help of a ventilation or larynx mask may occasionally be necessary, in particular, in severe OSA. In cases with marked oxygen desaturation on sleep study, oxygen insufflation (such as 2–4 L/min via blow by face mask or nasal cannula) may help to prevent undesirable desaturations. Saliva aspiration can occur, but it is rare and usually not dangerous. However, it may compromise the procedure, due to extreme coughing. Laryngospasm is rare. Regurgitation and aspiration acid reflux are theoretically possible and might need specific treatment. The authors did not encounter such cases. To prevent complications in high-risk patients such as those with body mass index greater than 35 kg/m^2 and problematic anatomical features (short neck, modified Mallampati position IV), DISE may be performed at the same time with positive airway pressure administration.

Reliability and Validity

Questions and concerns that arose about reliability of DISE have been elegantly addressed by two studies. Indeed, Rodriguez-Bruno et al. concluded that sleep endoscopy has good reliability, particularly in the evaluation of hypopharyngeal structures [12]. The investigators looked at test-retest reliability, comparing the results from two distinct exams analyzed by one person. Furthermore, when comparing assessments by two independent reviewers of prerecorded sleep endoscopy procedures, Kezirian et al. demonstrated moderate to substantial interrater reliability [13]. This was significant in the identification of primary structures involved in obstruction versus individual structures. This same study demonstrated a higher interrater reliability for assessment of the palatal region for obstruction in general versus assessment of individual structures that cause obstruction in the palatal region. The authors stated that the lower reliability in assessing individual structures is less important in palatal obstruction, because traditional uvulopalatopharyngoplasty (UPPP) treatment is the same regardless of the structure involved, be it the soft palate or velopharynx lateral pharyngeal wall. Kezirian et al.'s study also mentions that the tongue, epiglottis, and lateral pharyngeal walls are the three structures most commonly involved in obstruction in the hypopharynx [13]. At this site, there is a moderate to substantial interrater reliability in assessing individual hypopharyngeal structures that cause obstruction. Because there are varying treatment options for the different structures that are involved, sleep endoscopy can help to determine which hypopharyngeal and oropharyngeal procedure will be the most efficacious.

Lastly, the validity of DISE has been tested by Berry et al. [14]. The authors found that none of asymptomatic patients snored or obstructed during target controlled infusion with propofol, whereas all of symptomatic patients presented snoring/obstruction during the same circumstances.

Sleep Position

More than half of patients with OSA have positional-dependent OSA, defined as an AHI in the worst sleeping position twice or more compared to the AHI in the other positions. Previous studies have already shown that difference head positions can influence collapsibility of the passive pharynx in patients with sleep-disordered breathing. Van Kesteren et al. have provided additional evidence that head position, separately from trunk position, is an additional important factor in the occurrence of apnea-hypopnea in a subpopulation of OSA patients (discussed in chapter "The Contribution of Head Position to the Apnea/Hypopnea Index in Patients with Position-Dependent Obstructive Sleep Apnea") [15]. Intuitively, these head positions could influence the outcome of DISE. Although DISE is predominantly performed in supine position, when physicians consider positional therapy in combined treatment with surgery, it would make more sense to assess levels of obstruction in other sleeping positions. It is possible that positional OSA patients have distinct anatomical characteristics whereby the gravitational effects could have a higher effect on the upper airway by displacing anterior pharyngeal structures and the pharynx. DISE performed in different positions could further help to elucidate the pathophysiology of non-positional and positional apneics.

We have recently shown that the severity of upper airway collapse in the DISE of patients with OSA decreases significantly when the head is rotated to the lateral side (data submitted for publication) [16]. There is however no significant difference between rotation of the head to the right or left side. Head rotation improves the airway significantly more in patients with positional OSA than in patients with non-positional OSA. Indeed, patients with positional OSA have significantly more complete anteroposterior collapse at the palate and tongue base level than non-positional OSA patients.

Furthermore, we have recently demonstrated that rotation of the head and lateral positions have similar types of upper airway collapse during DISE [17]. This could be of clinical relevance. When applying positional therapy, it could be more important to place the sensor on the neck in order to rotate the head than to place the sensor on the trunk. And perhaps even more important, when positional therapy will be an integral part of treatment, it makes more sense to perform DISE in lateral position, than in supine position.

Our method of utilizing DISE is validated since we obtain comparable results to Isono et al. [18]. Another research shows that the head posture has a marked effect on the collapsibility and site of collapse of the passive upper airway (measured by electromyogram), and thus manipulating head posture during propofol sedation may assist with identification of pharyngeal regions vulnerable to collapse during sleep and may be useful for guiding surgical intervention. Although this study was not performed in OSA patients, it is a guide that head position is an important factor in assessing upper airway patency and could be important during DISE.

These findings are of clinical importance as it may not be necessary for patients during DISE to rotate to the lateral side but that the head rotation is enough to improve the AHI. In addition, patients who cannot tolerate positional therapy due to back complaints could potentially benefit from head rotation only. Currently, positional therapy devices are placed on the trunk of the body. The device could also be placed at the back of the neck or on the head in order to independently rotate the patients head. Further studies are ongoing to investigate whether this will be an effective way of treating positional OSA patients.

Based on the results of the aforementioned studies, we recommend that DISE should include lateral and not only supine position especially in patients with positional OSA, when positional therapy is considered in the treatment plan.

Conclusions

DISE is a valid addition to polysomnography and clinical assessment of the OSA patient. Correct technique and performance presumed, it is a reliable and safe tool to detect and analyze the phenomena of the upper airway during sleep visually and acoustically. The anatomical structures that are involved in sound generation and obstruction of the upper airway can be identified individually. By identifying specific structures that mediate collapse, surgeons may potentially be able to develop targeted, effective treatment plans. Individual therapeutic planning concerning choice and extent of surgical procedures can be optimized. With the help of passive maneuvers, the potential efficacy of mandibular repositioning devices can be estimated. The shared use of the VOTE classification can facilitate the scientific evaluation of DISE in individual centers and also the collection of data across multiple centers. With these data, we can compare results across studies and find supporting evidence whether DISE is indeed beneficial to assess the outcomes of existing and novel treatments for snoring and OSA. Head rotation during DISE improves upper airway collapse. This improvement is predominantly seen in positional OSA patients. In addition, there was no difference in upper airway collapse between right and left head rotation and also no difference between rotation of the head and lateral positions. We recommend that in positional patients, when positional therapy is considered as only treatment or as combined treatment, DISE should be performed in not only in the supine but also in the lateral position.

References

1. Croft CB, Pringle M. Sleep endoscopy: a technique of assessment in snoring and obstructive sleep apnoea. Clin Otolaryngol. 1991;16:504–9.
2. Kotecha BT, Hannan SA, Khalil HM, Georgalas C, Bailey P. Sleep nasendoscopy: a 10-year retrospective audit study. Eur Arch Otorhinolaryngol. 2007;264:1361–7.
3. Soares D, Sinawe H, Folbe AJ, Yoo G, Badr S, Rowley JA, Lin HS. Lateral oropharyngeal wall and supraglottic airway collapse associated with failure in sleep apnea surgery. Laryngoscope. 2012;122:473–9.
4. Koutsourelakis I, Safruddin F, Ravesloot MJL, Zakynthinos S, de Vries N. Surgery for obstructive sleep apnea: sleep endoscopy determinants of outcome. Laryngoscope. 2012;122: 2587–91.
5. Maurer JT, Hörmann K. Endoscopy in sleep medicine. HNO. 2010;58:341–7.
6. Johal A, Battagel JM, Kotecha BT. Sleep nasendoscopy: a diagnostic tool for predicting treatment success with mandibular advancement splints in obstructive sleep apnoea. Eur J Orthod. 2005;27:607–14.
7. Hessel NS, de Vries N. Diagnostic work-up of socially unacceptable snoring. II. Sleep endoscopy. Eur Arch Otorhinolaryngol. 2002;259:158–61.
8. Hillman DR, Walsh JH, Maddison KJ, Platt PR, Kirkness JP, Noffsinger WJ, et al. Evolution of changes in upper airway collapsibility during slow induction of anesthesia with propofol. Anesthesiology. 2009;111:63–71.
9. Rabelo FA, Braga A, Kupper DS, et al. Propofol-induced sleep: polysomnographic evaluation of patients with obstructive sleep apnea and controls. Otolaryngol Head Neck Surg. 2010;142:218–24.
10. Ravesloot MJ, de Vries N. One hundred consecutive patients undergoing drug-induced sleep endoscopy: results and evaluation. Laryngoscope. 2011;121:2710–6.
11. Kezirian EJ, Hohenhorst W, de Vries N. Drug-induced sleep endoscopy: the VOTE classification. Eur Arch Otorhinolaryngol. 2011;268:1233–6.
12. Rodriguez-Bruno K, Goldberg AN, McCulloch CE, Kezirian EJ. Test-retest reliability of drug-induced sleep endoscopy. Otolaryngol Head Neck Surg. 2009;140:646–51.
13. Kezirian EJ, White DP, Malhotra A, Ma W, McCulloch CE, Goldberg AN. Interrater reliability of drug-induced sleep endoscopy. Arch Otolaryngol Head Neck Surg. 2010;136:393–7.
14. Berry S, Roblin G, Williams A, Watkins A, Whittet H. Validity of sleep nasendoscopy in the investigation of sleep related breathing disorders. Laryngoscope. 2005;115:538–40.
15. Van Kesteren ER, van Maanen JP, Hilgevoord AA, Laman DM, de Vries N. Quantitative effects of trunk and head position on the apnea hypopnea index in obstructive sleep apnea. Sleep. 2011;34:1075–81.
16. Safiruddin F, Koutsourelakis I, de Vries N. Analysis of the influence of head rotation during drug-induced sleep endoscopy in obstructive sleep apnea. Laryngoscope. 2014. doi:10.1002/lary.24598
17. Safirrudin F, Koutsourelakis I, de Vries N. Upper airway collapse during drug induced sleep endoscopy: head rotation in supine position compared with lateral head and trunk position. Eur Arch Otorhinolaryngol. doi:10.1007/s00405-014-3215-z.
18. Isono S, Remmers JE, Tanaka A, Sho Y, Sato J, Nishino T. Anatomy of pharynx in patients with obstructive sleep apnea and in normal subjects. J Appl Physiol. 1997;82:1319–26.

Changes in Site of Obstruction in Obstructive Sleep Apnea Patients According to Sleep Position

Tae-Bin Won, Chul Hee Lee, and Chae-Seo Rhee

Introduction

Obstructive sleep apnea (OSA) is a manifestation of upper airway instability during sleep. The unstable airway results from a combination of a structurally vulnerable upper airway and a physiologic loss of muscle tone that occurs during sleep. Adequate treatment of OSA is imperative considering its impact on quality of life and numerous complications this disease is associated with.

The severity of the disease varies and is determined by multiple factors that are still not completely understood. It is well known that sleep position affects the occurrence and severity of sleep apnea [1, 2]. OSA worsens in terms of apnea frequency, duration, desaturation, and duration of arousals in the supine position. Positional dependency defined as having a supine AHI two times greater than a non-supine AHI [3] can be seen in as many as 50–70 % of OSA patients [3, 4].

The mechanism responsible for worsening of OSA in the supine position is not clear. Most likely it relates to the effect of gravity on the size or shape of the upper airway [5]. A smaller pharyngeal airway in the supine posture making it more vulnerable to collapse is an intuitive explanation [6]. However, reports are inconsistent in this regard, with some studies reporting the pharynx to be smaller in the supine than in the lateral recumbent posture [5, 7, 8] and others reporting a similar pharyngeal size in the two postures [9–11]. Until now the effect of posture on the upper airway during sleep in OSA patients is largely unknown.

T.-B. Won, M.D., Ph.D.
Department of Otorhinolaryngology, Seoul National University College of Medicine, Seoul National University Hospital, Seongnam, South Korea

C.H. Lee, M.D., Ph.D. • C.-S. Rhee, M.D., Ph.D. (✉)
Department of Otorhinolaryngology, Seoul National University Bundang Hospital, 300 Gumi-dong, Bundang-gu, Seongnam-si, Gyeonggi-do 463-707, South Korea
e-mail: csrhee@snu.ac.kr

N. de Vries et al. (eds.), *Positional Therapy in Obstructive Sleep Apnea*,
DOI 10.1007/978-3-319-09626-1_10

Various efforts have been made to elucidate the effect of positional dependency using tools such as acoustic reflection [9, 11], lateral cephalometry [12–14], computed tomography [10], magnetic resonance imaging [15], and optical coherence tomography [16, 17]. However, these studies have limitations as they are performed while awake and/or during only the supine position.

In this chapter, we introduce a unique study in which we evaluated the changes of site and pattern of obstruction of the upper airway according to sleep position by the use of dynamic airway evaluation during drug-induced sleep.

Patient Characteristics

Eighty-five patients were included in this study. The inclusion criteria were patients who had performed full-night attended nocturnal polysomnography (PSG), patients who underwent drug-induced sleep endoscopy in the supine and lateral position, and patients with an AHI greater than 15. Patients with a previous history of upper airway surgery were excluded from this study.

Subgroup analysis was performed according to severity and lateral AHI. They were divided into two groups according to severity: moderate OSA (AHI = 15–30) and severe OSA (AHI > 30) groups. Among the 85 patients, 78 patients who had at least 30 min of lateral sleep were divided into two groups according to the lateral AHI (average of AHI in the left and right decubitus position): lateral obstructor group (LO, lateral AHI ≥ 10) and lateral nonobstructor group (LNO, lateral AHI < 10).

There were 61 males and 24 females with a mean age of 47.8 ± 6.7 years. Body mass index (BMI) was 26.9 ± 2.7 kg/m^2. Mean AHI, mean supine AHI, and mean lateral AHI (average of right and left lateral AHI) were 33.3 ± 16.0, 44.3 ± 22.4, and 21.3 ± 22.4, respectively. The lowest oxygen saturation was 80.02 ± 13.8 %, and proportion of oxygen saturation below 90 % was 7.5 ± 13.1 % (Table 1).

Drug-Induced Sleep Endoscopy

Drug-induced sleep endoscopy (DISE) was performed in the following manner. The patient lied down comfortably in the supine position. Heart rate and oxygen saturation were monitored throughout the examination. Examination started in the awake state after unilateral nasal topical anesthesia and decongestion using cotton pledges placed at the middle meatus. Thereafter, sleep was induced by intravenous administration of midazolam (initial dose of 3 mg for adult patients over 50 kg; 0.06 mg/kg). After the patient fell asleep, endoscopy was performed through the same nostril. Desaturation events (drop of basal saturation during sleep of more than 3 %) were analyzed for obstruction level, structure, pattern, and degree and representative findings recorded. If there was no desaturation, changes during snoring were analyzed. Additional bolus of 0.5 mg of midazolam was administered in the

Table 1 Demographic and polysomnographic findings

PSG parameters	$n=85$
M:F	61:24
Age	47.8±6.7
BMI	26.9±2.7
AHI	33.3±16.0
Supine AHI	44.3±22.4
Lateral AHI	21.3±22.4
O_2 saturation min	80.2±13.8
O_2 saturation<90 %	7.5±13.1

BMI body mass index, *AHI* apnea-hypopnea index

event of awakenings. Target level of sedation was upper muscle relaxation producing obstruction (i.e., snoring or apnea) without respiratory depression. Level of sedation was maintained to a modified Ramsay score of 5 (sluggish response to a light glabellar tap or loud auditory stimulus) or 70–80 in selected patients in which BIS monitoring was used.

After observing the airway in the supine position, the patients were positioned in the right lateral decubitus position. Body and head was moved simultaneously so that axis of the body and the Frankfort plane of the head were perpendicular to the bed.

At least three obstructive events were observed in each position, and the most severe event was determined as the obstruction site of the patient. After the conclusion of the examination, 2 mg of flumazenil was administered intravenously as an antidote. The average examination time was 40 min.

Midazolam-induced sleep endoscopy (MISE) findings were classified according to obstruction structures (soft palate (SP), lateral wall (LW) including palatine tonsils, tongue base (TB), and larynx (LX) including epiglottis). The degree of obstruction was determined as 0, no obstruction; 1, partial obstruction (vibration with desaturation); and 2, complete obstruction (total collapse of airway with desaturation). For obstruction in the tongue base more than >50 % displacement compared to the awake state was determined as grade 1, while grade 2 obstruction was attributed for more than 75 % obstruction.

DISE Findings According to Sleep Position

In the supine position, the most common structure contributing to obstruction was the soft palate which was observed in 87.6 % of patients ($n=74$) followed by TB ($n=65$, 76.5 %), LW ($n=60$, 70.6 %), and LX ($n=18$, 21.2 %) (Table 2). When the patients were positioned in the lateral decubitus position, the most frequent anatomical structure contributing to obstruction changed from the SP to the LW which was seen in 51 patients (60 %), followed by SP ($n=19$, 22.3 %), TB ($n=6$, 7.1 %),

Table 2 Changes of obstruction site according to sleep position ($n=85$)

Obstruction site	Supine position, patient number (%)	Lateral position, patient number (%)
Soft palate		
Total ($n=85$)	74 (87.6)	19 (22.3)*
Mod OSA ($n=47$)	43 (91.5)	9 (19.1)*
Severe OSA ($n=38$)	31 (81.6)	10 (26.3)*
Lateral wall		
Total	60 (70.6)	51 (60.0)
Mod OSA	29 (61.7)	17 (36.2)*
Severe OSA	31 (81.6)	34 (89.5)
Tongue base		
Total	65 (76.5)	6 (7.1)*
Mod OSA	38 (80.1)	4 (8.5)*
Severe OSA	27 (71.1)	2 (5.0)*
Larynx		
Total	18 (21.2)	1 (1.2)*
Mod OSA	11 (23.4)	0 (0)*
Severe OSA	7 (18.4)	1 (2.6)*
No obstruction		
Total	0 (0)	21 (24.7)*
Mod OSA	0 (0)	14 (29.8)*
Severe OSA	0 (0)	2 (5.3)*

OSA obstructive sleep apnea
**p*-value<0.05

and LX ($n=1$, 1.4 %). A patent airway with no discernible site of obstruction was found in 25.3 % of patients in the lateral position. The degree of obstruction of the six patients who showed TB obstruction in the lateral position was all grade 1, indicating partial obstruction (Table 2). The prevalence of obstruction in the SP, TB, and LX showed statistically significant decrease when sleep position was changed from supine to lateral position ($p<0.05$), while overall prevalence of LW obstruction was not affected by position change ($p>0.05$).

Changes in Obstruction Site According to Severity of OSA

Among the 85 patients, 47 patients had moderate OSA (AHI = 15–29) and 38 patients had severe OSA (AHI ≥ 30). In moderate OSA patients, the prevalence of all the anatomic structures contributing to obstruction (SP, LW, TB, LX) showed significant improvement ($p<0.05$) when position was changed from supine to lateral, with no airway obstruction in 29.8 % of patients (Table 2).

In severe OSA patients, the prevalence of obstruction in the SP, TB, and LX showed significant improvement (SP changed from 81.6 % to 26.3 %, TB from

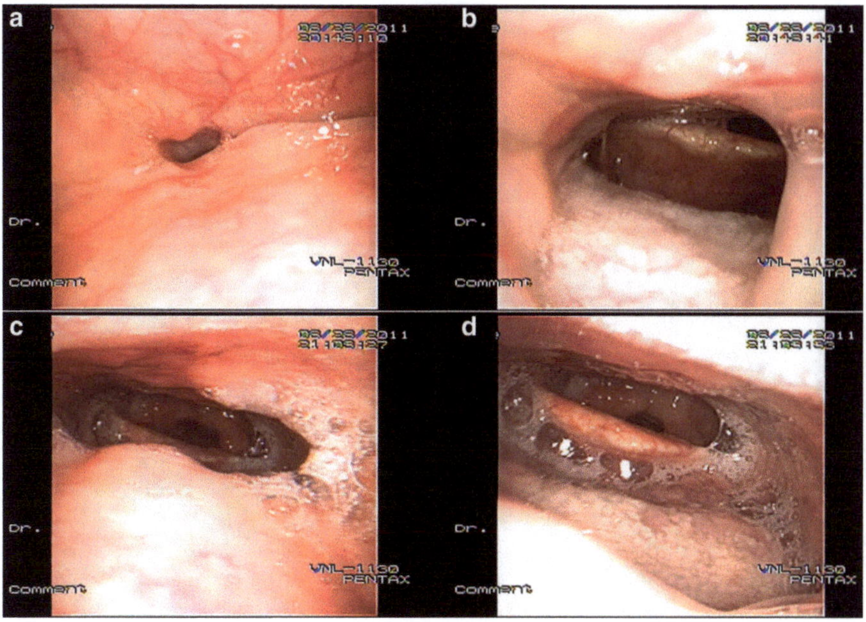

Fig. 1 Representative DISE findings from our series showing changes in site of obstruction according to sleep position. In the supine position (**a, b**), the patient shows obstruction at the soft palate (**a**) and tongue base resulting in secondary epiglottis obstruction (**b**). When the patient changed position to the lateral decubitus position (**c, d**) a patent airway was observed in the retropalatal and retroglossal airway. The AHI for this particular patient was 44.2 (total), 52.6 (supine), 7.4 (lateral). The patient was classified as lateral nonobstructor

71.1 % to 5.0 %, LX from 18.4 % to 2.6 %) after position is changed to the lateral position ($p<0.05$). However, there was no change in the prevalence of obstruction in the LW. The incidence of LW obstruction in the lateral position was significantly higher in the severe OSA patients (89.5 %) compared to the moderate OSA patients (36.2 %) ($p<0.05$).

Representative DISE findings in the supine and lateral positions are shown in Figs. 1 and 2.

Changes in Obstruction Site in Lateral Obstructors and Lateral Nonobstructors

Subgroup analysis was carried out in 78 patients whose sleep time spent in lateral position was greater than 30 min. Among them, 50 patients were position dependent (PD), while 28 were non-position dependent (NPD). Patients with a lateral AHI equal or below 10 were regarded as lateral nonobstructors (LNO), while those who had a lateral AHI equal or above 10 were regarded as lateral obstructors (LO). Characteristics of the two groups are summarized in Table 3.

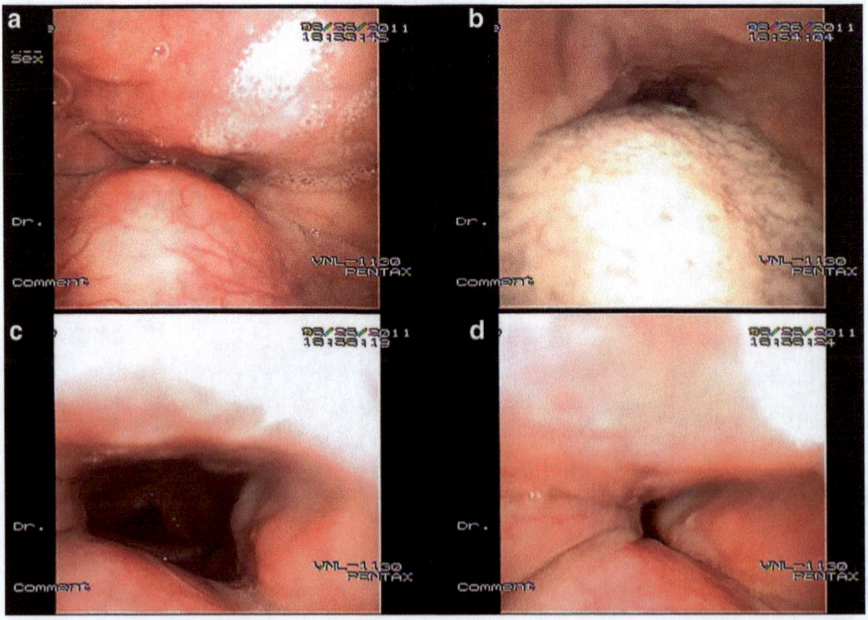

Fig. 2 Representative DISE findings from our series showing changes in site of obstruction according to sleep position. In the supine position (**a**, **b**), the patient shows obstruction at the soft palate (**a**), oropharyngeal lateral wall, and tongue base (**b**). When the patient changed position to the lateral decubitus position (**c**, **d**), there was no obstruction observed in the soft palate and tongue base (**c**); however, there was persistent obstruction in the lateral walls (**b**). The AHI for this particular patient was 63.8 (total), 89.7 (supine), and 32.2 (lateral). The patient was classified as lateral obstructor

Table 3 Demographic and polysomnographic findings of LO and LNO

	LO ($n=42$)	LNO ($n=36$)
M:F	34:8	25:11
Age	46.7±8.3	48.8±5.7
BMI	28.8±3.2	25.2±2.3*
AHI total	46.9±13.6	22.3±4.24*
Supine AHI	58.3±25.4	31.3±18.4*
Lateral AHI	29.4±19.7	7.8±5.3*
Position dependency	14 (33.3 %)	36 (100 %)*

LO lateral obstructor, *LNO* lateral nonobstructor
*p-value <0.05

According to this criteria, 42 patients (53.8 %) were classified as LO group. Mean age was 46.7±5.3 years, with 34 males and 8 females. Body mass index was 28.8±3.2 kg/m^2 and mean AHI was 46.9±13.6. Positional dependency was found in 33.3 % of patients. Changes in obstruction site are shown in Table 4. When position was changed from supine to lateral, prevalence of obstruction in the SP, TB,

Table 4 Changes of obstruction site according to sleep position in LO and LNO patients

Obstruction site	SP	LW	TB	LX	No
LO ($n=42$)					
Supine	35 (83.3)	36 (85.7)	30 (71.5)	11 (26.2)	0 (0)
Lateral	13 (31.0)*	35 (83.3)[a]	4 (9.5)*	1 (2.6)[b,*]	1 (2.4)
LNO ($n=36$)					
Supine	32 (88.9)	19 (52.8)	30 (83.3)	8 (22.2)	0
Lateral	6 (16.7)*	12 (33.3)	1 (2.8)*	0 (0)*	19 (52.8)*

Value represents number and (%); numbers are not mutually exclusive
LO Lateral obstructor, *LNO* lateral nonobstructor
*p-value <0.05
[a]Significant difference between LO and LNO in the lateral position
[b]Due to redundant arytenoid mucosa

and LX was significantly reduced ($p<0.05$). However, LW obstruction showed no significant change (85.7 % in supine position to 83.3 % in lateral position).

Thirty-six patients (46.2 %) were classified as LNO group. Mean age was 48.8±3.4 years, with 25 males and 11 females. Body mass index was 25.2±2.3 kg/m^2 and mean AHI was 22.3±4.24. Positional dependency was found in all (100 %) patients. Changes in obstruction site are shown in Table 4. When position was changed from supine to lateral, 19 of 36 patients (52.8 %) showed a patent airway. Prevalence of obstruction in the SP, TB, and LX was significantly reduced ($p<0.05$). LW obstruction also showed reduction (52.8 % in supine position to 33.3 % in lateral position) in LNO group, but it failed to show statistical significance. In the 12 patients who still showed obstruction in the LW in the lateral position, 6 patients showed only partial obstruction (grade 1). Only one patient showed TB obstruction in the lateral position and this was grade 1.

When the prevalence of obstruction in the lateral position was compared between the LO and LNO groups, only LW obstruction was significantly different between the LO and LNO groups.

Discussion

Airway obstruction during sleep which occurs in OSA patients is not a continuous and constant process attesting that the obstruction is dynamic. Among various factors, sleep position is a major determinant that affects severity of OSA [3].

The mechanism responsible for worsening of OSA in the supine position or improvement in the lateral position is not clear. Previous studies have suggested that the airway shape (a more elliptically shaped airway) may contribute to its propensity to collapse [15]. Shortcomings of these studies include limited number of patients, size (CSA) or shape of the airway evaluated using static images without information on the site, or anatomic structure contributing to obstruction. Furthermore, evaluation was performed while awake which can be a major limitation since upper airway muscle tone show marked differences when asleep.

Evaluating the upper airway of OSA patients has been an elusive task. Recent implementation of dynamic evaluation of the airway during sleep (DAES) techniques such as sleep videofluoroscopy (SVF) or DISE have greatly enhanced our knowledge of the dynamic changes which occurs in the upper airway during sleep. Numerous studies have shown that it is a safe, feasible, and valid tool for dynamic assessment of the upper airway [18–21]. Using sleep videofluoroscopy, we have already shown that position dependency can be associated with obstruction site [2]. However, previous SVF and DISE studies that evaluate the upper airway during sleep have only been performed in the supine position.

Our results show that in the supine position, the most prevalent obstruction site was the SP (87.6 %) followed by the TB (76.5 %) which is comparable to other reports [22–24]. When sleep posture was changed to the lateral recumbent position, obstruction at the SP, TB, and LX improved significantly, with 24.7 % ($n = 21$) of patients showing no overall obstruction. Improvement of obstruction at the TB and LX was most prominent (TB 76.5–7.1 % and LX from 21.2 % to 1.2 %). This pattern of improvement was maintained when stratified according to severity of AHI. The one patient who showed persistent obstruction at the larynx in the lateral position was a patient whose redundant arytenoid mucosa was causing the obstruction at the laryngeal inlet irrespective of sleep posture.

Obstruction at the lateral walls (LW), on the other hand, did not show significant improvement after position change (70.6 % in supine vs. 60.0 % in lateral). When severity of AHI was taken into consideration, improvement was seen in the moderate OSA group (61.7–36.2 %), while there was no change in the severe OSA group (81.6–89.5 %). Lateral wall obstruction is considered to be the most dynamic structure of the upper airway and thus a major contributor of upper airway collapse in OSA patients. Soares and colleagues have shown that patients with lateral wall obstruction are associated with surgical failure [25]. Overall frequency of lateral wall collapse in our study was 70.6 % in the supine position which is higher than other reports with DISE (51.2 %) [18]. We believe that this is due to exclusion of mild OSA patients in our study. When the mild OSA patients are taken into account, the rate of LW obstruction was 48 % which is comparable to other reports. Our study shows that LW obstruction is prominent in severe OSA patients, and this finding is accentuated in the lateral sleep position.

Prevalence of TB obstruction in the supine position was 71.1 %. However, there was a dramatic decrease in frequency of TB obstruction in the lateral sleep position. Only 6 out of 85 patients (7.1 %) showed TB obstruction in the lateral position. Furthermore, all six patients showed partial (grade 1) obstruction. This finding of improvement in obstruction of the TB with position change was consistently seen irrespective of age, sex, BMI, and severity.

We have observed a dramatic change in the upper airway during sleep when sleep position is changed from supine to lateral. This change is mainly focused in the TB and LX. Most OSA patients show improvement in TB and LX obstruction, irrespective of severity. Therefore, we can think that LW collapsibility will determine if the patient will still have persistent obstruction in the lateral position. Severe OSA patients or patients with a high BMI tend to have increased LW collapsibility which will cause persistent obstruction in the lateral position. This is one of the reasons why the number of position-dependent (PD) patients decrease with increasing severity [2]. In the same context, we can speculate that most PD patients are patients who have TB obstruction without severe LW collapse. In a previous study, we have shown that UP3 can change non-PD patients into PD patients rendering them candidates for positional therapy [26, 27]. This is in agreement with our current study because UP3 can reduce LW collapsibility and thus decrease the lateral AHI making these patients PD.

Positioning the patient laterally and evaluating the changes in the airway can give us additional useful clinical information. As shown in our study, in the lateral position, most of the TB and LX components can be nullified. Therefore, a more accurate assessment of the SP and LW collapsibility can be achieved. In the supine position, obstructions at the SP and LW are frequently influenced by obstruction at the TB. We can commonly encounter patients whose SP is posteriorly displaced secondarily due to a retrodisplaced tongue. Displacement of the TB can also alter LW tension and can cause secondary LW collapse. In the lateral position, primary LW collapse can be assessed because the influence of the TB has been taken away. In the case of primary LW collapse, treatment options should be determined accordingly. If surgery is planned, techniques targeting the LW collapse should be implemented for increased success.

Conclusion

The upper airway changes according to sleep posture, and this change accounts for the varying severity of apneic events in OSA patients. We have provided another insight into the upper airway mechanics involved in positional dependency of OSA patients. When sleep posture is changed from supine to lateral, obstruction due to structures such as the tongue base and larynx improves dramatically. Obstruction in lateral position is mostly due to obstruction at the oropharyngeal lateral walls. Therefore, position dependency is mostly determined by lateral wall collapsibility. Evaluating the changes of the upper airway according to sleep position can further characterize the upper airway collapsibility and can be used for tailored treatment planning.

References

1. Cartwright RD. Effect of sleep position on sleep apnea severity. Sleep. 1984;7(2):110–4.
2. Sunwoo WS, Hong SL, Kim SW, et al. Association between positional dependency and obstruction site in obstructive sleep apnea syndrome. Clin Exp Otorhinolaryngol. 2012;5(4): 218–21.
3. Oksenberg A, Silverberg DS, Arons E, Radwan H. Positional vs nonpositional obstructive sleep apnea patients: anthropomorphic, nocturnal polysomnographic, and multiple sleep latency test data. Chest. 1997;112(3):629–39.
4. Pevernagie DA, Shepard Jr JW. Effects of body position on upper airway size and shape in patients with obstructive sleep apnea. Acta Psychiatr Belg. 1994;94(2):101–3.

5. Isono S, Tanaka A, Nishino T. Lateral position decreases collapsibility of the passive pharynx in patients with obstructive sleep apnea. Anesthesiology. 2002;97(4):780–5.
6. Oksenberg A, Silverberg DS. The effect of body posture on sleep-related breathing disorders: facts and therapeutic implications. Sleep Med Rev. 1998;2(3):139–62.
7. Litman RS, Wake N, Chan LM, et al. Effect of lateral positioning on upper airway size and morphology in sedated children. Anesthesiology. 2005;103(3):484–8.
8. Ono T, Otsuka R, Kuroda T, Honda E, Sasaki T. Effects of head and body position on two- and three-dimensional configurations of the upper airway. J Dent Res. 2000;79(11):1879–84.
9. Jan MA, Marshall I, Douglas NJ. Effect of posture on upper airway dimensions in normal human. Am J Respir Crit Care Med. 1994;149(1):145–8.
10. Pevernagie DA, Stanson AW, Sheedy II PF, Daniels BK, Shepard Jr JW. Effects of body position on the upper airway of patients with obstructive sleep apnea. Am J Respir Crit Care Med. 1995;152(1):179–85.
11. Martin SE, Marshall I, Douglas NJ. The effect of posture on airway caliber with the sleep-apnea/hypopnea syndrome. Am J Respir Crit Care Med. 1995;152(2):721–4.
12. Miyamoto K, Ozbek MM, Lowe AA, Fleetham JA. Effect of body position on tongue posture in awake patients with obstructive sleep apnoea. Thorax. 1997;52(3):255–9.
13. Saigusa H, Suzuki M, Higurashi N, Kodera K. Three-dimensional morphological analyses of positional dependence in patients with obstructive sleep apnea syndrome. Anesthesiology. 2009;110(4):885–90.
14. Yildirim N, Fitzpatrick MF, Whyte KF, Jalleh R, Wightman AJ, Douglas NJ. The effect of posture on upper airway dimensions in normal subjects and in patients with the sleep apnea/hypopnea syndrome. Am Rev Respir Dis. 1991;144(4):845–7.
15. Rodenstein DO, Dooms G, Thomas Y, et al. Pharyngeal shape and dimensions in healthy subjects, snorers, and patients with obstructive sleep apnoea. Thorax. 1990;45(10):722–7.
16. Armstrong JJ, Leigh MS, Sampson DD, Walsh JH, Hillman DR, Eastwood PR. Quantitative upper airway imaging with anatomic optical coherence tomography. Am J Respir Crit Care Med. 2006;173(2):226–33.
17. Walsh JH, Leigh MS, Paduch A, et al. Effect of body posture on pharyngeal shape and size in adults with and without obstructive sleep apnea. Sleep. 2008;31(11):1543–9.
18. Kezirian EJ, Hohenhorst W, de Vries N. Drug-induced sleep endoscopy: the VOTE classification. Eur Arch Otorhinolaryngol. 2011;268(8):1233–6.
19. Kezirian EJ, White DP, Malhotra A, Ma W, McCulloch CE, Goldberg AN. Interrater reliability of drug-induced sleep endoscopy. Arch Otolaryngol Head Neck Surg. 2010;136(4):393–7.
20. Lee CH, Mo JH, Kim BJ, et al. Evaluation of soft palate changes using sleep videofluoroscopy in patients with obstructive sleep apnea. Arch Otolaryngol Head Neck Surg. 2009;135(2):168–72.
21. Lee CH, Hong SL, Rhee CS, Kim SW, Kim JW. Analysis of upper airway obstruction by sleep videofluoroscopy in obstructive sleep apnea: a large population-based study. Laryngoscope. 2012;122(1):237–41.
22. Ravesloot MJ, de Vries N. One hundred consecutive patients undergoing drug-induced sleep endoscopy: results and evaluation. Laryngoscope. 2011;121(12):2710–6.
23. Eichler C, Sommer JU, Stuck BA, Hormann K, Maurer JT. Does drug-induced sleep endoscopy change the treatment concept of patients with snoring and obstructive sleep apnea? Sleep Breath. 2013;17(1):63–8.
24. Steinhart H, Kuhn-Lohmann J, Gewalt K, Constantinidis J, Mertzlufft F, Iro H. Upper airway collapsibility in habitual snorers and sleep apneics: evaluation with drug-induced sleep endoscopy. Acta Otolaryngol. 2000;120(8):990–4.
25. Soares D, Sinawe H, Folbe AJ, et al. Lateral oropharyngeal wall and supraglottic airway collapse associated with failure in sleep apnea surgery. Laryngoscope. 2012;122(2):473–9.
26. Lee CH, Kim SW, Han K, et al. Effect of uvulopalatopharyngoplasty on positional dependency in obstructive sleep apnea. Arch Otolaryngol Head Neck Surg. 2011;137(7):675–9.
27. Lee CH, Shin HW, Han DH, et al. The implication of sleep position in the evaluation of surgical outcomes in obstructive sleep apnea. Otolaryngol Head Neck Surg. 2009;140(4):531–5.

Part IV
Initial Work Up: General

Towards a Clinical Classification System for Position-Dependent Obstructive Sleep Apnea

Madeline Ravesloot, Michaël H. Frank, J. Peter van Maanen, E.A. Verhagen, Jan de Lange, and Nico de Vries

Treatment of position-dependent obstructive sleep apnea (POSA) has advanced dramatically recently with the introduction of a new generation of positional therapy (PT), a small device attached to either the neck or chest which corrects the patient from adopting the supine position through a vibrating stimulus. Encouraging data have been published suggesting that this simple therapy successfully prevents patients with POSA from adopting the supine position without negatively influencing sleep efficiency, as well as allowing for good adherence [1–3]. Unfortunately, evaluating the efficacy of PT and comparing results are hindered by the fact that there are no universally used POSA criteria.

M. Ravesloot, M.D., Ph.D. (✉)
Department of Otorhinolaryngology, Sint Lucas Andreas Ziekenhuis,
Jan Tooropstraat 164, Amsterdam 1061 AE, The Netherlands
e-mail: m.ravesloot@slaz.nl

M.H. Frank, D.M.D., M.D. • J. de Lange, D.M.D., M.D., Ph.D.
Department of Oral and Maxillofacial Surgery, Academic Medical Centre, University of Amsterdam, Amsterdam, The Netherlands

J.P. van Maanen, M.D.
Department of Otolaryngology, Sint Lucas Andreas Ziekenhuis, Amsterdam, The Netherlands

E.A. Verhagen, Ph.D.
Department of Public and Occupational Health, EMGO Institute for Health and Care Research, VU Medical Center, Amsterdam, The Netherlands

N. de Vries, M.D., Ph.D.
Department of Otolaryngology, Sint Lucas Andreas Ziekenhuis, Amsterdam, The Netherlands

Department of Otolaryngology, University Hospital Antwerp, Antwerp, Belgium

N. de Vries et al. (eds.), *Positional Therapy in Obstructive Sleep Apnea*,
DOI 10.1007/978-3-319-09626-1_11

Current Definitions of Position-Dependent Obstructive Sleep Apnea

Various definitions of POSA have been applied in literature. In 1984, Cartwright suggested that physicians should differentiate between patients with either positional or non-positional obstructive sleep apnea. She described the arbitrary cut-off point of *a difference of 50 % or more in apnea index between supine and non-supine positions* [4–6].

Despite being the most common classification system and definition used to date, various modified versions of Cartwright's criteria have been applied in the literature. In 1998, Marklund et al. defined supine-dependent sleep apnea as follows: *a supine AHI ≥10, together with a lateral AHI <10* [7]. Both Mador and Permut's groups defined POSA as follows: *an apnea-hypopnea index (AHI) of fewer than 5 events per hour whilst in the non-supine position as well as a decrease in the AHI between the supine and non-supine postures* [8, 9]. In Bignold et al.'s study, when patients met the following criteria, they were deemed position dependent: *overall AHI ≥ 15/h, supine AHI ≥ twice the non-supine AHI; ≥20 min of sleep in supine and non-supine postures and non-supine AHI <15* [10].

Current Developments

The application of various classifications hinders the comparison of the studies on PT. Furthermore, it can be questioned which classification is best suited to identify ideal candidates for new-generation PT. For example, Mador et al. felt that their definition was more clinically relevant, given that avoidance of the supine sleeping position by patients who fit their description would result in normalisation of the AHI and subsequent relief of symptoms of OSA [8]. Bignold et al. were the first to include a minimum sleeping time per position [10].

Bearing this in mind, a new clinically relevant positional OSA classification system was developed, named the Amsterdam Positional OSA Classification (APOC) [11]. It aims to accurately identify candidates who will benefit from a clinically significant improvement of their OSA with PT. The APOC criteria evolve around the percentage of total sleep time spent in either worst sleeping position (WSP) or best sleeping position (BSP) and the AHI in BSP. On applying APOC, one discriminates between the true positional patient, the non-positional patient and the multifactorial patient, whose OSA severity is influenced in part by sleep position.

A panel of three field experts developed the APOC criteria. These criteria are based on three major observations.

1. Insufficient distribution of the various sleeping positions

They advocated that, although an arbitrary cut-off value, a patient should sleep more than 10 % of the total sleep time (TST) in the WSP before PT should be considered. This was based on the question: how long must a patient sleep in a certain position for the AHI measured to be valid and representative.

2. Self-correction of the WSP

The panel hypothesised that certain patients "self-correct". These patients have a high AHI in WSP but spend the majority of the night in BSP. Although these patients are classified as position dependent according to Cartwright's criteria, they would have very limited benefit from PT.

3. Clinical relevance of elimination of the WSP

The panel discussed that in rare cases, despite a ≤50 % difference between the AHI in the WSP and BSP, elimination of the WSP would still be clinically relevant; PT might make a clinically relevant difference. By lowering the OSA severity category, patients could be eligible for less aggressive primary therapy (for example, lower CPAP pressure, less invasive surgery), especially since PT is simple, cheap, well tolerated and reversible. In patients who do not tolerate (or refuse) CPAP or oral appliances, PT can be considered as salvage therapy.

In contrast to earlier classification systems, when applying APOC, one discriminates between the true positional patient, the non-positional patient and the multifactorial patient, whose OSA severity is influenced in part by sleep position. The patients with true POSA could be cured by PT alone and are categorised as APOC I, whilst patients classified as APOC II or III can benefit from PT, but not cured.

The majority of previous POSA classification systems do not take the TST spent in different positions into account but used the differential advantage of the non-supine AHI over the supine AHI calculated as a ratio. In the APOC classification, the TST is taken into consideration by requesting that a patient should sleep more than 10 % of the TST in the WSP before PT should be considered and by means of the expected decrease of the overall AHI. Since the overall AHI is directly related to the TST, the APOC gives a more thorough evaluation of the potential role of PT.

In clinical practice, patients meeting the following criteria can be diagnosed with POSA, according to the APOC criteria (see Fig. 1 flowchart):

1. Diagnosed with OSA according to the American Academy of Sleep Medicine (AASM) criteria [12]
2. <10 % of the TST in both BSP and WSP
3. Have a BSP AHI of less than 5
4. Have a BSP AHI in a lower OSA severity category
5. Have an overall AHI of at least 40 and at least a 25 % lower BSP AHI

In Table 1, we describe the best possible outcome per category of the APOC. The APOC criteria were found to be more effective in identifying patients, shown by an increase in sensitivity, specificty and predictive value, that will (not) benefit from PT, thus resulting in a more cost-efficient treatment.

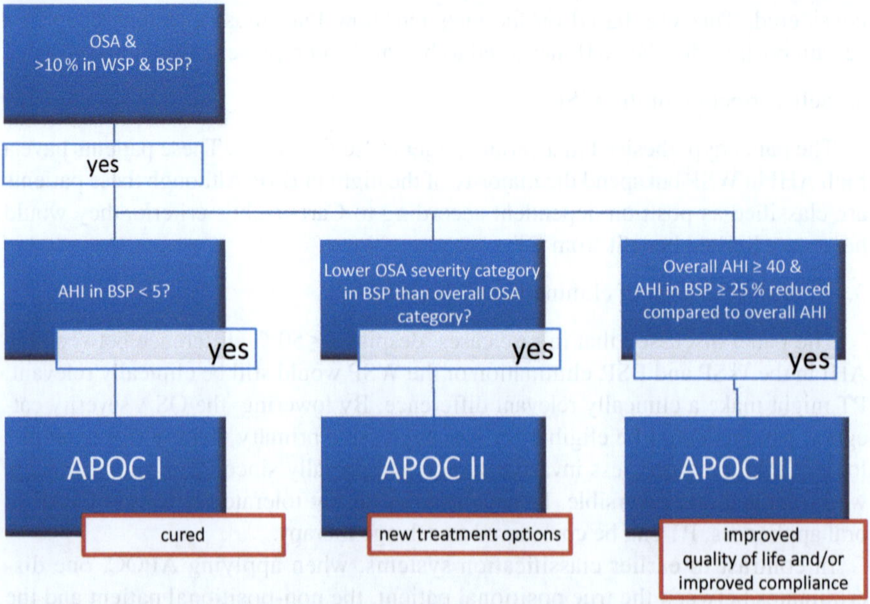

Fig. 1 Flowchart for the APOC. The *red boxes* show the best possible outcome for these patients with successful positional therapy (PT). *AHI apnea-hypopnea index, APOC Amsterdam positional OSA Classification, BSP best sleeping position, OSA obstructive sleep apnea, WSP worst sleeping position*

Table 1 Best possible outcome per category of the APOC

APOC I: Patients who theoretically can be cured with PT only (resulting in an AHI < 5)
• Patients are diagnosed APOC 1 if the BSP AHI < 5
APOC II: Patients who theoretically can decrease an OSA severity category through treatment with PT, rendering other treatment options available
• Patients are diagnosed APOC II if the AHI in the BSP falls into a lower OSA severity category than the overall AHI
APOC III:
• Patients with an overall AHI ≥ 40, who can theoretically achieve a >25 % reduction of their AHI with PT only, thereby improving compliance of existing therapies

AHI apnea-hypopnea index, *APOC* Amsterdam positional OSA Classification, *OSA* obstructive sleep apnea, *BSP* best sleeping position, *PT* positional therapy, *WSP* worst sleeping position

Considerations

It is important to stress that even though new-generation PT devices are not internationally available as yet, APOC was developed with new-generation PT devices in mind rather than conventional PT (TBT). New-generation PT can be defined as follows: a well-tolerated device which prevents a patient from adopting the supine position without negatively influencing sleep efficiency, as objectified by a full-night PSG. It is to be expected that PT will gain momentum in the scope of OSA treatment.

Future Perspectives

Submitted to a peer-reviewed journal, results are reported of a retrospective, single-centre, cohort study aiming to measure the prevalence of POSA according to APOC in a consecutive series of patients referred for polysomnography (PSG) and its association with certain patient characteristics. Approximately two-thirds of the patients were diagnosed with POSA according to APOC, the majority with APOC I. The most common WSP was the supine position. In confirmation to previous studies, statistical analysis suggests that POSA is inversely related to a higher AHI and BMI.

It is hoped that the shared use of this classification can facilitate collection of data across multiple centres and comparison of results across studies.

References

1. van Maanen JP, Meester KA, Dun LN et al. The sleep position trainer: a new treatment for positional obstructive sleep apnoea. Sleep Breath. 2013;17:771–9.
2. van Maanen JP, Richard W, Van Kesteren ER et al. Evaluation of a new simple treatment for positional sleep apnoea patients. J Sleep Res. 2012;21:322–9.
3. Bignold JJ, Mercer JD, Antic NA, McEvoy RD, Catcheside PG. Accurate position monitoring and improved supine-dependent obstructive sleep apnea with a new position recording and supine avoidance device. J Clin Sleep Med. 2011;7(4):376–83.
4. Cartwright RD. Effect of sleep position on sleep apnea severity. Sleep. 1984;7(2):110–4.
5. Oksenberg A, Khamaysi I, Silverberg DS, Tarasiuk A. Association of body position with severity of apneic events in patients with severe nonpositional obstructive sleep apnea. Chest. 2000;118(4):1018–24.
6. Cartwright RD, Diaz F, Lloyd S. The effects of sleep posture and sleep stage on apnea frequency. Sleep. 1991;14(4):351–3.
7. Marklund M, Persson M, Franklin KA. Treatment success with a mandibular advancement device is related to supine-dependent sleep apnea. Chest. 1998;114(6):1630–5.
8. Permut I, Diaz-Abad M, Chatila W, Crocetti J, Gaughan JP, D'Alonzo GE, Krachman SL. Comparison of positional therapy to CPAP in patients with positional obstructive sleep apnea. J Clin Sleep Med. 2010;6(3):238–43.
9. Mador MJ, Kufel TJ, Magalang UJ, Rajesh SK, Watwe V, Grant BJB. Prevalence of positional sleep apnea in patients undergoing polysomnography. Chest. 2005;128(4):2130–7.
10. Bignold JJ, Mercer JD, Antic NA, McEvoy RD, Catcheside PG. Accurate position monitoring and improved supine-dependent obstructive sleep apnea with a new position recording and supine avoidance device. J Clin Sleep Med. 2011;7(4):376–83.
11. Frank MH, Ravesloot MJL, van Maanen JP, Verhagen E, de Lange J, de Vries N. Positional OSA part 1: towards a clinical classification system for position-dependent obstructive sleep apnoea. Sleep Breath. 2014 [Epub ahead of print].
12. Iber C, Ancoli-Israel S, Chesson Jr AL, Quan SF, for the American Academy of Sleep Medicine. The AASM manual for the scoring of sleep and associated events: rules, terminology and technical specifications. 1st ed. Westchester, IL: American Academy of Sleep Medicine; 2007.

Correlation Between Calculated/Predicted and Actual AHI After Positional Therapy

Linda B.L. Benoist and Anneclaire V. Vroegop

Introduction

Prediction of treatment outcome is crucial for all OSA treatment modalities, as this may prevent unnecessary costs and "trial and error" treatment choices. This is an important item of the clinical reality involving OSA patients. With this in mind, the crucial question that still remains unanswered is: Can the effect of positional therapy be predicted from the (baseline) sleep study? What treatment outcome is to be expected in which patient? What is the predictive value of the baseline non-supine AHI? This item is subject to different theories and hypotheses and will be discussed in the following paragraphs.

Different types of sleep study recording systems are available. Some systems include sleeping position analysis; others do not. Most provide information on time spent per position and the AHI distribution per position. Some polysomnography (PSG) systems calculate the non-supine AHI. When the non-supine AHI is not available in the PSG report, this value can be calculated as follows:

$$\frac{\left(\mathrm{AHI}_{\mathrm{prone}} \times \mathrm{TST}_{\mathrm{prone}}\right) + \left(\mathrm{AHI}_{\mathrm{left}} \times \mathrm{TST}_{\mathrm{left}}\right) + \left(\mathrm{AHI}_{\mathrm{right}} \times \mathrm{TST}_{\mathrm{right}}\right)}{\mathrm{TST}_{\mathrm{prone}} + \mathrm{TST}_{\mathrm{left}} + \mathrm{TST}_{\mathrm{right}}}$$

L.B.L. Benoist, M.D. (✉)
Ear Nose and Throat, Sint Lucas Andreas Ziekenhuis,
Jan Tooropstraat 164, Amsterdam 1061 AE, The Netherlands
e-mail: l.benoist@slaz.nl

A.V. Vroegop, M.D., Ph.D.
ENT Department and Head and Neck Surgery, Antwerp University Hospital,
Edegem, Antwerp, Belgium

Saint Lucas Andreas Hospital, Amsterdam, The Netherlands

N. de Vries et al. (eds.), *Positional Therapy in Obstructive Sleep Apnea*,
DOI 10.1007/978-3-319-09626-1_12

Hypotheses on Treatment Prediction with Positional Therapy

1. Calculated Non-supine AHI
   According to the first hypothesis, the calculated baseline non-supine AHI is equal to the actual AHI with positional therapy. However, in literature this theory has proven to be incorrect [1, 2].
2. Averaging
   The second hypothesis is based on the theory that the remaining percentage of total sleep time in the other sleeping positions per position can be proportionally divided. Two different examples are given in Fig. 1.

   If a patient is treated with positional therapy, it can be expected that the % TST in supine is reduced to 0. Following this theory, the remaining percentages of sleeping positions with positional therapy can be proportionally divided according to the baseline distribution. However, this relies on the assumption that these percentages remain similar compared to the baseline study.
3. Fixed Correction
   The final theory is based on the assumption that with positional therapy, the percentage of supine sleeping position is not likely to be reduced to 0. This implies that one should take into account, for instance, a fixed percentage of the residual percentage of supine sleeping position with positional therapy and should correct for this in advance. In chapters "Results of a First-Generation New Device for Positional Therapy" and "Long-Term (6 Months) Effectiveness, Compliance, and Subjective Sleep Outcomes of Treatment with the Sleep Position Trainer in

Example 1

	Supine	Right	Left	Non-supine
AHI	40	5	20	11
% TST	50	30	20	50

Baseline PSG

	Supine	Right	Left	Non-supine
AHI	0	5	20	11
% TST	0	60	40	100

PSG with SPT

Example 2

	Supine	Right	Left	Non-supine
AHI	20	4	1	3
% TST	70	20	10	30

Baseline PSG

	Supine	Right	Left	Prone	Non-supine
AHI	0	4	1	2	3
% TST	0	60	30	10	100

PSG with SPT

Fig. 1 Examples of treatment prediction based on averaging

a Large Cohort of Position-Dependent OSA Patients", percentages of 3–5 % are mentioned. The baseline AHI in supine position must be thoroughly assessed, as a high supine AHI can have a large impact on the total AHI with positional therapy even though the residual percentage of supine sleeping position has been drastically reduced to less than 5 %.

Future research on the validity of these various theories is needed. Selection of reliable prediction of success of therapy per patient increases maximal individual treatment effectiveness.

References

1. van Maanen JP, Richard W, Van Kesteren ER, et al. Evaluation of a new simple treatment for positional sleep apnoea patients. J Sleep Res. 2012;21(3):322–9.
2. van Maanen JP, Meester K, Dun L, et al. The sleep position trainer: a new treatment for positional obstructive sleep apnoea. Sleep Breath. 2013;17(2):771–9.

Part V
Sleep Position in Specific Patient Groups

Influence of Sleep Position on Snoring

Linda B.L. Benoist, Sharon Morong, J. Peter van Maanen, Anthony A.J. Hilgevoord, and Nico de Vries

Introduction

Snoring is an acoustic phenomenon that affects approximately 20–40 % of the general population [1]. It is caused by vibration of tissue structures in the upper airway during sleep [2, 3]. Non-apneic snoring has been shown to be associated with clinical conditions such as depression and excessive daytime sleepiness in adults and may also have clinical implications in the development of hypertension, ischemic heart disease, and cerebrovascular diseases [1, 4]. In this chapter, the prevalence of position dependency in non-apneic snorers and the influence of various factors such as BMI, neck circumference, age, gender, and sleep efficiency on sleeping position will be discussed.

This chapter is a modified version of the article "Evaluation of position dependency in non-apneic snorers" 2014. The final publication is available at link.springer.com.

L.B.L. Benoist, M.D. (✉)
Ear Nose and Throat, Sint Lucas Andreas Ziekenhuis,
Jan Tooropstraat 164, Amsterdam 1061 AE, The Netherlands
e-mail: l.benoist@slaz.nl

S. Morong, M.D., M.Sc., F.R.C.S.C.
Department of Otolaryngology, Sint Lucas Andreas Ziekenhuis, Amsterdam, The Netherlands

J.P. van Maanen, M.D.
Department of Otolaryngology, Sint Lucas Andreas Ziekenhuis, Amsterdam, The Netherlands

A.A.J. Hilgevoord, M.D., Ph.D.
Department of Neurology and Clinical Neurophysiology, St. Lucas Andreas Hospital, Amsterdam, The Netherlands

N. de Vries, M.D., Ph.D.
Department of Otolaryngology, Sint Lucas Andreas Ziekenhuis, Amsterdam, The Netherlands

Department of Otolaryngology, University Hospital Antwerp, Antwerp, Belgium

N. de Vries et al. (eds.), *Positional Therapy in Obstructive Sleep Apnea*,
DOI 10.1007/978-3-319-09626-1_13

Snoring and Position Dependency

Snoring is known to be the most frequently reported symptom in obstructive sleep apnea (OSA), and non-apneic snoring is thought to be a precursor to the development of OSA [5]. Fiz et al. described a 3.2 times higher risk of developing OSA in patients with complaints of non-apneic snoring when compared with non-snorers [6].

Non-apneic snoring has also been shown to have negative impacts on the individual's bed partners, family members, and their general quality of life [7]. Armstrong et al. [8] found a statistically significant improvement in marital relations after snoring was treated. In children, there is increasing evidence that neurocognitive impairments are much more frequent in children with non-apneic snoring when compared with non-snorers [9].

Many studies have looked at position dependency in patients with OSA and potential therapeutic options for this population [2, 5, 10–16]. One study reported that the effect of sleep position in patients with OSA is inversely related to the severity of the disease; in other words, the lower a patient's apnea-hypopnea index (AHI), the more often they were found to be position dependent [13]. Very few studies, however, have addressed these issues in non-apneic snorers. The AASM guidelines are used to accurately define non-apneic snorers (AHI<5).

Methods

Patients

A cohort of consecutive patients was screened for complaints of excessive snoring or symptoms suspicious for sleep-disordered breathing. Overnight polysomnographic data were collected, and non-apneic snorers who met all the inclusion criteria were selected for statistical analysis. Hypnograms were screened from subjects aged 18 years or older in whom a polysomnography was performed for suspicion of OSA or excessive snoring. Subjects with an apnea-hypopnea index (AHI) <5 and total sleep time >3 h and subjects who slept in supine position between 10 and 90 % of the total sleep time (TST) were selected [17].

Polysomnography

Polysomnography (PSG) was performed during an overnight visit in the hospital. Recordings were performed using a digital PSG (Embla A10, Broomfield, CO, USA). A position sensor (Sleepsense, St Charles, IL, USA) attached to the midline of the abdominal wall was used to differentiate between supine, prone, right lateral, left lateral, and upright positions. The system allowed continuous monitoring and analysis of snoring throughout the night. Snoring sounds with a minimum duration of 300–3,000 ms were automatically detected based on both the signal of the nasal cannula and a piezoelement sensor taped to the skin over the cricoid. The amplitudes of the snoring signals were known to be very variable.

Definitions

The term non-apneic snorers will be used in this chapter to define snorers without any apneic events. The total snoring index is defined as the number of snore events in any body position (prone, supine, left, right, and upright) per hour of sleep. Non-apneic snorers were defined as patients with a snoring index >1 and an AHI<5 [4].

The supine snoring index is the number of snore events per hour of sleep while lying in supine position. Supine-dependent snoring patients are patients whose supine snoring index is higher than their total non-supine snoring index. (These patients may not necessarily have slept the majority of the night in a supine position.)

Results

76 patients were eligible for statistical analysis. Prevalence of position dependency in non-apneic snorers was 65.8 % ($p<0.008$). A stepwise regression showed that only BMI had a significant effect ($p<0.003$) on the supine snore index.

Patient demographic data and PSG results are presented in Table 1. Of the patients, 51 % were male and 49 % were female. Mean age was 43 ± 13 (range 22–91), and mean BMI was 27.2 ± 5.3 (range 18.6–43.9). Mean supine snore index was 485.51 ± 269.9, and a mean non-supine snore index of 432.1 ± 275.8 was shown. Supine-dependent patients comprised 65.8 % of our sample group with a statistical significance of 0.008 using the Wilcoxon signed-rank test. Table 2 shows no statistical demographic differences between patients who are supine dependent and those who are not. A logistic regression also confirms this. The influence of factors such

Table 1 Patient demographics and polysomnographic results

Characteristics	Mean ± SD
Age	43.0 ± 13.04
BMI	27.18 ± 5.26
Neck circumference (cm)	37.64 ± 3.05
AHI	2.13 ± 1.44
Sleep efficiency (%)	87.90 ± 10.01
Total sleep time (min)	440.29 ± 3.79

SD standard deviation, *BMI* body mass index, *AHI* apnea-hypopnea index

Table 2 Comparison of demographics between supine-dependent and non-supine-dependent patients

Characteristics	SDS ($n=50$, 65.8 %) Mean ± SD	NSDS ($n=26$, 34.2 %) Mean ± SD	Mann–Whitney (p-value)
Age	44.26 ± 13.66	40.58 ± 11.64	0.208
BMI	27.26 ± 5.71	27.03 ± 4.36	0.844
Neck circumference (cm)	37.41 ± 3.14	38.08 ± 2.87	0.334
Sleep efficiency (%)	87.43 ± 10.92	88.82 ± 8.27	0.917

SD standard deviation, *SDS* supine dependent snorers, *NSDS* non-supine-dependent snorers

as BMI, age, gender, neck circumference, and sleep efficiency on the supine snore index was addressed using a stepwise regression analysis. This analysis demonstrated that only BMI had a significant effect on the supine snore index ($p<0.003$).

Discussion

Prior studies have addressed the issue of position dependence when looking at patients with OSA. It has been well proven that many patients suffering from OSA have a different rate of apneic events in the lateral position, when compared with the supine position [11]. Position-dependent OSA (POSA) is defined as an AHI which is at least twice as high in supine sleeping position compared to the AHI during sleep in other positions [10, 14–16]. Although the criteria for POSA where AHI is used as a parameter are not comparable with supine-dependent snoring, the results from Mador et al.'s study suggest that the proportion of patients with non-apneic snoring (AHI < 5), who are position dependent, may be even higher than 50 % [13].

The aim of this study was to address the issue of position dependence in patients who have non-apneic snoring, given the prevalence of this condition in the general population; the impact of snoring on an individual's neurocognitive, physical, and psychosocial well-being [7, 9]; and the significant potential for therapeutic intervention.

Position Dependency

From our study, 65.8 % of our non-apneic snorers were supine dependent. Other studies have tried to look at position dependence and snoring in apneic and non-apneic snorers with differing results. Braver et al. [2] found that in a combined group of 20 male apneic and non-apneic snorers, snoring was not influenced by changes in sleep position. Nakano et al. [5] reported that while position dependence was seen in patients with non-apneic snoring, variable results were seen in apneic snorers. A more recent study by Koutsourelakis et al. [1], however, found that position dependence was noted in both apneic and non-apneic snorers. The possible reasons for these variable results are a lack of a standardized definition for position-dependent snoring, which will be further discussed in our limitations, and differences in study design and definitions of apnea. In Braver et al.'s study, no attempt was made to separate non-apneic from apneic snorers before assessing position dependence. The latter two studies did attempt to separate apneic snorers from non-apneic snorers, but, based on the AASM guidelines [4], the AHI criteria used in these studies to define the non-apneic group actually included patients with mild OSA [1, 5]. Our study objectively measured the influence of position dependence on non-apneic snorers, adhering to the AASM guidelines for sleep apnea.

We also found that the higher a patients' BMI, the more likely they were to be position-dependent snorers. This result, however, is within a sample group of non-apneic patients. Other studies looking at the association of BMI with position in apneic patients found that POSA seemed to correlate with a slightly reduced BMI [4, 15, 18]. In these studies, however, an increased BMI also correlated with an increased AHI or AI. These findings, therefore, corroborate Mador et al.'s [13] findings that patients with less OSA were more likely to be position dependent.

Measurement of Snoring

There were a few limitations to our study. One such limitation is the lack of a quantitative definition for position-dependent snoring. This, however, is seen in the majority of the literature looking at position dependence in non-apneic patients. One study defined position-dependent snoring as a >50 % reduction in snoring rate in the lateral position when compared with the supine position [19]. There are, however, no standardized guidelines defining criteria for position-dependent snoring. As such, comparisons made between position-dependent non-apneic and apneic snorers should take this into consideration. Various parameters have been used to measure snoring in the literature. Such methods include snore intensity (decibels), snoring frequency (snores/h), snoring rate (% TST), or duration (seconds or milliseconds) [20]. Our parameter of choice for the measurement of snoring, the snore index, does not give information regarding the loudness or duration of snoring. While the snore index may not be as comprehensive a research tool when compared with other snoring parameters, it confers the advantage of clinical applicability, as it can be easily obtained from sleep polysomnograms and has also been used in other studies [2]. Also, risk factors such as alcohol consumption, ingestion of tranquilizers/sedatives, and smoking, which can influence snoring habits, sleeping quality, and body position during sleep, were not included in this study. Lastly, the only position individually analyzed for position dependence was the supine position. We have especially chosen for this sleeping position, because in the criteria for POSA, sleeping mostly in supine position is also used to define position dependence.

Positional Therapy

The results of our study potentially have significant implications for the role of positional therapy in non-apneic snorers. As discussed in other chapters of this volume, the effectiveness of positional therapy in patients with POSA has been tested since the 1980s [14–16, 21–23] and compared with other therapeutic approaches [24–27]. Several attempts to decrease the severity of OSA by influencing supine sleep position have been reported and show that positional therapy can reduce AHI to normal values in patients with POSA [15, 16, 21–24]. The tennis ball technique (TBT) was the first technique to be implemented, but several other methods have also been used as positional therapy in POSA [28]. While all these techniques may have been successful at reducing the AHI, its limiting factor was a lack of compliance secondary to discomfort and the occurrence of arousals while turning from one lateral position to the other, thereby disturbing the patient's sleep quality and sleep architecture [17]. Long-term (6 months) compliance has been reported to be only 10 % [29].

In chapters "Short-Term (4 Weeks) Results of the Sleep Position Trainer for Positional Therapy", "Long-Term (6 Months) Effectiveness, Compliance, and Subjective Sleep Outcomes of Treatment with the Sleep Position Trainer in a Large Cohort of Position-Dependent OSA Patients", and "10 Problems and Solutions for Positional Therapy: Technical Aspects of the Sleep Position Trainer", a new product for positional therapy will be discussed, the sleep position trainer (SPT) [30]. The SPT is a sensor that measures the sleeping position and gives the user feedback with a soft vibration when adopting a supine sleeping posture. The sleep position trainer has been able to overcome the major limitations of positional therapy, with its high compliance rates and lack of change in sleep efficiency. Since we have discovered that the majority of non-apneic snorers are supine dependent, such a device has great potential for the implementation in future therapy.

Conclusion

In this chapter, the AASM guidelines are used to accurately define non-apneic snorers ($AHI<5$) and provide scientific evidence that the majority of non-apneic snorers are supine dependent. Furthermore, our results show that patients within this population who had a higher BMI snored more frequently in the supine position. Given the prevalence of snoring in the general population and its impact on an individual's neurocognitive, physical, and psychosocial well-being, there is a tremendous potential for the use of positional therapy. Future studies will look at the efficacy of this device in snorers.

References

1. Koutsourelakis I, Perraki E, Zakynthinos G, Minaritzoglou A, Vagiakis E, Zakynthinos S. Clinical and polysomnographic determinants of snoring. J Sleep Res. 2012;21(6):693–9.
2. Braver HM, Block AJ, Perri MG. Treatment for snoring. Combined weight loss, sleeping on side, and nasal spray. Chest. 1995;107(5):1283–8.
3. Wilson K, Stoohs RA, Mulrooney TF, Johnson LJ, Guilleminault C, Huang Z. The snoring spectrum: acoustic assessment of snoring sound intensity in 1,139 individuals undergoing polysomnography. Chest. 1999;115(3):762–70.
4. American Academy of Sleep Medicine. International classification of sleep disorders: diagnostic and coding manual. 2nd ed. Westchester, NY: American Academy of Sleep Medicine; 2005.
5. Nakano H, Ikeda T, Hayashi M, Ohshima E, Onizuka A. Effects of body position on snoring in apneic and nonapneic snorers. Sleep. 2003;26(2):169–72.
6. Fiz JA, Jane R, Sola-Soler J, Abad J, Garcia MA, Morera J. Continuous analysis and monitoring of snores and their relationship to the apnea-hypopnea index. Laryngoscope. 2010;120(4):854–62.
7. Beninati W, Harris CD, Herold DL, Shepard Jr JW. The effect of snoring and obstructive sleep apnea on the sleep quality of bed partners. Mayo Clin Proc. 1999;74(10):955–8.
8. Armstrong MW, Wallace CL, Marais J. The effect of surgery upon the quality of life in snoring patients and their partners: a between-subjects case-controlled trial. Clin Otolaryngol Allied Sci. 1999;24(6):510–22.
9. Brockmann PE, Urschitz MS, Schlaud M, Poets CF. Primary snoring in school children: prevalence and neurocognitive impairments. Sleep Breath. 2012;16(1):23–9.
10. Cartwright RD, Diaz F, Lloyd S. The effects of sleep posture and sleep stage on apnea frequency. Sleep. 1991;14(4):351–3.
11. Cartwright RD. Effect of sleep position on sleep apnea severity. Sleep. 1984;7(2):110–4.
12. Hoffstein V. Snoring. Chest. 1996;109(1):201–22.
13. Mador MJ, Kufel TJ, Magalang UJ, Rajesh SK, Watwe V, Grant BJ. Prevalence of positional sleep apnea in patients undergoing polysomnography. Chest. 2005;128(4):2130–7.
14. Oksenberg A, Silverberg DS. The effect of body posture on sleep-related breathing disorders: facts and therapeutic implications. Sleep Med Rev. 1998;2(3):139–62.
15. Oksenberg A, Silverberg DS, Arons E, Radwan H. Positional vs nonpositional obstructive sleep apnea patients: anthropomorphic, nocturnal polysomnographic, and multiple sleep latency test data. Chest. 1997;112(3):629–39.
16. Richard W, Kox D, den Herder C, Laman M, van Tinteren H, de Vries N. The role of sleep position in obstructive sleep apnea syndrome. Eur Arch Otorhinolaryngol. 2006;263(10):946–50.
17. van Maanen JP, Richard W, Van Kesteren ER, et al. Evaluation of a new simple treatment for positional sleep apnoea patients. J Sleep Res. 2012;21(3):322–9.
18. Itasaka Y, Miyazaki S, Ishikawa K, Togawa K. The influence of sleep position and obesity on sleep apnea. Psychiatry Clin Neurosci. 2000;54(3):340–1.
19. Choi JH, Park YW, Hong JH, et al. Efficacy study of a vest-type device for positional therapy in position dependent snorers. Sleep Biol Rhythms. 2009;7:181–7.
20. Ravesloot MJL, van Maanen JP, Dun L, de Vries N. The undervalued potential of positional therapy in position-dependent snoring and obstructive sleep apnea-a review of the literature. Sleep Breath. 2013;17(1):39–49.
21. Cartwright RD, Lloyd S, Lilie J, Kravitz H. Sleep position training as treatment for sleep apnea syndrome: a preliminary study. Sleep. 1985;8(2):87–94.
22. Maurer JT, Stuck BA, Hein G, Verse T, Hörmann K. Treatment of obstructive sleep apnea with a new vest preventing the supine position. Dtsch Med Wochenschr. 2003;128(3):71–5.
23. Wenzel S, Smith E, Leiacker R, Fischer Y. Efficacy and longterm compliance of the vest preventing the supine position in patients with obstructive sleep apnea. Laryngorhinootologie. 2007;86(8):579–83.

24. Cartwright R, Ristanovic R, Diaz F, Caldarelli D, Alder G. A comparative study of treatments for positional sleep apnea. Sleep. 1991;14(6):546–52.
25. Jokic R, Klimaszewski A, Crossley M, Sridhar G, Fitzpatrick MF. Positional treatment vs continuous positive airway pressure in patients with positional obstructive sleep apnea syndrome. Chest. 1999;115(3):771–81.
26. Permut I, az-Abad M, Chatila W, et al. Comparison of positional therapy to CPAP in patients with positional obstructive sleep apnea. J Clin Sleep Med. 2010;6(3):238–43.
27. Skinner MA, Kingshott RN, Filsell S, Taylor DR. Efficacy of the 'tennis ball technique' versus nCPAP in the management of position-dependent obstructive sleep apnoea syndrome. Respirology. 2008;13(5):708–15.
28. Oksenberg A, Silverberg D, Offenbach D, Arons E. Positional therapy for obstructive sleep apnea patients: a 6-month follow-up study. Laryngoscope. 2006;116(11):1995–2000.
29. Bignold JJ, ans-Costi G, Goldsworthy MR, et al. Poor long-term patient compliance with the tennis ball technique for treating positional obstructive sleep apnea. J Clin Sleep Med. 2009;5(5):428–30.
30. van Maanen JP, Meester K, Dun L, et al. The sleep position trainer: a new treatment for positional obstructive sleep apnoea. Sleep Breath. 2013;17(2):771–9.

The Effect of Body Position on Sleep Apnea in Children

Amal Isaiah and Kevin D. Pereira

Abbreviations

OSA	Obstructive sleep apnea
PSG	Polysomnogram, polysomnography
CPAP	Continuous positive airway pressure
AT	Adenotonsillectomy
MRI	Magnetic resonance imaging
SDB	Sleep-disordered breathing
CFD	Computational fluid dynamics
AHI	Apnea-hypopnea index
RDI	Respiratory disturbance index

Introduction

In recent years, the increasing trend of childhood obstructive sleep apnea syndrome (OSA) has generally followed the increasing prevalence of obesity in that age group. Accordingly, between 1980 and 2000, the prevalence of obesity has doubled in the age group 6–11 and tripled among children 12–17 years of age [1, 2], ultimately emerging as a leading cause for morbidity associated with OSA [3, 4], and thus sowing the seeds for ill health and loss of economic productivity later in adulthood [5].

A. Isaiah, M.D., D.Phil.
Department of Otorhinolaryngology-HNS, University of Maryland, Baltimore, MD, USA

K.D. Pereira, M.D., M.S. (✉)
University of Maryland School of Medicine,
16 S Eutaw St Ste 500, Baltimore, MD 21201, USA
e-mail: kevindpereira@gmail.com

N. de Vries et al. (eds.), *Positional Therapy in Obstructive Sleep Apnea*,
DOI 10.1007/978-3-319-09626-1_14

Adenotonsillectomy has generally been accepted as standard of care for remediation of PSG-proven OSA, in line with observed findings related to mechanical obstruction caused by extra-luminal soft tissues on the pediatric airway [6–8]. However, despite this, adenotonsillectomy fails to completely address OSA-related symptoms in certain children [9, 10] in whom altered tone [11, 12] and adiposity [13] play a significant role. Besides these factors, body position appears to modulate airflow significantly and is dependent on the stage of sleep [14]. Thus far, there is data to show both in adults and children that the chief metric of severity of OSA, the apnea-hypopnea index (AHI), is worse in the supine position. Both OSA severity and physiologic indicators of airflow, such as critical closing pressure and the optimum level of CPAP required seem to increase during the supine position during sleep [15].

Despite the observed relationship between fixed anatomic factors such as size of pharyngeal soft tissues and the degree of sleep apnea, dynamic control of airway lumen during sleep—particularly *dependence* of oropharyngeal and nasopharyngeal soft tissues due to the effect of gravity in the supine position—may be difficult to quantify, and thus the purpose of this chapter is to lay a foundation for understanding the modulation of the *physiologic* airway by position of the body.

Pathophysiology of Upper Airway Obstruction

The upper aerodigestive tract in humans maintains similarity to other mammals at birth. However, at about 18 months postnatally, there is a gradual drive towards compartmentalization of function for the pharyngeal and laryngeal musculatures [16, 17]. During sleep, pharyngeal dilators that oppose narrowing of the oropharyngeal airway during wakefulness have decreased tonic activity. In normal individuals, this decrease does not reach the critical closing pressure resulting in maintenance of patency at all times. However, in individuals with OSA, the tonic activation of pharyngeal dilators is enhanced during the awake condition compared to those without OSA. During sleep, the lack of this tonic activation leads to marked reduction in airway patency. Both neurologic and anatomic factors modulate this sleep-related reduction in airway patency. The *neural* hypothesis suggests that in the presence of OSA, there is a tendency towards general reduction of pharyngeal tone, especially within the genioglossus [18]. Alternatively, the anatomic hypothesis favors normal sleep-related reduction of tone within the upper airway that potentiates lack of stability within the pharyngeal musculature [19]. Thus the decreased tonic activation of pharyngeal dilators poses an anatomically unfavorable circumstance eventually enhancing dependent collapsibility in children with OSA.

Subsequent to formation of discrete channels within the upper aerodigestive tract, anomalous anatomic factors related to development can contribute to OSA in infants. It is to be noted that in very young infants, physiologic factors such as central nervous system immaturity can contribute significantly to the pathogenesis of OSA. Craniofacial syndromes, such as Crouzon's and Apert's, and mandibulofacial dysostoses, such as Treacher Collins and Pierre Robin sequence, have distinct roles in changing the upper airway collapsibility either anatomically or by altering the neuromuscular tone [20, 21]. In this age group, full-term neonates who are obligate nasal breathers are susceptible to limitation of airflow following nasal obstruction due to anatomical anomalies or in the presence of an upper respiratory tract infection.

Thus far, the role of adenotonsillar hypertrophy in the pathogenesis of OSA in children has been validated by consensus statements from the American Academy of Pediatrics who recommends adenotonsillectomy as the gold standard initial treatment [22, 23]. Indeed, many authors have reported improvement in nasal airflow subsequent to adenotonsillectomy, resulting in both resolution of symptoms and improvement in quality of life in these children [24]. These changes are directly contingent upon the extent of volumetric reduction of naso- and oropharyngeal soft tissues, and is equivalent to a decompression of static obstructive pathology, as confirmed by polysomnographic and MRI-derived information [25].

Given this information, the success of adenotonsillectomy in remediation of symptoms in obese children with OSA is suboptimal. For example, while the success rate is in excess of 80 % in non-obese children with OSA, it drops to less than 40 % in overweight and obese children, with the accepted norm that adenotonsillectomy improves, yet does not resolve, OSA-related symptoms in the second group [26].

Immaturity correlates significantly with the severity of OSA, with spontaneous neck flexion, glottic closure, and a highly compliant chest wall contributing to events associated with cessation of airflow in more than half of infants presenting with apneic events [27] that are very responsive to CPAP-based treatment. These events are known to occur with increased association and frequency with sleep and are most pronounced in deep stages.

While both adenotonsillar hypertrophy and extraluminal adiposity represent static factors that change the size and shape of airway lumen, dependence and position aggravate sleep-disordered breathing in a dynamic fashion. A schematic of the relative contributions of these factors are shown in Fig. 1. Based on the structural model suggested by Isono and colleagues [15], less force is required in an anteroposterior dimension to compress the airway in the supine position compared with that in a lateral position, thus increasing the tendency towards collapse.

Various authors have highlighted fluid dynamics that are passively altered in association with increased upper airway collapsibility in children with OSA. Some understanding of fluid-volume physics of the upper airway is of potential importance to determine the poor response seen in some children with OSAS to adenotonsillectomy.

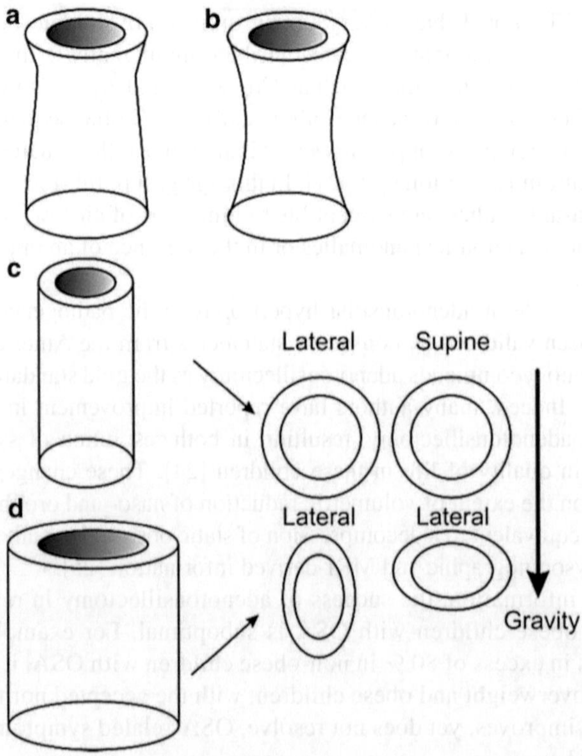

Fig. 1 Influences of dynamic and static forces on the airway (cylinder). (**a**) and (**b**) show, respectively, the focally obstructed airway in adenotonsillar *vs.* an airway that is attenuated along its entire length. Shape of the airway also constitutes a risk—specifically, a more *elliptical* or *eccentric shape*. Similarly, a larger cross-sectional area in a representative airway as shown in (**d**) is more prone to collapse when compared to (**c**). Differences in the tendency to collapse are illustrated to the right

Biomechanics of Upper Airway Obstruction

History of Fluid Models

Historically, fluid models have found use in the analysis of nasal airway obstruction and for preoperative planning prior to functional septorhinoplasty in adults. In addition, inspiratory peak flow limitation has been found to correlate very well with functional limitations in allergic rhinitis. A significant, negative, nonlinear relationship was also found between minimum cross-sectional area and intranasal resistance. Furthermore, acoustic rhinometry demonstrated that small intrusions into the lumen of the nose that might be missed by rhinoscopy produce an exponentially greater increase in nasal resistance measurements by rhinomanometry [28].

Computational fluid dynamics is a branch of fluid physics that uses computer-based mathematical algorithms to model and determine the parameters affecting

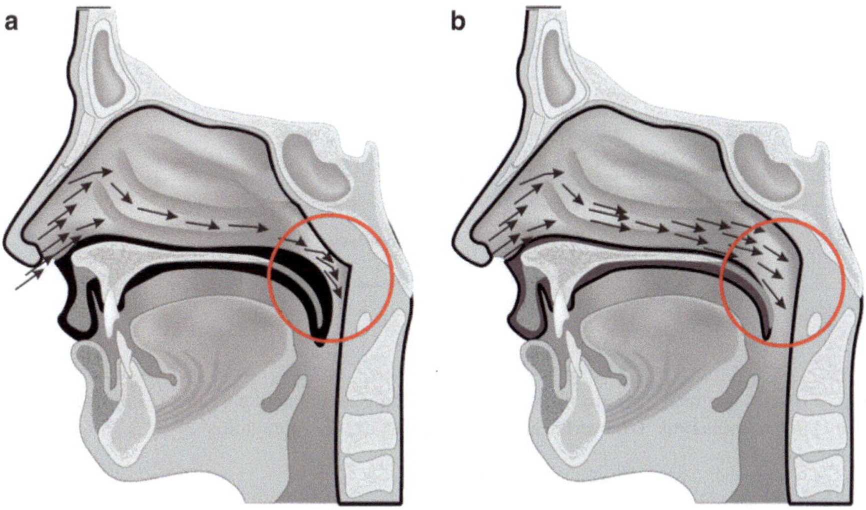

Fig. 2 Upper airway models of an OSA airway (**a**) and a normal control (**b**) signifying the overlap area (*red*) with the palatine tonsils below and lateral to the oropharynx and nasopharynx overlap the adenoids superior and posterior to the nasopharynx. In this location, there is a significant drop in cross-sectional area. This leads to both increases in turbulence and reduction of airflow. For data from reconstructed MR images, see Xu et al. [31]

fluid flow. With advances in computational power and distributed processing, airflow characteristics in a geometrically altered airway can be delegated to the individual subunits of a central processing unit (CPU) of a computer.

Historically, the upper airway and its associated flow resistance has been modeled either as an elliptical orifice with local airway obstruction in a 2-D model of pharyngeal airflow [29] or that of a 3-D conduit to study the effects of area variation and turbulence [30] as a function of pressure exerted by extraluminal soft tissues. Indeed, as discussed in the following sections, effects of dependence (gravity) on luminal collapsibility are shown by computational models of the upper airway and confirmed by clinical and PSG-derived data from pediatric populations.

Techniques for Modeling the Obstructed Airway

Modeling the obstructed airway encompasses several parameters that may be incorporated into two broad types (Fig. 2). In most models [31, 32], various fluid dynamic parameters such as pressure drops, velocity distribution, wall shear stress, and distribution of wall force induced by pressure at various locations within the airway are calculated with various inspiratory flow rates. However, in these models, deformability of the airway wall—either induced by gravity or by extra luminal soft tissues—is not taken into account, and thus, the rendition of data from this

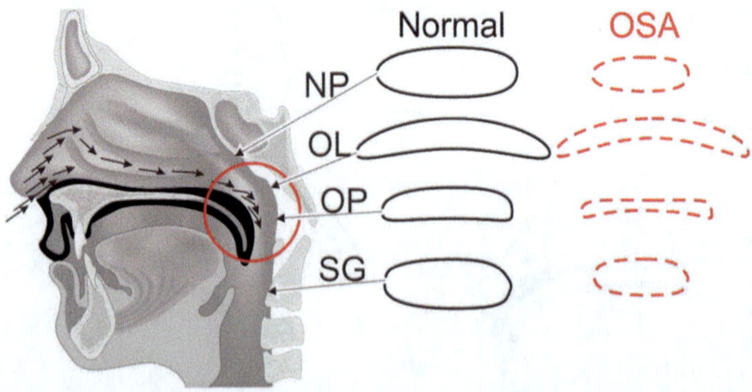

Fig. 3 Cross-sectional anatomy from normal breathing and apneic episodes (*solid* and *broken loops*). *NP* nasopharynx, *OL* overlap area, *OP* oropharynx, *SG* supraglottis

technique suffers from oversimplification. In the second type of approach that is also computationally intensive, a finite element model (FEM)[1] may be established with contribution from luminal variability as a function of deformability and material stress providing more realistic anatomical models. In either of these types of models, both CT- or MRI-based volumetric data may be acquired for computational reconstructions.

The central theme of simulations of fluid dynamics of the airway is the Navier-Stokes (NS) equation, with or without Reynolds averaging, among others, such as the Spalart-Allmaras model. A detailed description of all the mathematical models is beyond the scope of this section. Briefly, NS equations are useful for describing behavior of fluids and have found applications to model weather, ocean currents, and vascular flow patterns. One of the fundamental characteristics of biological flow patterns is that of *turbulence*, which is the time-dependent chaotic behavior seen in fluid flow. This is relevant to flow within the upper airway in children with OSA, which is characteristically turbulent, with worsening seen in focally narrowed sections such as the nasal valve area and the retropalatal and retroglossal segments.

Xu et al. [31] studied computational fluid models of the upper airway using MRI-derived volumetric information and showed luminal restriction as shown within an overlap area in Fig. 3. This illustrates the airflow patterns as derived from the data shown by the same authors, re-rendered two dimensionally. The highlighted area points to the site of maximum obstruction and is enhanced during sleep. The overlap area is normally located between the adenoids posterosuperiorly within the nasopharynx and palatine tonsils inferolaterally within the oropharynx in patients with OSA. Importantly, a turbulent jet is expected downstream of the site of obstruction [33]. The authors concluded that in children, area restriction in the pharynx may be

[1] FEM involves replacement of continuous geometry with a set of objects with a fixed number of simple components. Elements connected at nodal points that may be common to two or more adjacent elements. A set of elements is referred to as *mesh*.

as important as nasal resistance in driving airway collapse in OSA. Thus, respiratory system models that include apnea mechanics may benefit from including pharyngeal restriction along with airway collapse properties. These CFD models may also be used as a benchmark for building simplified models of pressure drop in the pharynx to analyze larger numbers of subjects or for incorporation into dynamic system models.

Impact of Dependence on Airway Collapsibility: Theoretic Models

As described in the previous section, the upper airway is susceptible to collapse from extraluminal pressure exerted within the retroglossal and retropalatal areas with considerable reduction of luminal diameter at the overlap area. Huang et al. [34] recently completed a FEM modeling study to understand the circumferential deformability of the airway using material properties such as Young's modulus and Poisson ratio. In this study, the lumen is characteristically an ellipse that has variable material properties anteroposteriorly and laterally (Fig. 4). The pharynx in a patient with OSA is analogous to a collapsible conduit when the pharyngeal constrictors are completely relaxed. The degree of structural collapse during sleep is inversely proportional to the diameter of the awake airway due to increase in kinetic energy of fluid flow through these segments.

When deformability across the longitudinal plane is considered, the material properties including compliance and stiffness of the airway are opposed by extraluminal, compressive force exerted by gravity. In this scenario, it is critical to understand that the airway patency is maintained as a balance between intrinsic mechanical properties of the pharynx and the neural control of pharyngeal dilators.

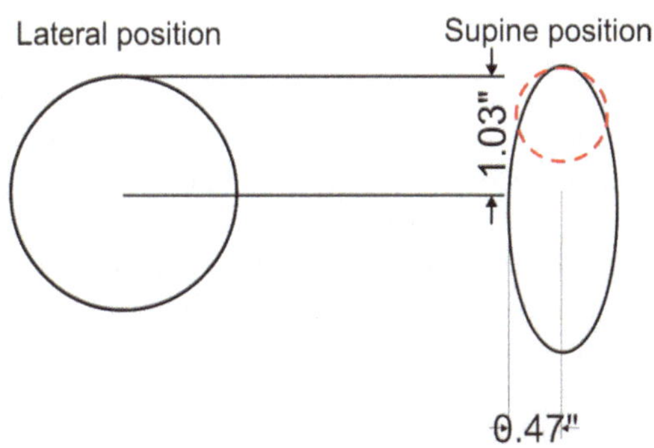

Fig. 4 Influence of dependence on change in shape and structural collapsibility of the pharyngeal airway. Here, lateral position causes the airway to be more *circular* in shape with a larger pressure gradient required to collapse compared to the supine position. In the latter, the radius of curvature (*red*) is 50 % that of a circular airway inducing a collapse in the longitudinal axis

It may thus be postulated that the improvement of pharyngeal luminal diameter due to the lateral position may be due to structural change or increase in dilator tone. Using optical coherence tomography, the physical changes in shape and orientation have been studied before [35]. In this study, the authors report that the airway changes from a transversely oriented elliptical shape when supine to a more circular shape when in the lateral recumbent posture. Laplace's law states that at equilibrium, the pressure gradient across a concave surface is directly proportional to the wall tension and inversely proportional to its radius of curvature. It follows that the pressure gradient required to compress the airway varies inversely as a function of its radius of curvature. Hence, as the transverse elliptical airway changes to a more circular shape with change to the lateral posture, its propensity to collapse decreases as a function of the reduction in radius of curvature of its anterior and posterior walls. In proportions, this can be expressed as ratio of the lengths of the major and minor axes of the elliptical cross section.

Clinical Correlates of Theoretic models

For several years, it has been known that sleeping in prone position can increase the amount of time spent sleeping, particularly the duration of quiet sleep [36]. In addition, it has also been known that prone sleeping is associated with reduced responsiveness to arousal stimuli [37]. Using the theoretic and modeling-derived data described in the previous section, we review the correlation of sleep position with clinically derived data, specifically in children, OSA parameters.

Pereira et al. [38] examined the variability of respiratory disturbance index (RDI) in children less than 3 years of age with sleep position from PSG data. The authors found that RDI positively correlated with the amount of time spent in the supine position, thus raising questions about PSGs that underestimate the severity of OSA by not sampling the postural variability of sleep apnea. This data is in agreement with theoretic models that show enhanced collapsibility in the supine position caused by dependent forces that act on the extraluminal soft tissues.

In another study from the same institution and authors, infants aged 8–12 months [39] referred for suspicion of sleep-disordered breathing were retrospectively reviewed. AHI variation was determined as a function of body position. This study attempted to characterize the relationship between the hypoxic episodes associated with OSA and the age at which infants begin to change body position. This study showed that there was no significant effect of body position on sleep-disordered breathing, although REM sleep represented a significant risk factor for OSA. This result assumes significance as sudden infant death syndrome (SIDS) is currently the most common cause of postnatal death in the United States and has known association with OSA [40].

Isono and colleagues [15] determined atonic properties of the human pharynx by inducing a deep plane of anesthesia and examining the effectiveness of lateral position in improving structural properties of each pharyngeal segment, consequently eliminating neuromuscular factors. Although the study was in adults, their results showed a convincing reduction in pharyngeal closing pressures in the lateral position. However, this is not in agreement with findings from patients with artificially occluded nasal airways where there is a small yet nonsignificant reduction in pharyngeal closing pressures.

Effect of Body Position on OSA: Role of Current Therapies

In summary, a number of studies have evaluated the effect of body position during sleep on OSA and have not effectively agreed on a consensus. While one study showed an increase in AHI in the supine position [38], another showed the opposite [41]. Some of these differences may be related to study design. This is a fundamental difference when compared with adults in prone position that improves OSA by reduction of tongue prolapse. Given the multitude of results, no recommendations can be made for maintaining a particular position of sleep other than to avoid the supine position which results in the maximum amount of airway obstruction. There is need for more data in this regard to establish firmer guidelines.

The gold standard for treatment of OSAS in children continues to be adenotonsillectomy. There is overwhelming evidence to support adenotonsillectomy in remediation of OSA symptoms showing uniform improvement in PSG criteria in majority of the children undergoing the procedure. Obesity appears to limit the usefulness of this procedure. A meta-analysis of adenotonsillectomy in obese children showed that 88 % of obese patients still had a postoperative AHI ≥ 1 per hour [26]. It is thus of critical importance to stress on weight management in these children including referrals as indicated.

Intranasal corticosteroids are useful for initial trial in children with mild OSA. They cause a dose-dependent reduction of proliferation of nasopharyngeal soft tissue, and this is supported by both level I clinical and histopathologic evidence shown in tonsils harvested from children with OSA [42]. In children with orthodontic abnormalities that are directly related to OSA, use of dental appliances is controversial. Thus far, the data is very limited with one study showing a reduction of snoring and restless sleep in the background of a small sample size and non-blinded study design. Despite this, dental appliances may be useful in reduction of anomalous occlusion and consequently improve OSA. Other therapies such as high-flow oxygen that circumvents the inspiratory flow limitation and hypoxic spells may provide a physiologic solution, but the use and transport of such a device would be cumbersome. Typically, it is thought that children requiring lower levels of CPAP could potentially be candidates for high-flow oxygen delivery devices such as Vapotherm™.

Thus far, a number of anatomic and neuromotor aspects of airflow within the upper airway have been discussed for critical analysis of positional changes associated with OSA. Despite the few studies performed that investigated PSG-derived information to assess changes during sleep, there has been no consensus, although age and the stage of sleep appear to affect the severity. Obesity indeed plays a role in OSA treatment and alters the response to adenotonsillectomy. Weight management remains a critical issue that prevents and reduces the extraluminal compression of the upper airway during sleep. Computational tools have helped us understand the physical changes in flow that take place as a function of apneic episodes. Despite this, more level I clinical evidence is necessary at this stage to establish firm recommendations for alteration of posture during sleep in children >1 year of age.

References

1. Ogden CL, et al. Centers for disease control and prevention 2000 growth charts for the United States: improvements to the 1977 National Center for Health Statistics version. Pediatrics. 2002;109:45.
2. Flegal KM, Wei R, Ogden C. Weight-for-stature compared with body mass index–for-age growth charts for the United States from the Centers for Disease Control and Prevention. Am J Clin Nutr. 2002;75:761.
3. Redline S, et al. Risk factors for sleep-disordered breathing in children associations with obesity, race, and respiratory problems. Am J Respir Crit Care Med. 1999;159:1527.
4. Wing Y, et al. A controlled study of sleep related disordered breathing in obese children. Arch Dis Child. 2003;88:1043.
5. Bixler EO, et al. Sleep disordered breathing in children in a general population sample: prevalence and risk factors. Sleep. 2009;32:731.
6. Brouillette RT, Fernbach SK, Hunt CE. Obstructive sleep apnea in infants and children. J Pediatr. 1982;100:31.
7. Greenfeld M, Tauman R, DeRowe A, Sivan Y. Obstructive sleep apnea syndrome due to adenotonsillar hypertrophy in infants. Int J Pediatr Otorhinolaryngol. 2003;67:1055.
8. Brouilette R, et al. A diagnostic approach to suspected obstructive sleep apnea in children. J Pediatr. 1984;105:10.
9. Fregosi RF, et al. Sleep-disordered breathing, pharyngeal size and soft tissue anatomy in children. J Appl Physiol. 2003;95:2030.
10. Lam Y-Y, et al. The correlation among obesity, apnea-hypopnea index, and tonsil size in children. Chest. 2006;130:1751.
11. Marcus CL, et al. Upper airway dynamic responses in children with the obstructive sleep apnea syndrome. Pediatr Res. 2005;57:99.
12. Goh DY, Galster P, Marcus CL. Sleep architecture and respiratory disturbances in children with obstructive sleep apnea. Am J Respir Crit Care Med. 2000;162:682.
13. Kaditis AG, et al. Adiposity in relation to age as predictor of severity of sleep apnea in children with snoring. Sleep Breath. 2008;12:25.
14. Litman RS, et al. Effect of lateral positioning on upper airway size and morphology in sedated children. Anesthesiology. 2005;103:484.
15. Isono S, Tanaka A, Nishino T. Lateral position decreases collapsibility of the passive pharynx in patients with obstructive sleep apnea. Anesthesiology. 2002;97:780.
16. Laitman J, Crelin E, Conlogue G. The function of the epiglottis in monkey and man. Yale J Biol Med. 1977;50:43.
17. Laitman JT, Reidenberg JS. The human aerodigestive tract and gastroesophageal reflux: an evolutionary perspective. Am J Med. 1997;103:2S.
18. Mezzanotte WS, Tangel DJ, White DP. Waking genioglossal electromyogram in sleep apnea patients versus normal controls (a neuromuscular compensatory mechanism). J Clin Invest. 1992;89:1571.

19. Horner R, Shea S, McIvor J, Guz A. Pharyngeal size and shape during wakefulness and sleep in patients with obstructive sleep apnoea. QJM. 1989;72:719.
20. Pijpers M, et al. Undiagnosed obstructive sleep apnea syndrome in children with syndromal craniofacial synostosis. J Craniofac Surg. 2004;15:670.
21. Lauritzen C, Lilja J, Jarlstedt J. Airway obstruction and sleep apnea in children with craniofacial anomalies. Plast Reconstr Surg. 1986;77:1.
22. Gozal D. Sleep-disordered breathing and school performance in children. Pediatrics. 1998;102:616.
23. Chervin RD, et al. Sleep-disordered breathing, behavior, and cognition in children before and after adenotonsillectomy. Pediatrics. 2006;117:e769.
24. Tarasiuk A, Simon T, Tal A, Reuveni H. Adenotonsillectomy in children with obstructive sleep apnea syndrome reduces health care utilization. Pediatrics. 2004;113:351.
25. Mihaescu M, Murugappan S, Gutmark E, Donnelly LF, Kalra M. Computational modeling of upper airway before and after adenotonsillectomy for obstructive sleep apnea. Laryngoscope. 2008;118:360.
26. Costa DJ, Mitchell R. Adenotonsillectomy for obstructive sleep apnea in obese children: a meta-analysis. Otolaryngol Head Neck Surg. 2009;140:455.
27. Dransfield DA, Spitzer AR, Fox WW. Episodic airway obstruction in premature infants. Arch Pediatr Adolesc Med. 1983;137:441.
28. Roithmann R, et al. Acoustic rhinometry, rhinomanometry, and the sensation of nasal patency: a correlative study. J Otolaryngol. 1994;23:454.
29. Leiter J. Analysis of pharyngeal resistance and genioglossal EMG activity using a model of orifice flow. J Appl Physiol. 1992;73:576.
30. Shome B, et al. Modeling of airflow in the pharynx with application to sleep apnea. Trans ASME-K-J Biomech Eng. 1998;120:416.
31. Xu C, et al. Computational fluid dynamics modeling of the upper airway of children with obstructive sleep apnea syndrome in steady flow. J Biomech. 2006;39:2043.
32. Mylavarapu G, et al. Validation of computational fluid dynamics methodology used for human upper airway flow simulations. J Biomech. 2009;42:1553.
33. Young DF, Tsai FY. Flow characteristics in models of arterial stenoses—I. Steady flow. J Biomech. 1973;6:395.
34. Huang R, Li X, Rong Q. Control mechanism for the upper airway collapse in patients with obstructive sleep apnea syndrome: a finite element study. Sci China Life Sci. 2013;56(4):366–72.
35. Walsh JH, et al. Evaluation of pharyngeal shape and size using anatomical optical coherence tomography in individuals with and without obstructive sleep apnoea. J Sleep Res. 2008;17:230.
36. Kahn A, et al. Prone or supine body position and sleep characteristics in infants. Pediatrics. 1993;91:1112.
37. Skadberg B, Markestad T. Behaviour and physiological responses during prone and supine sleep in early infancy. Arch Dis Child. 1997;76:320.
38. Pereira KD, Roebuck JC, Howell L. The effect of body position on sleep apnea in children younger than 3 years. Arch Otolaryngol Head Neck Surg. 2005;131:1014.
39. Pereira KD, Rathi NK, Fatakia A, Haque SA, Castriotta RJ. Body position and obstructive sleep apnea in 8–12-month-old infants. Int J Pediatr Otorhinolaryngol. 2008;72:897.
40. Engelberts AC. The role of obstructive apnea in sudden infant death syndrome and apparent life threatening event. Int J Pediatr Otorhinolaryngol. 1995;32:S59.
41. Zhang X-W, Li Y, Zhou F, Guo C-K, Huang Z-T. Association of body position with sleep architecture and respiratory disturbances in children with obstructive sleep apnea. Acta Otolaryngol. 2007;127:1321.
42. Kheirandish-Gozal L, Gozal D. Intranasal budesonide treatment for children with mild obstructive sleep apnea syndrome. Pediatrics. 2008;122:e149.

Sleep Position and Pregnancy

Sharon Morong, Brenda Hermsen, and Nico de Vries

Introduction

Sleep-disordered breathing (SDB) has been shown to be associated with negative clinical sequelae such as systemic hypertension and cardiovascular disease. Pregnant patients can also be diagnosed with SDB, the negative consequences of which not only pertain to the patient but to the unborn fetus as well. Despite this, however, SDB is underdiagnosed in pregnant patients. In this chapter, we will discuss the physiologic respiratory changes that occur during pregnancy, SDB in pregnancy, supine hypotensive syndrome (SHS), the complications and current treatments for these events, and the potential role for positional therapy in pregnant women whose problems may be specifically position dependent.

Respiration Changes During Pregnancy

During pregnancy, several changes occur in the upper and lower airways, both anatomically and physiologically. Many of these changes occur early in gestation and can continue into the immediate postpartum period.

S. Morong, M.D., M.Sc., F.R.C.S.C. (✉)
Department of Otolaryngology, Sint Lucas Andreas Ziekenhuis,
Jan Tooropstraat 164, Amsterdam 1061 AE, The Netherlands
e-mail: sharon.morong@gmail.com

B. Hermsen, M.D.
Department of Gynecology, Sint Lucas Andreas Ziekenhuis, Amsterdam, The Netherlands

N. de Vries, M.D., Ph.D.
Department of Otolaryngology, Sint Lucas Andreas Ziekenhuis,
Jan Tooropstraat 164, Amsterdam 1061 AE, The Netherlands

Department of Otolaryngology, University Hospital Antwerp, Antwerp, Belgium

N. de Vries et al. (eds.), *Positional Therapy in Obstructive Sleep Apnea*,
DOI 10.1007/978-3-319-09626-1_15

During the first trimester, many changes occur in the upper respiratory tract. Patients often experience mucosal edema, capillary congestion, and hyperemia, which are said to be, in part, secondary to increased estrogen levels. As such, many pregnant women are diagnosed with estrogen-induced rhinitis. These changes typically peak in the third trimester but can continue throughout pregnancy. Another change reported during the first trimester is a reduction in pharyngeal size using the Mallampati scoring system [1]. This reduction in pharyngeal size is reportedly worse in women with preeclampsia [2].

Thoracic changes noted in the pregnant patient are an elevated diaphragm, increased diaphragmatic excursion, and an increase in the diameter of the chest with decreased chest wall compliance. These anatomic changes account for approximately 20 % decrease in functional residual capacity (FRC) [3]. Physiologically, respiratory drive is noted to increase secondary to increased progesterone levels. Minute ventilation increases with an increase in tidal volume, which results in a decrease in partial pressure of carbon dioxide ($PaCO_2$). Alveolar oxygen tension, however, increases with partial pressure of oxygen (PaO_2), with pressures reaching as high as 106 mmHg [4]. These changes in CO_2 and O_2 levels enable differential gradients to be created between the mother and fetus, which allow for delivery of O_2 to the fetus and excretion of CO_2 from the fetus.

Pregnant women experience physiologic anemia that results in a decrease in the arterial O_2 content. This, however, is counteracted by an increase in cardiac output. Pregnant women are thus more dependent on cardiac output for maintenance of O_2 delivery.

Because of these physiologic changes, up to 75 % pregnant women have physiologic dyspnea [4], rendering both mother and fetus more susceptible to respiratory compromise with changes in position [5–7]. During respiratory compromise, maternal O_2 consumption and desaturations are much more rapid, which can result in fetal hypoxia [5, 8]. At a PaO_2 of 60 mmHg or O_2 saturation of 90 %, with an alveolar arterial (A-a) gradient of 15 or less, fetal oxygenation can be maintained. The PaO_2 and A-a gradient, however, can be affected when the mother is in a supine position. Potential desaturations that can occur in the supine position may be secondary to positionally induced changes in cardiac output and/or early airway closure during tidal breathing secondary to reduced pharyngeal size and increased airway collapsibility [6, 7]. Other studies have postulated that the strong ventilatory drive that occurs in response to increased progesterone levels can have a “suction effect” on an already edematous upper airway leading to airway obstruction [9, 10]. This effect would be exacerbated in the supine position. These changes may be even more readily seen in the obese pregnant patient. In patients who are obese, ventilation perfusion (V/Q) mismatches may occur secondary to the upper lung zones being preferentially ventilated with perfusion to the lower lung fields being maintained. This mismatch worsens in the supine position [4].

Sleep-Disordered Breathing During Pregnancy

In addition to the physiologic respiratory changes pregnant women undergo, some experience additional SDB. Changes in sleep patterns can be quite normal during pregnancy and typically start during the first trimester. Such changes include decreased rapid eye movement (REM) sleep secondary to increased estrogen levels and increased non-REM sleep secondary to increased progesterone levels [11–13]. Decreased FRC can become worse during sleep and some pregnant women may be more likely to have central sleep apnea secondary to an increased sensitivity threshold to CO_2 levels, with subsequent hyperventilation [4]. Oxytocin levels, noted to increase at night, may cause increased contractions with interruption of sleep [9, 14, 15]. Other factors affecting sleep include gastroesophageal reflux, nocturia, and leg cramps [16].

SDB comprise many disorders such as snoring, upper airway resistance syndrome, OSA, and obesity-hyperventilation syndrome. The American academy of sleep medicine has coined the term "pregnancy-associated sleep disorders" [17]. The incidence of SDB in nonpregnant women and obese nonpregnant women is approximately 6–8 % and 37 %, respectively [14]. Although the incidence of SDB in pregnant women is unknown, they are found to be more susceptible to SDB, with obese patients more likely to develop SDB when pregnant. A recent prospective observational study by Louis et al. reported an SDB prevalence of 15.4 % in obese pregnant women [18]. There are various factors that can increase the risk of SDB in pregnancy such as weight gain, upper airway changes, diaphragm elevation, decreased FRC, hyperventilation, and an increase in non-REM sleep. Factors that have been found to decrease the risk of SDB are increases in minute ventilation, decreases in REM sleep, and sleeping in a lateral position as gestation advances [4].

Studies comparing snoring in pregnant versus nonpregnant women have found that approximately 4 % of nonpregnant women snore, while 14–52 % of pregnant women snore by the third trimester [19–22]. The incidence of snoring in women with preeclampsia has been reportedly up to 85 % [2].

The incidence of OSA in women of childbearing age is approximately 5 %. Its incidence in pregnancy is still unclear. Symptoms of OSA tend to differ in women compared with men. Women may often present with symptoms of fatigue, insomnia, morning headaches, and depression. Daytime hypersomnolence has been shown to increase during pregnancy with Epworth Sleepiness Scale (ESS) scores of more than 10 seen in up to 25 % pregnant patients [20, 23]. One study reported a significant correlation between ESS scores and snoring and gasping at night [23]. Pregnant women are less likely, however, to have witnessed apneas, and their most common presenting complaint is snoring [4]. OSA, if left untreated, often worsens during pregnancy. The physiologic sequelae of OSA include hypercapnia, hypoxemia, increased sympathetic tone, and peripheral vascular resistance with tachycardia [9, 14]. OSA in this population is likely underestimated given that the presenting symptoms may not be classic for OSA and may be mistaken as physical, mental, or emotional manifestations of changes occurring during pregnancy.

Complications of Sleep-Disordered Breathing During Pregnancy

In nonpregnant women, the association between SDB and hypertension, cardiorespiratory, and metabolic dysfunction has been well established [4]. Studies have reported possible relationships between SDB and gestational hypertension, preeclampsia, and intrauterine growth restriction (IUGR) in pregnant women [4]. Louis et al. reported that within a cohort of obese pregnant patients, OSA was significantly associated with preeclampsia and more frequent cesarean deliveries [18]. One study reported that pregnant women who are sleep deprived closer to term are more likely to have a longer duration of labor and higher rates of cesarean section [24]. During pregnancy, snoring has been found to have independent associations with hypertension, preeclampsia, and IUGR [19, 25]. Franklin et al. reported that in 502 women, snoring was an independent risk factor for both hypertension and preeclampsia after adjusting for age and weight [19]. There are various theories that exist regarding the association between snoring and preeclampsia. Such theories include a decrease in antioxidant activity and increases in oxidative stress markers [4]. Significant associations have also been found between symptoms of SDB during pregnancy and poorly controlled blood pressure up to 2 weeks postpartum [2]. Other complications that have been noted in pregnant patients with sleep apnea are right-sided heart failure and pulmonary hypertension [2].

The adverse outcomes of SDB on neonates are still unclear. One prospective observational study reported that OSA in obese pregnant women is significantly associated with more frequent neonatal intensive care unit admissions [18]. Some case reports have documented acute fetal decelerations during clinically detected maternal apneic episodes [26–28]. A review of various case reports looking at maternal and fetal complications associated with SDB in pregnancy found that most complications were either not treated at all or treatment was initiated quite late after complications had occurred. Patients, however, who were treated prior to or during their first trimester had fewer maternal and fetal complications. The above review, however, summarizes case reports. Randomized controlled trials would be needed to confirm these findings [29].

Current Treatment for SDB During Pregnancy

The management of SDB for pregnant patients is slightly different to their nonpregnant counterparts. For pregnant patients, advocating weight loss to alleviate SDB is not recommended. While there may be some consensus recommending treatment to nonpregnant patients with an apnea-hypopnea index (AHI) >5, there are no such specific recommendations for pregnant women. Continuous positive airway pressure (CPAP) is currently used to treat OSA in pregnant women, despite the theoretical risk of aspiration from its use. It has been found to have an associated decrease in nocturnal blood pressure levels and improvement in cardiac output throughout all sleep stages in patients with preeclampsia [2]. Smaller studies have reported that patients who were at risk for preeclampsia were placed on CPAP until delivery. None of these patients developed preeclampsia, and all patients had low systolic and diastolic pressure readings [2]. Treatment with CPAP has also been reported to have an associated lower incidence of IUGR than untreated women [4].

Guilleminault et al. reported on the effects of nasal CPAP in 12 non-obese pregnant patients, 7 of whom were diagnosed with SDB prior to pregnancy. In the five patients diagnosed after conception, CPAP was initiated, on average, at approximately 10 weeks gestation age (GA). All women in this study were known to be chronic snorers before pregnancy. The average AHI was 21 and the average respiratory disturbance index (RDI) was 33. Clinical improvement was noted with CPAP, using various scales such as the Epworth Sleepiness Scale (ESS), the fatigue scale, and the visual analogue scale (VAS). All subjects had full-term pregnancies and healthy infants. Six women required increases in nCPAP pressure at 24–26 weeks GA, while four patients reported morning nasal congestion with CPAP use [21].

Complications and Treatment of Supine Hypotensive Syndrome During Pregnancy

Sixty percent of women experience supine symptoms at some point during their pregnancy [30]. In some patients, these supine signs and symptoms were noted to be associated with hypotension. Some of the signs and symptoms were nausea and dizziness, dyspnea or Cheyne-Stokes respiration, restlessness and muscle twitching, headaches, numb or cold legs, tinnitus, fatigue, loss of consciousness, incontinence, convulsions, and a desire to flex their hips and knees. Howard et al. coined the term supine hypotensive syndrome to characterize these events [31]. There have been several definitions for this syndrome. Calvin et al. defined it as a decrease in mean arterial pressure of greater than 15 mmHg in the supine position together with a sustained increase in heart rate of at least 20 beats per minute [32]. Other definitions cited are a decrease of 15–30 mmHg in systolic pressure to be significant but not severe hypotension [33]. One study classified the syndrome as mild (decrease >30 and <80 mmHg), moderate (same pressure with intolerable symptoms), or severe (presents in a shock state) [30]. The time of onset of symptoms after being in a supine position has varied from 3 to 30 min [34–36]. The incidence of SHS ranges from 2.5 % to 20.6 % [37, 38]. Although there are several reported symptoms as part of this syndrome, there are various reports that have documented patients who have been asymptomatic during supine hypotension. Sluder et al. reported a patient who remained asymptomatic at an arterial pressure of 80/60 mmHg until she became syncopal with a further decrease in pressure [39]. Another report by Oxorn et al. documented findings of a patient with a systolic pressure of 80 mmHg and a heart rate of 120–160 with no symptoms. Her blood pressure rose to 130/70 mmHg when placed in a lateral position [39, 40]. Kato and Tanako also reported an asymptomatic patient with a blood pressure of 80/40 mmHg who eventually became dyspneic at 60/30 mmHg [30].

Several cases of SHS have been reported prenatally [39, 41, 42], during prenatal exercises [35, 43], vaginal exams [35, 44], ultrasound scanning [38], induction of and during labor, and cesarean sections [45]. Some authors have reported that SHS typically occurs during the eighth and ninth months of pregnancy; however, other studies have noted a much earlier onset. One report noted the development of supine symptoms from the onset of the perception of fetal movements [46]; another study reported supine symptoms from the fifth month of gestation [47].

Theories for this syndrome include pathologic elevation of the diaphragm; aortic and inferior vena cava (IVC) compression, now often combined to be termed aorto-caval compression; or a utero-cardiac neurologic reflex. IVC compression reduces venous return, which subsequently causes hypotension. Aortic compression caused by a supine position initially increases systemic arterial pressure and can lead to a baroreceptor-mediated vagal bradycardia and eventual hypotension [48]. The neurogenic cause of SHS is said to be a sympathetic reflex following uterine pressure on posterior structures. Aortocaval compression is currently the most favored theory. Several maneuvers such as leg flexion [46, 49] and hyperpnea [31, 50] have been reported to alleviate SHS caused by aortocaval compression. Switching from a supine to lateral position is, however, the most effective at reversing symptoms caused by SHS [36, 51].

Complications associated with SHS are placental abruption and amniotic fluid embolism. Placental abruption has been reportedly associated with this syndrome both with patients with preeclampsia [44] and patients who had normal pregnancies [42, 52, 53]. Studies have also reported that prolonged periods in a supine position can potentially lead to fetal complications [54, 55]. Dumont et al. suggested avoiding the supine position throughout late pregnancy [35].

Position Dependence and Sleep Disordered Breathing

POSA is defined, according to Cartwright's criteria, as an AHI that is at least twice as high in the supine position when compared with other sleeping positions [56]. Based on these criteria, it is reported that 53–56 % of nonpregnant women and men with OSA have positional OSA, known as POSA [56–60]. One study specifically looking at an Asian population with OSA found that 67 % of patients met the criteria for POSA [61]. It is possible, however, that the criteria currently being used may in fact underestimate the true prevalence of POSA. One study, for example, reported that 80 % of patients had a positional component to their OSA, with 56 % meeting Cartwright's criteria and the rest having a supine AHI higher than in other positions, but not twice as high [62]. It has also been reported that an inverse relationship exists between position dependency and the severity of OSA. The less severe a patient's OSA, the more likely they were to be position dependent [63]. The lateral sleep position has been reported to protect against apneic and hypopneic events [2].

One study further stated that when comparing the AHI in both right and left lateral positions in patients with OSA, a decrease in AHI was noted when sleeping on the right side. This was particularly seen in patients with moderate and severe OSA [64].

Positional Therapy

Positional therapy for patients with POSA was first developed in the 1980s as a conservative management option [57–59, 65–67] and has since been included in clinical practice guidelines [68]. This form of therapy has been shown to reduce the AHI in patients with POSA [57, 59, 65, 67, 69]. Various techniques have been employed to implement positional therapy. One such technique is the tennis ball technique. This technique involves placing a tennis ball into the pocket of a cloth band or belt and wrapping this device around the abdomen with the tennis ball positioned at the center of the back. The pressure of the tennis ball is felt in the supine position, alerting the patient to move to another sleeping position [70]. A slight modification of this technique involved patients wearing a vest filled with semirigid foam on the back [66]. These techniques were successful at reducing the AHI in patients with POSA, but the compliance rates, however, have been low. One study looked at compliance rates in 67 patients using the tennis ball technique, approximately 2.5 years after treatment was initiated. Less than 10 % of these patients remained compliant. This was found to be secondary to back discomfort and the occurrence of arousals when changing sleeping positions [71].

A new positional therapy device, the sleep position trainer (SPT), has been developed which incorporates a sensor that detects sleeping position and softly vibrates when the patient is in a supine position. The vibration intensity increases until the patient moves from a supine to another sleeping position [72]. Van Maanen et al. reported 92.7 % compliance rate with the SPT and associated reductions in AHI (significant decrease from 16.4 to 5; $p<0.001$). He also reported reductions in subjective sleepiness and improvements noted in sleep-related quality of life. The median percentage of sleeping time in the supine position decreased from 49.9 % to 0.0 % ($p<0.001$) [73].

Role of Positional Therapy During Pregnancy

Through physiologic changes in respiration during pregnancy, SDB, and, for some pregnant women, the supine position itself, respiratory compromise to both mother and fetus can ensue. OSA in the pregnant population is likely underdiagnosed because symptoms of daytime sleepiness and fatigue may wrongly be attributed to the pregnancy itself. The correct diagnosis for these patients can potentially prevent complications of preeclampsia and IUGR with early treatment.

Currently, for pregnant patients who are diagnosed with OSA and treated, nasal CPAP is administered. While this form of treatment has shown success, there is a theoretical risk of aspiration with its use. Close follow-up is required to ensure CPAP pressures continue to be effective as a patient progresses during pregnancy, and CPAP may also cause discomfort and nasal congestion, which may affect compliance with this modality of treatment. Concerns regarding CPAP compliance pertain not only to pregnant women but also to the general population. Although no standardized definition for CPAP compliance exists, a criterion of 4-h usage per night for at least 5 nights per week has generally been used in the literature [74–76]. A literature review reported that 29–83 % patients were noncompliant with CPAP therapy, using the device for less than 4 h per night [75].

In the general population, 56 % of patients with OSA were found to be position dependent. It is possible that many pregnant patients with OSA may also be position dependent and thus be candidates for positional therapy, a simple, noninvasive alternative to CPAP, which may render less discomfort to the patient.

Another event that may cause respiratory compromise in the pregnant patient is SHS. While SHS has been associated with very severe symptoms and signs requiring position change in conjunction with resuscitative measures, there have been cases where patients have been asymptomatic or reported mild symptoms of supine intolerance. It is still unclear what effect prolonged, intermittent hypotension and hypoxia in the supine position during pregnancy can have on the fetus, but some authors have recommended that patients noted to have any form of SHS should avoid the supine position throughout their pregnancy. These patients would be good candidates for positional therapy.

Conclusion

SDB is currently underdiagnosed in pregnant women, and with treatment, complications such as preeclampsia and IUGR may be prevented. Many of these patients may have position-dependent SDB, which would render them appropriate candidates for positional therapy. Pregnant patients, who experience symptoms in a supine position and are diagnosed with or at risk of SHS, may also be good candidates for positional therapy. Further research is needed to better determine the prevalence of OSA and POSA during pregnancy and to investigate optimal treatment modalities for this population.

References

1. Pilkington S, Carli F, Dakin MJ, Romney M, De Witt KA, Dore CJ, Cormack RS. Increase in Mallampati score during pregnancy. Br J Anaesth. 1995;74(6):638–42.
2. Bourjeily G. Sleep disorders in pregnancy. Obstet Med. 2009;2:100–6.

3. Wise RA, Polito AJ, Krishnan V. Respiratory physiologic changes in pregnancy. Immunol Allergy Clin North Am. 2006;26(1):1–12.
4. Bobrowski RA. Pulmonary physiology in pregnancy. Clin Obstet Gynecol. 2010;53(2): 285–300.
5. Archer Jr GW, Marx GF. Arterial oxygen tension during apnoea in parturient women. Br J Anaesth. 1974;46(5):358–60.
6. Garrard GS, Littler WA, Redman CW. Closing volume during normal pregnancy. Thorax. 1978;33(4):488–92.
7. White DP. Pathogenesis of obstructive and central sleep apnea. Am J Respir Crit Care Med. 2005;172(11):1363–70.
8. Cheun JK, Choi KT. Arterial oxygen desaturation rate following obstructive apnea in parturients. J Korean Med Sci. 1992;7(1):6–10.
9. Santiago JR, Nolledo MS, Kinzler W, Santiago TV. Sleep and sleep disorders in pregnancy. Ann Intern Med. 2001;134(5):396–408.
10. Edwards N, Middleton PG, Blyton DM, Sullivan CE. Sleep disordered breathing and pregnancy. Thorax. 2002;57(6):555–8.
11. Colvin GB, Whitmoyer DI, Lisk RD, Walter DO, Sawyer CH. Changes in sleep-wakefulness in female rats during circadian and estrous cycles. Brain Res. 1968;7(2):173–81.
12. Branchey M, Branchey L, Nadler RD. Effects of estrogen and progesterone on sleep patterns of female rats. Physiol Behav. 1971;6(6):743–6.
13. Fang J, Fishbein W. Sex differences in paradoxical sleep: influences of estrus cycle and ovariectomy. Brain Res. 1996;734(1–2):275–85.
14. Edwards N, Sullivan CE. Sleep-disordered breathing in pregnancy. Sleep Med Clin. 2008;3: 81–95.
15. Kapsimalis F, Kryger M. Obstructive sleep apnea in pregnancy. Sleep Med Clin. 2007;2: 603–13.
16. Gunderson EP, Rifas-Shiman SL, Oken E, Rich-Edwards JW, Kleinman KP, Taveras EM, Gillman MW. Association of fewer hours of sleep at 6 months postpartum with substantial weight retention at 1 year postpartum. Am J Epidemiol. 2008;167(2):178–87.
17. Medicine AAoS. International classification of sleep disorders, revised: diagnostic and coding manual. Westchester, IL: Medicine AAoS; 2000.
18. Louis J, Auckley D, Miladinovic B, Shepherd A, Mencin P, Kumar D, Mercer B, Redline S. Perinatal outcomes associated with obstructive sleep apnea in obese pregnant women. Obstet Gynecol. 2012;120(5):1085–92.
19. Franklin KA, Holmgren PA, Jonsson F, Poromaa N, Stenlund H, Svanborg E. Snoring, pregnancy-induced hypertension, and growth retardation of the fetus. Chest. 2000;117(1): 137–41.
20. Pien GW, Fife D, Pack AI, Nkwuo JE, Schwab RJ. Changes in symptoms of sleep-disordered breathing during pregnancy. Sleep. 2005;28(10):1299–305.
21. Guilleminault C, Kreutzer M, Chang JL. Pregnancy, sleep disordered breathing and treatment with nasal continuous positive airway pressure. Sleep Med. 2004;5(1):43–51.
22. Schutte S, Gross A, Segal J. Self reported snoring and sleep in high risk pregnancies. Sleep Res. 1995;24:342.
23. Bourjeily G, Raker C. Epworth sleepiness score in pregnancy. Toronto: American Thoracic Society; 2008.
24. Lee KA, Gay CL. Sleep in late pregnancy predicts length of labor and type of delivery. Am J Obstet Gynecol. 2004;191(6):2041–6.
25. Bourjeily G, Habr F, Miller M, Rosene-Montella K. Symptoms of sleep disordered breathing, BMI and pregnancy outcomes. Accepted for slide presentation at the American College of Chest Physicians for 2007 meeting, Chicago, IL. Chest 2007;132:463a.
26. Joel-Cohen SJ, Schoenfeld A. Fetal response to periodic sleep apnea: a new syndrome in obstetrics. Eur J Obstet Gynecol Reprod Biol. 1978;8(2):77–81.
27. Roush SF, Bell L. Obstructive sleep apnea in pregnancy. J Am Board Fam Pract. 2004; 17(4):292–4.

28. Charbonneau M, Falcone T, Cosio MG, Levy RD. Obstructive sleep apnea during pregnancy. Therapy and implications for fetal health. Am Rev Respir Dis. 1991;144(2):461–3.
29. Champagne KA, Kimoff RJ, Barriga PC, Schwartzman K. Sleep disordered breathing in women of childbearing age and during pregnancy. Indian J Med Res. 2010;131:285–301.
30. Kato J, Tanaka T. Shock due to supine hypotensive syndrome. Sanfujinka No Jissai. 1967;16(2):118–23.
31. Howard BK, Goodson JH, Mengert WF. Supine hypotensive syndrome in late pregnancy. Obstet Gynecol. 1953;1(4):371–7.
32. Calvin S, Jones III OW, Knieriem K, Weinstein L. Oxygen saturation in the supine hypotensive syndrome. Obstet Gynecol. 1988;71(6 Pt 1):872–7.
33. Quilligan EJ, Tyler C. Postural effects on the cardiovascular status in pregnancy: a comparison of the lateral and supine postures. Am J Obstet Gynecol. 1959;78:465–71.
34. Mc Jr RW. Postural shock in pregnancy. Am J Obstet Gynecol. 1951;62(3):627–32.
35. Dumont M, Peyre M, Villard JP. Dorsal decubitus postural hypotensive shock in pregnant women. Presse Med. 1962;70:622–4.
36. Brigden W, Howarth S, Sharpey-Schafer EP. Postural changes in the peripheral blood flow of normal subjects with observations on the vaso-vagal fainting reactions as a result of tilting, the lordotic posture, pregnancy, and spinal anesthesia. Clin Sci. 1950;9:79–91.
37. Skachedub RG. Hypotensive syndrome in pregnant women in supine position. Akush Ginekol (Mosk). 1969;45(4):57–61.
38. Blanda F. Sulla possibilie in sorgenza di una shock posturale ipotensivo, dopo prolungato decubito dorsale, nella donna gravida [On the possible occurrence of hypotensive postural shock in pregnant women after prolonged dorsal decubitus]. Clin Ginec (Catania). 1963;5: 373–86.
39. Sluder HM. The supine hypotensive syndrome of pregnancy. N C Med J. 1956;17(9):420–2.
40. Oxorn H. Postural hypotension in pregnancy. Can Med Assoc J. 1960;83:436.
41. Arnold Jr ET. Syncopal seizures in recumbent position in late pregnancy. J Med Assoc Ga. 1953;42(5):246–7.
42. Smith K, Fields H. The supine hypotensive syndrome; a factor in the etiology of abruptio placentae. Obstet Gynecol. 1958;12(4):369–72.
43. Lemtis H, Seger R. Supine hypotension syndrome and premature separation of the normally implanted placenta (author's transl). Geburtshilfe Frauenheilkd. 1974;34(3):175–80.
44. Sullivan Jr WM, Grossbard P. Supine hypotensive syndrome producing abruptio placentae. J Med Soc N J. 1954;51(11):470–1.
45. Kinsella SM, Lohmann G. Supine hypotensive syndrome. Obstet Gynecol. 1994;83(5 Pt 1): 774–88.
46. Tumova Z. Clinostatic hypotensive syndrome in pregnancy. Ceska Gynekol. 1962;27:651–6.
47. Sensing H. Supine hypotensive syndrom [Supine hypotensive syndrome]. Dtsch Med Wochenschr. 1963;23:2226–8.
48. Milsom I, Forssman L. Factors influencing aortocaval compression in late pregnancy. Am J Obstet Gynecol. 1984;148(6):764–71.
49. Holmes F. Incidence of the supine hypotensive syndrome in late pregnancy. A clinical study in 500 subjects. J Obstet Gynaecol Br Emp. 1960;67:254–8.
50. Ahltorp G. Uber Ruckenlagebeschwerden bei Graviden [On problems in the supine position in pregnant women]. Acta Obstet Gynecol Scand. 1935;15:295–341.
51. Leighton B. Anaesthetic complications: intraoperative. In: Obstetric anesthesia. Philadelphia, PA: JB Lippincott; 1993. p. 616–8.
52. Pyorala T, Pyorala K. Supine hypotensive syndrome of late pregnancy and premature separation of the placenta. Acta Obstet Gynecol Scand. 1960;39:100–5.
53. Robbins RA, Estrara T, Russell C. Supine hypotensive syndrome and abruptio placentae. A case report. Am J Obstet Gynecol. 1960;80:1207–8.
54. Erofeev Iu N, Kiseleva KS. The significance of the syndrome of compression of the inferior vena cava at the last stage of pregnancy. Akush Ginekol (Mosk). 1969;45(9):72–4.

55. Courtney L. Supine hypotension syndrome during caesarean section. Br Med J. 1970;1(5699): 797–8.
56. Cartwright RD. Effect of sleep position on sleep apnea severity. Sleep. 1984;7(2):110–4.
57. Oksenberg A, Silverberg DS, Arons E, Radwan H. Positional vs nonpositional obstructive sleep apnea patients: anthropomorphic, nocturnal polysomnographic, and multiple sleep latency test data. Chest. 1997;112(3):629–39.
58. Oksenberg A, Silverberg DS. The effect of body posture on sleep-related breathing disorders: facts and therapeutic implications. Sleep Med Rev. 1998;2(3):139–62.
59. Richard W, Kox D, den Herder C, Laman M, van Tinteren H, de Vries N. The role of sleep position in obstructive sleep apnea syndrome. Eur Arch Otorhinolaryngol. 2006;263(10): 946–50.
60. Sunnergren O, Brostrom A, Svanborg E. Positional sensitivity as a confounder in diagnosis of severity of obstructive sleep apnea. Sleep Breath. 2013;17(1):173–9.
61. Teerapraipruk B, Chirakalwasan N, Simon R, Hirunwiwatkul P, Jaimchariyatam N, Desudchit T, Charakorn N, Wanlapakorn C. Clinical and polysomnographic data of positional sleep apnea and its predictors. Sleep Breath. 2012;16(4):1167–72.
62. van Maanen JP, Richard W, Van Kesteren ER, Ravesloot MJ, Laman DM, Hilgevoord AA, de Vries N. Evaluation of a new simple treatment for positional sleep apnoea patients. J Sleep Res. 2012;21(3):322–9.
63. Mador MJ, Kufel TJ, Magalang UJ, Rajesh SK, Watwe V, Grant BJ. Prevalence of positional sleep apnea in patients undergoing polysomnography. Chest. 2005;128(4):2130–7.
64. Ozeke O, Erturk O, Gungor M, Hizel SB, Aydin D, Celenk MK, Dincer H, Ilicin G, Ozgen F, Ozer C. Influence of the right- versus left-sided sleeping position on the apnea-hypopnea index in patients with sleep apnea. Sleep Breath. 2012;16(3):617–20.
65. Cartwright RD, Lloyd S, Lilie J, Kravitz H. Sleep position training as treatment for sleep apnea syndrome: a preliminary study. Sleep. 1985;8(2):87–94.
66. Maurer JT, Stuck BA, Hein G, Verse T, Hormann K. Treatment of obstructive sleep apnea with a new vest preventing the supine position. Dtsch Med Wochenschr. 2003;128(3):71–5.
67. Wenzel S, Smith E, Leiacker R, Fischer Y. Efficacy and longterm compliance of the vest preventing the supine position in patients with obstructive sleep apnea. Laryngorhinootologie. 2007;86(8):579–83.
68. Veasey SC, Guilleminault C, Strohl KP, Sanders MH, Ballard RD, Magalang UJ. Medical therapy for obstructive sleep apnea: a review by the Medical Therapy for Obstructive Sleep Apnea Task Force of the Standards of Practice Committee of the American Academy of Sleep Medicine. Sleep. 2006;29(8):1036–44.
69. Cartwright R, Ristanovic R, Diaz F, Caldarelli D, Alder G. A comparative study of treatments for positional sleep apnea. Sleep. 1991;14(6):546–52.
70. Oksenberg A, Silverberg D, Offenbach D, Arons E. Positional therapy for obstructive sleep apnea patients: a 6-month follow-up study. Laryngoscope. 2006;116(11):1995–2000.
71. Bignold JJ, Deans-Costi G, Goldsworthy MR, Robertson CA, McEvoy D, Catcheside PG, Mercer JD. Poor long-term patient compliance with the tennis ball technique for treating positional obstructive sleep apnea. J Clin Sleep Med. 2009;5(5):428–30.
72. Ravesloot MJ, van Maanen JP, Dun L, de Vries N. The undervalued potential of positional therapy in position-dependent snoring and obstructive sleep apnea-a review of the literature. Sleep Breath. 2013;17(1):39–49.
73. van Maanen JP, Meester KA, Dun LN, Koutsourelakis I, Witte BI, Laman DM, Hilgevoord AA, de Vries N. The sleep position trainer: a new treatment for positional obstructive sleep apnoea. Sleep Breath. 2013;17(2):771–9.
74. Ravesloot MJ, de Vries N. Reliable calculation of the efficacy of non-surgical and surgical treatment of obstructive sleep apnea revisited. Sleep. 2011;34(1):105–10.
75. Weaver TE, Grunstein RR. Adherence to continuous positive airway pressure therapy: the challenge to effective treatment. Proc Am Thorac Soc. 2008;5(2):173–8.
76. Richard W, Venker J, den Herder C, Kox D, van den Berg B, Laman M, van Tinteren H, de Vries N. Acceptance and long-term compliance of nCPAP in obstructive sleep apnea. Eur Arch Otorhinolaryngol. 2007;264(9):1081–6.

Positional OSA in Down Syndrome

Marjolein A.J. van Looij

Down syndrome (DS) is the most common genetic cause of developmental disability, affecting the entire human population independent on geography, race, or socioeconomic standing. The rate of live births may vary over time depending on changing trends in average maternal age, legislation, and personal and religious views on pregnancy termination and changes in health care. Today about 1 of every 691 babies in the USA is born with the syndrome [1].

In 95 % of cases, DS is caused by trisomy 21, in 4 % by a (unbalanced) translocation, and in 1 % by mosaicisms. The impact of these genetic abnormalities may be very variable in different individuals, resulting in a wide range of phenotypes.

The syndrome is characterized by a variety of dysmorphic features mostly affecting the head and neck and extremities, such as upslanting palpebral fissures; epicanthic folds; flat nasal bridge or facial profile; dysplastic, low-set, small ears; brachycephaly; small white or grayish/brown spots on the periphery of the iris (Brushfield spots); a furrowed, protruding tongue; a short neck with excessive skin at the nape of the neck; abnormal dentition; a narrow palate; short, broad hands; clinodactyly; a transverse palmar (Simian) crease; a sandal gap; and hyperflexibility of the joints.

Cognitive impairment affects almost all individuals with DS, although the extent to which it does so is very variable. Psychiatric and behavioral problems such as ADHD, conduct/oppositional disorder, and aggressive behavior are more common in children with DS as compared to typical children; however, they are less common than in children with most other causes of mental retardation. Adults are at risk of developing major depressive illness or aggressive behavior.

Apart from the apparent dysmorphic characteristics described above, physical problems that commonly occur in DS comprise heart disease, either congenital

M.A.J. van Looij, M.D., Ph.D. (✉)
Ear Nose and Throat Surgery, Sint Lucas Andreas Ziekenhuis,
Jan Tooropstraat 164, Amsterdam 1061 AE, The Netherlands
e-mail: m.vanlooij@slaz.nl

N. de Vries et al. (eds.), *Positional Therapy in Obstructive Sleep Apnea*,
DOI 10.1007/978-3-319-09626-1_16

(complete or partial atrioventricular septal defects, VSD, ASD, tetralogy of Fallot, or a patent ductus arteriosus) or acquired (valve abnormalities); pulmonary disease (asthma, parenchymal lung disease, chronic aspiration); endocrine disorders (hypothyroidism, diabetes); gastrointestinal tract abnormalities (e.g., celiac disease, duodenal atresia, or stenosis); growth retardation; obesity; ophthalmologic disorders (refraction errors, strabismus, nystagmus, or cataracts); sensorineural, mixed, or conductive hearing loss; hematologic disorders (polycythemia, macrocytosis, decreased white blood cell counts, increased risk of leukemia); skin disorders; urologic abnormalities; infertility; arthropathy; atlantoaxial instability; and immune deficiency.

Sleep and OSA in Down Syndrome

Several reports on sleep characteristics in DS children have been published over the past 50 years. When reviewing the literature, it is important to consider the outcomes of the studies in, as Churchill et al. clearly stated in a 2012 review, "the context of advancing technology, varying research methodologies and research ethics" [2]. Normal polysomnographic values for children and adolescent were not described until 1992 [3], and over time criteria used for diagnosing pediatric obstructive sleep apnea (OSA) have not always been entirely clear or consistent. Furthermore, numbers of DS patients included in studies are usually small.

It is, however, clear, even taking the above into consideration, that whereas OSAS is a fairly common sleep disorder affecting an estimated 1–3 % of the general pediatric population, the prevalence in DS is much higher.

In a 2012 review paper, Churchill et al. describe a prevalence of OSA in DS between 24 and 97 %. Several studies report on the falling short of parents and/or caregivers in identifying all children with sleep problems (e.g., [2, 4, 5]). Also, habitual snoring does not necessarily coincide with OSA in DS patients; in fact in a study by Ng et al., it was absent in a large proportion—61.5 %—of DS OSA patients [6]. Hence, it has been recommended that all children with DS, regardless of history, should undergo PSG at a certain age.

Although, like in the general population, most authors describe a relation between body weight and OSA, there is no strict concordance on the relationship between BMI and OSA in DS in literature. OSA in DS is more common in male than in female individuals. The prevalence of OSA in DS seems to increase with age [2].

Polysomnography in Down Syndrome

As with the above epidemiologic findings, there is no absolute concordance on polysomnographic findings in DS in literature. Reported data especially disagree on the presence or absence of central apneas and abnormalities in (N)REM sleep in DS. A high frequency of movements, awakenings, and arousals is often mentioned.

Levanon et al., for example, found a normal distribution of sleep stages in 11 children with DS, when comparing them to controls. However, stage two sleep was significantly shorter in DS, and a higher number of stage shifts from "deeper" to "lighter" sleep stages occurred. Moreover, they also found sleep in children with DS to be significantly fragmented, with frequent awakenings and arousals. These disturbances were only partially related to OSAS (8.6 %), but there was an association with jerks appearing in clusters. Leg movements occurred significantly more often in the Down group than in the comparison group. Sleep technicians also described frequent and abrupt changes in body positions as well as awkward sleeping positions in the subjects with DS. They reported patients sleeping in a sitting position in bed or resting the legs straight up against the wall [7].

More recently, Senthilvel et al. compared sleep characteristics of a group of DS patients to those of controls that underwent PSG for suspected sleep apnea; no significant differences could be demonstrated in total sleep time, sleep efficiency, REM time, mean O_2 saturation, O_2 nadir, total AHI, arousal index, number of position changes, or percentage of time spent in each sleep position [8].

Whereas OSA in healthy children is usually caused by adenoidal and/or tonsillar hypertrophy, several clinical features may exist in DS that potentially lead to sleep-disordered breathing (SDB) or OSA. These features do not necessarily all affect every child with the syndrome, and if present, the effect on sleep may be somewhat varying in intensity.

The upper airway may be compromised by a relative, rather than absolute, macroglossia [9], glossoptosis, maxillary hypoplasia, underdeveloped midface, pharyngeal crowding by a posteriorly placed tongue, pterygoid and parapharyngeal fat pads, lymphoid hyperplasia, and a generalized hypotonia, also affecting the muscles surrounding the upper airways. Furthermore, children with DS are at increased risk for many comorbidities that could be associated with disrupted sleep such as gastroesophageal reflux disease; laryngo-, tracheo-, or bronchomalacia; obesity; congenital heart disease; pulmonary hypertension; leukemia; ear infections; and scoliosis (e.g., [2, 10]).

Fung et al. studied drug-induced sleep endoscopy results of 23 DS children in a retrospective case-control study. As compared to age-, gender-, and BMI percentile-matched peers, DS patients manifested significantly less adenoidal obstruction but more pharyngeal and lingual collapse. This is consistent with inherent hypotonia and possibly relative macroglossia [10].

Therapeutic Options for OSA in DS

The most commonly identified risk factor for OSA in otherwise healthy children is adenotonsillar hypertrophy; the primary treatment is adenotonsillectomy [11]. To assess the effect of early adenotonsillectomy as compared to watchful waiting on cognition, behavior, quality of life, and polysomnographic findings in school-age children with the obstructive sleep apnea syndrome, Marcus et al. recently conducted a multicenter, single-blind, randomized, controlled trial. Although no significant differences in change from baseline values in attention and executive function scores could be demonstrated between groups, polysomnographic findings normalized in a larger proportion of children in the early adenotonsillectomy group than in the control group (79 % and 46 %, respectively). In addition in the surgical group, there were significantly greater improvements in behavioral and quality of life findings. Besides, symptoms of OSAS as measured by PSQ-SRDB and the Epworth Sleepiness Scale and PedsQL and OSA-18 were significantly more reduced in the surgical than the watchful waiting group [12].

Results of adenotonsillectomy in DS are markedly worse. Shete et al. studied pre- and post-adenotonsillectomy polysomnography parameters in 11 DS patients and found a total AHI improvement in the DS group that, although significant, was not as marked as in a control group of non-DS patients. In fact, 73 % of DS patients required further treatment, being either CPAP, BiPAP, or nocturnal oxygen for residual OSA [13]. Likewise, in the group of DS children studied by Marcus et al., polysomnograms improved in all of eight children who underwent tonsillectomy and adenoidectomy but normalized in only three [4].

Lingual tonsils may play an important role in the coming about of persistent OSA after adenotonsillectomy in DS children. Enlarged lingual tonsils were found using cine MRI in 35 % of DS patients with persistent OSA despite previous surgery [14].

Treatment of OSA in general includes CPAP, oral device therapy, and surgery. Although exact data are lacking, it is a clinical reality that the compliance of CPAP in children with DS is often low. Oral device therapy in small children is not possible and only becomes an option after approximately 12 years of age, and here low compliance remains a concern as well. In case of failure of surgery for adenotonsillar hypertrophy, the surgical therapeutic armamentarium in children with DS is much smaller than in adults. Surgical interventions, such as tracheostomy, mandibular distraction osteotomy, genioglossus advancement, rapid maxillary advancement, lingual tonsillectomy, tongue reduction, hyoid advancement or suspension, uvulopalatopharyngoplasty, tonsillar pillar application, and laryngotracheoplasty, should be performed with the most reluctance in growing children [15]. A new development in general is neuromodulation, stimulation of the hypoglossal nerve. Results in adults are promising [16]. In theory, this intervention could be of value in children with DS, because of the combination of relative macroglossia and hypotonia. The treatment is patient friendly, causing little pain, and the device can be activated with a time delay by parents or other caregivers. The costs, however, are high. So far, hypoglossal nerve stimulation has not been investigated in children with DS.

When considering surgery in DS patients, the high risks of complications should always be carefully weighed against the expected benefits of the intervention.

To ascertain the risks of postoperative complications when performing adenoidectomy and tonsillectomy in patients with DS, Goldstein et al. performed a retrospective review of medical records over a 10-year period of time in a tertiary children's hospital.

During tonsillectomies and adenoidectomy, there is a significantly higher amount of estimated intraoperative blood loss in Down patients as compared to controls. Moreover, anesthetic complications (such as postextubation stridor, upper airway obstruction, laryngospasm, and apnea) occurred significantly more often in the DS group. Postoperative respiratory complications requiring intervention occurred five times more often in the DS group. The length of hospitalization was significantly increased in the DS group, and as many as 25 % of DS patients were admitted to the pediatric intensive care unit postoperatively. Significantly more controls were discharged from the same-day surgery unit. During the postoperative course, the time to recover from incisional pain was longer in the DS group, as was the median time until intake of clear liquids, the median duration of intravenous therapy, and the median time until out of bed [17].

Furthermore, it should be taken into account that induction of anesthesia may worsen some of the previously described features in DS, such as hypotonia, predisposing patients for complications. Intubation of DS patients may be difficult due to the presence of laryngeal or tracheal stenosis, both of which have an increased incidence in the population. Besides, atlantoaxial instability is probably present in 10–20 % of the Down population. For this reason, hyperextension and hyperflexion should be prevented, both during intubation and surgery.

Finally, maintaining a steady anesthetized state in pediatric DS patients may be difficult due to frequently occurring comorbidities such as an increased pulmonary vascular resistance secondary to cardiac disease.

The increased risk of postoperative complications in DS patients even in relative "straightforward" surgery such as adenotonsillectomy as well as the lower success rates for solving OSA by adenotonsillectomy and low compliance to CPAP in this population warrants the search for alternative therapeutic options in this vulnerable group of patients.

Even more so, when we take into consideration:

1. The fact that the 1-year survival of live births with DS (especially in babies with cardiovascular malformations) has increased dramatically over the last 20 years, reaching almost 100 % [18], means that more patients will reach the age at which OSA in this population might lead to a range of adverse effects.
2. The fact that successful treatment of OSA may result in beneficial effects on cardiovascular, pulmonary, and urologic disease as well as on cognition and psychiatric disorders such as depression.

   For example, OSAS may cause chronic intermittent hypoxemia and respiratory acidosis, leading to pulmonary hypertension and eventually cor pulmonale and congestive heart failure. Early intervention might reverse this pathway and serious cardiovascular sequelae may be prevented.

Positional OSA in DS

Disturbed sleep is a common feature in DS and DS patients have been reported to assume uncommon sleep positions (see previously).

In 2011 Senthilvel et al. first described a peculiar body position assumed by some DS children during sleep. Nine out of 17 DS patients described in the paper spent a proportion of their total sleep time sitting crossed legged, torso flopped forward. Although no significant differences could be demonstrated in percentage of time spent in each sleep position, there seemed to be a tendency for DS patients to spend a larger percentage of total sleep time in supine position ($p=0.06$). Interestingly, however, AHI in DS children was lowest in prone and the previously described leaning forward position as compared to other body positions [8]. As was previously suggested for obese pediatric patients [19], adopting the prone or leaning forward position may promote upper airway patency.

A nationwide surveillance about the relationship between sleeping posture and symptoms of SDB among patients with DS in Japan was performed in 2012 by Sawatari et al. 75 % of caregivers who filled out the questionnaire reported unusual sleep positions, and significantly more so in younger than older patients [20] (data presented at X world congress on sleep apnea, Rome 2012). In addition, Rahmawati et al. recorded pulse oximetry in a group of 13 Japanese DS patients and found that peculiar sleep positions in these patients significantly improved the nocturnal desaturation index. The patients assuming the peculiar positions tended to be of younger age than those who did not [21] (data presented at X world congress on sleep apnea, Rome 2012).

To study the effect of body position on OSA in pediatric DS patients, we did a retrospective chart study.

We performed 21 PSGs in 12 DS patients under 20 over a period of 2 years and 5 months (see Table 1). The male to female ratio in our population was 5:7. Ages ranged from 2 years and 8 months to 19 years and 7 months.

OSA (AHI>1) was found in 17/24 (71 %) polysomnographies and in 10/12 (83 %) children. In only two of our DS children OSA could not be demonstrated. One was a girl of Mediterranean descent; she was tested at 2 years and 8 months and at 4 years and 1 month of age. The other was a Caucasian boy; he was tested at the age of 6 years and 1 month.

Central apneas and PLMs were rare.

Pre- and post-adenotonsillectomy PSGs were available in two patients. In patient 3, the AHI improved from being 6.7 preoperatively to 4.8 postoperatively. In patient 8, however, AHI increased dramatically from 8.7 preoperatively to 28.4 postoperatively.

Information on sleep position was available in 66.7 % of patients; in this group 100 % of parents/caretakers reported abnormal sleeping positions, such as the previously described “legs crossed, torso flopped forward position”, but also a baby-like position, with the knees pulled up toward the armpits and the torso leaning forward, and a sitting position (see Fig. 1).

Table 1 Patient characteristics and PSG outcomes

Pat	G	Etn	Age (y, m)	His	BMI	AHI	AHI s	% s	AHI ns	% ns	Pos	Abnpos	C	PLM
1	F	med	3, 3	Blank	19.4	18.7	31.9	49.8	7.1	50.2	+	u.	2.2	3.7
2	F	med	2, 8	Blank	17.8	0.2	0.3	65.2	0	34.8	+	u.	0.2	0
			4, 10	A	n.a.	0.4	0.2	62.1	0.7	37.9	–		0.2	2.4
3	F	cre	4, 0	Blank	16.3	0.7	1.6	45.1	0	51.9	+	+(b)	0	n.a.
			5, 3	Blank	16.5	6.7	6.9	81.3	4.8	18.8	–		0	0
			5, 5	AT	16.5	4.8	1.8	14	n.a.	86	–		1.1	n.a.
			6, 3	AT	13.9	5	n.a.	0	5	100	u.		0	5.6
4	M	cau	1, 11	A	17.2	15	n.a.	0	15	54.1	u.	u.	0	0
5	F	med	19, 2	AT/rA	31.6	51.2	51.4	100	n.a.	0	u.	u.	0.2	0.8
			19, 7	AT/rA	30.3	37.5	65.7	21.9	29.8	78.1	+		2.8	1.7
6	F	med	10, 2	AT	n.a.	14.8	40.4	14.6	8.6	80.7	+	+	0	1.2
			11, 6	AT	n.a.	6.6	7.2	31	6.1	69	–		6.1	0
7	M	cau	6, 10	Blank	14.5	0.5	1.6	23.9	0.1	75.4	+	+	0	n.a.
8	M	afr	4, 2	Blank	18.3	8.7	n.a.	0	8.7	100	u.	+	0	n.a.
			4, 8	AT	n.a.	28.4	0	0.3	28.6	99.8	u.		0.3	n.a
9	M	cau	10, 10	A	17.8	2	n.a.	0.2	2	99.8	u.	+	0	0.9
10	M	cau	14, 9	AT/TR	18	19.4	25.4	52.1	25.1	47.9	–	+ (s)	0.9	4
11	F	med	4, 5	Blank	17	12.2	58.6	17.2	1.1	82.8	+	+	0	5.2
			4, 8	SPT	16	27.5	29.7	48.8	26.1	51.2	–		2	6.7
12	F		5, 2	AT	n.a.	2.2	5.9	25.6	1.2	74.4	+	+	0.1	0.5
			5, 5	SPT	15	5.1	3.1	19.5	5.6	80.5	–		0.2	n.a.

Pat patient, *G* gender, *Etn* ethnicity, *Age* (*y*, *m*) age (years, months), *His* medical history, *BMI* body mass index, *AHI* apnea-hypopnea index, *s* supine, *% s* % of total sleep time spent in supine position, *ns* non-supine, *% ns* % of total sleep time spent in non-supine position, *Pos* positional OSA, *Abnpos* abnormal sleep position as reported by parents and/or caregivers, *C* central apneas, *PLM* periodic limb movements, *SPT* sleep position trainer, *F* female, *M* male, *med* Mediterranean, *cre* creole, *cau* Caucasian, *afr* African, *A* adenoidectomy, *AT* adenoidectomy and tonsillectomy, *rA* re-adenoidectomy, *TR* tongue reduction. *n.a.* not available, *u.* unknown (due to % AHI >90 % or <10 %), (*b*) baby-like position, legs pulled up and torso leaning forward, (*s*) sitting

OSA was positional in 5/21 PSGs and non-positional in 6/21. In 6/21, we were unable to classify OSA as positional or non-positional due to the fact that over 90 % of total sleep time was spent in either supine or non-supine position. In two PSGs, OSA criteria were not met due to a low AHI in non-supine position (patient 3 at age 4.0 and patient 7).

In some patients, the AHI in prone position was notably lower than in supine or overall non-supine position. The most distinct example of this is to be found in the second PSG of patient 5 (AHI supine, 65.7; AHI non-supine, 29.8; and AHI prone, 3.5). In these cases, there seemed to be a protective effect from being in prone position during sleep (see Table 2).

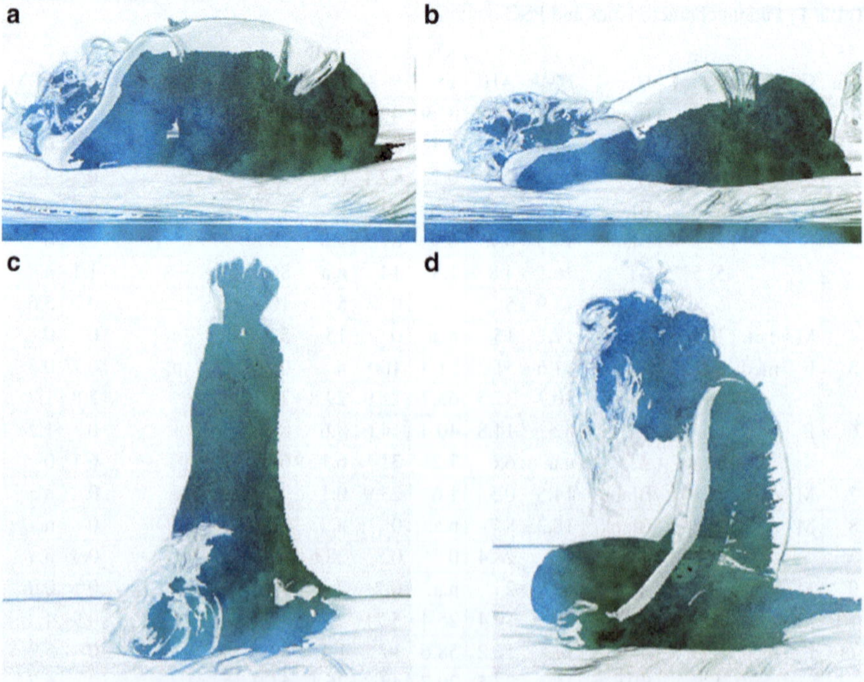

Fig. 1 Sleep positions frequently reported in DS. Panel (**a**) Crossed legged, torso flopped forward. Panel (**b**) "Baby position," knees pulled up toward armpits, torso leaning forward. Panel (**c**) Legs leaning up against the wall. Panel (**d**) Sitting position

We conclude that positional OSA in DS children is a common disorder. The health benefits that result from controlling OSA in this vulnerable group of patients, with high perioperative risks of complications, can be immense. Even considering the fact that SPT training in this population may take longer than in otherwise healthy patients, we feel that in selected DS patients, PT may be a promising non-invasive therapeutic option.

Table 2 PSG positional data

Pat	G	Age (y, m)	His	Abnpos	Pos	AHI	AHI s	% s	AHI ns	% ns	AHI p	% p
1	F	3, 3	Blank	u.	+	18.7	31.9	49.8	7.1	50.2	7.1	40.5
2	F	2, 8	Blank	u.	+	0.2	0.3	65.2	0	34.8	n.a.	0
		4, 10	A		–	0.4	0.2	62.1	0.7	37.9	n.a.	0
3	F	4, 0	Blank	+ (b)	+	0.7	1.6	45.1	0	51.9	0	25.4
		5, 3	Blank		–	6.7	6.9	81.3	4.8	18.8	12.3	1.1
		5, 5	AT		–	4.8	1.8	14	n.a.	86	4.8	32.5
		6, 3	AT		u.	5	n.a.	0	5	100	5.3	94.2
4	M	1, 11	A	u.	u.	15	n.a.	0	15	54.1	0	45.9[a]
5	F	19, 2	AT/rA	u.	u.	51.2	51.4	100	n.a.	0	n.a.	0
		19, 7	AT/rA		+	37.5	65.7	21.9	29.8	78.1	3.5	20[a]
6	F	10, 2	AT	+	+	14.8	40.4	14.6	8.6	80.7	7.1	39.2[a]
		11, 6	AT		–	6.6	7.2	31	6.1	69	0	7.1[a]
7	M	6, 10	Blank	+	+	0.5	1.6	23.9	0.1	75.4	0.3	35
8	M	4, 2	Blank	+	u.	8.7	n.a.	0	8.7	100	12.4	49.3
		4, 8	AT		u.	28.4	0	0.3	28.6	99.8	26.4	92
9	M	10, 10	A	+	u.	2	n.a.	0.2	2	99.8	3.7	50.6
10	M	14, 9	AT/TR	+ (s)	–	19.4	25.4	52.1	25.1	47.9	14.3	6.5[a]
11	F	4, 5	Blank	+	+	12.2	58.6	17.2	1.1	82.8	1.5	29.1
		4, 8	SPT		–	27.5	29.7	48.8	26.1	51.2	8.1	9.6[a]
12	F	5, 2	AT	+	+	2.2	5.9	25.6	1.2	74.4	0	14.7[a]
		5, 5	SPT		–	5.1	3.1	19.5	5.6	80.5	2.9	21.1[a]

[a]Patients with AHI prone < AHI supine

References

1. http://www.cdc.gov
2. Churchill SS, Kieckhefer GM, Landis CA, Ward TM. Sleep Med Rev. 2012;16(5):477–88.
3. Marcus CL, Omlin KJ, Basinki DJ, Bailey SL, Rachal AB, Von Pechmann WS, et al. Am Rev Respir Dis. 1992;146(5 Pt 1):1235–9.
4. Marcus CL, Keens TG, Bautista DB, Von Pechmann WS, Ward SL. Pediatrics. 1991;88(1):132–9.
5. Shott SR, Amin R, Chini B, Heubi C, Hotze S, Akers R. Arch Otolaryngol Head Neck Surg. 2006;132(4):432–6.
6. Ng DK, Hui HN, Chan CH, Kwok KL, Chow PY, Cheung JM, Leung SY. Singapore Med J. 2006;47(9):774–9.
7. Levanon A, Tarasiuk A, Tal A. J Pediatr. 1999;134(6):755–60.
8. Senthilvel E, Krishna JJ. Clin Sleep Med. 2011;7(2):158–62.
9. Guimaraes CV, Donnelly LF, Shott SR, Amin RS, Kalra M. Pediatr Radiol. 2008;38(10):1062–7.
10. Fung E, Witmans M, Ghosh M, Cave D, El-Hakim H. J Otolaryngol Head Neck Surg. 2012;41(2):138–44.
11. Marcus CL, Brooks LJ, Draper KA, Gozal D, Halbower AC, Jones J, et al. Am Acad Pediatr. 2012;130(3):e714–55.

12. Marcus CL, Moore RH, Rosen CL, Giordani B, Garetz SL, Taylor HG, et al. N Engl J Med. 2013;368(25):2366–76.
13. Shete MM, Stocks RM, Sebelik ME, Schoumacher RA. Int J Pediatr Otorhinolaryngol. 2010;74(3):241–4.
14. Fricke BL, Donnelly LF, Shott SR, Kalra M, Poe SA, Chini BA, Amin RS. Pediatr Radiol. 2006;36(6):518–23.
15. Rosen D. Curr Opin Pulm Med. 2011;17(6):431–6.
16. Strollo Jr PJ, Sooze RJ, Maurer JT, de Vries N, et al. Upper airway stimulation for obstructive sleep apnea. N Engl J Med. 2014;370(2):139–49.
17. Goldstein NA, Armfield DR, Kingsley LA, Borland LM, Allen GC, Post JC. Arch Otolaryngol Head Neck Surg. 1998;124(2):171–6.
18. Irving C, Basu A, Richmond S, Burn J, Wren C. Eur J Hum Genet. 2008;16(11):1336–40.
19. Dayyat E, Maarafeya MM, Capdevila OS, Kheirandish-Gozal L, Montgomery-Downs HE, Gozal D. Pediatr Pulmonol. 2007;42(4):374–9.
20. Sawatari et al. Presented at X world congress on sleep apnea, Rome; 2012.
21. Rahmawati et al. Presented at X world congress on sleep apnea, Rome; 2012.

Positional OSA in the Morbidly Obese and the Effect of Weight Loss on OSA Severity

Sharon Morong, Linda B.L. Benoist, and Nico de Vries

Introduction

Obesity has been shown to be a significant risk factor for OSA [1], yet screening for OSA in morbidly obese patients undergoing bariatric surgery is rarely performed. A study by Ravesloot et al. reported that approximately 70 % of patients undergoing bariatric surgery are diagnosed with OSA [2]. In this chapter we will discuss the prevalence of POSA in patients undergoing bariatric surgery and the influence of bariatric surgery on POSA. Furthermore, BMI, neck circumference, AHI, and age as predictors for POSA will be evaluated.

This chapter is a modified version of the article "The effect of weight loss on OSA severity and position dependence in the bariatric population." The final publication is available at link.springer.com.

S. Morong, M.D., M.Sc., F.R.C.S.C. (✉)
Department of Otolaryngology, Sint Lucas Andreas Ziekenhuis,
Jan tooropstraat 164, Amsterdam 1061 AE, The Netherlands
e-mail: sharon.morong@gmail.com

L.B.L. Benoist, M.D.
Ear Nose and Throat, Sint Lucas Andreas Ziekenhuis, Amsterdam, The Netherlands

N. de Vries, M.D., Ph.D.
Department of Otolaryngology, Sint Lucas Andreas Ziekenhuis,
Jan tooropstraat 164, Amsterdam 1061 AE, The Netherlands

Department of Otolaryngology, University Hospital Antwerp, Antwerp, Belgium

N. de Vries et al. (eds.), *Positional Therapy in Obstructive Sleep Apnea*,
DOI 10.1007/978-3-319-09626-1_17

Positional OSA

Studies looking more closely at OSA have reported that a subset of the general population of OSA patients is in fact position dependent. Cartwright's criteria defined a patient as having positional OSA (POSA) if the apnea-hypopnea index (AHI) in the supine position was at least twice as high as that in a non-supine position [3]. Approximately 53–56 % of OSA patients in the general population have POSA [4–6]. Another article looking specifically at the Asian population found the prevalence to be even higher at 67 % [7]. Oksenberg et al. found a correlation between the presence and absence of POSA in a general population of patients who lost or gained weight respectively [8]. Based on these findings, the authors hypothesize that the prevalence of POSA will be lower in obese patients undergoing bariatric surgery when compared with the general population and that a significant increase in POSA would be seen after bariatric surgery once these patients have lost weight.

Methods

A retrospective study was performed with data collected from a cohort of consecutive patients who were screened for OSA pre- and post-bariatric surgery from August 2008 to November 2012.

Patients were eligible for bariatric surgery if they were able to meet the International Federation for the Surgery of Obesity (IFSO) criteria. This criteria included patients aged 18–65 years and BMI from 35 kg/m^2 with associated comorbidity, i.e., hypertension, diabetes, OSA, or joint problems [2]. All patients who met the inclusion criteria for surgery were also screened for sleep-disordered breathing during preoperative workup. This diagnostic workup consisted of a visit to the otolaryngology clinic for a medical history intake, physical examination, and investigations, which included measurements of BMI, neck circumference, and a full overnight polysomnography (PSG).

Inclusion and Exclusion Criteria

Patients were included in the study if the following inclusion criteria were met: PSG was performed in our sleep clinic, a diagnosis of OSA (AHI>5), and supine sleeping position between 10 and 90 % of the total sleep time (TST) [5, 9]. They were excluded if non-supine sleeping positions were found to be less than 10 % of the TST.

Table 1 Patient demographics

Characteristics	Mean ± SD
Age (years)	47.2 ± 9.4
BMI	45.5 ± 7.3
Neck circumference (cm)	43.5 ± 4.8

BMI body mass index, *SD* standard deviation

Table 2 Polysomnographic results

Characteristics	Mean ± SD
Total AHI	31.5 ± 30.1
Desaturation index	31.4 ± 28.6
Sleep efficiency (%)	83.2 ± 11.0
Total sleep time (min)	420.8 ± 87.0

AHI apnea-hypopnea index, *SD* standard deviation

Polysomnography

In accordance with other studies, PSG was performed during an overnight visit in the hospital [2, 9]. Recordings were performed using a digital PSG (Embla A10, Broomfield, CO, USA). A position sensor (SleepSense, St Charles, IL, USA) attached to the midline of the abdominal wall was used to differentiate between supine, right lateral, and left lateral positions.

Definitions

According to the American Academy of Sleep Medicine (AASM), OSA can be classified as mild (AHI 5–14), moderate (AHI 15–30), or severe (AHI >30) [10]. We used Cartwright's definition for POSA where the AHI in supine position is at least two times higher than the non-supine AHI [3].

Results

Prevalence

Three hundred seventy patients were eligible for bariatric surgery, 80 patients were excluded for having only external PSG recordings, and 128 patients were excluded because they did not meet the inclusion criteria. To determine the prevalence of POSA, a total of 162 patients, 43 males and 119 females, with a mean age of 47.2 years (SD ± 9.4) were included in the analysis (Table 1).

Table 2 shows the polysomnographic results. Thirty-four percent (55 patients) had POSA. This was found to be significantly lower ($p < 0.001$) compared to the

Table 3 Comparison of demographics between positional and non-positional OSA patients before bariatric surgery

Characteristics	Positional OSA (n=55, 34.0 %) Mean±SD	Non-positional OSA (n=107, 76.0 %) Mean±SD	Mann–Whitney (p-value)
Age (years)	46.00±9.38	47.79±9.40	0.265
BMI	43.04±5.66	46.71±7.70	0.001
Neck circumference (cm)	41.85±3.75	44.28±5.01	0.006
Total AHI	19.26±15.42	37.82±33.69	<0.001

AHI apnea-hypopnea index, *SD* standard deviation, *OSA* obstructive sleep apnea

Table 4 Comparison of pre- and post-bariatric surgery results

Characteristics	Frequency (%)	Pre-BS (mean±SD)	Post-BS (mean±SD)	Wilcoxon signed ranks (p-value)
Gender				
Male	18 (19.8)			
Female	73 (80.2)			
BMI		45.2±6.7	36.0±5.8	<0.001
Neck circumference (cm)		43.1±4.4	39.5±4.0	<0.001
Total AHI		29.6±27.1	10.3±10.5	<0.001
Desaturation index		27.7±26.0	9.5±9.1	<0.001
Sleep efficiency (%)		84.3±11.3	90.1±8.5	0.001
Total sleep time (min)		418.5±76.8	429.4±64.0	0.052
Total	91			

AHI apnea-hypopnea index, *BMI* body mass index, *BS* bariatric surgery, *SD* standard deviation

53 % prevalence reported in the literature [5]. When comparing positional versus non-positional patients, BMI, neck circumference, and AHI were significantly different among these groups. Positional patients had a significantly lower BMI and neck circumference, and the AHI was lower in this group (Table 3).

Changes Following Bariatric Surgery

Of the 162 patients who underwent surgery, 43 patients were lost to follow-up or failed to obtain a postoperative PSG. Twenty-eight patients were excluded because they did not meet the inclusion criteria following surgery. In the remaining 91 patients, pre- and postsurgery PSG results were compared. There was an average follow-up interval of 7 months (SD±2.0) for PSG recording after surgery. Table 4 summarizes the comparison of both demographic and PSG results before and after surgery. A significant decrease in BMI, neck circumference, total AHI, and desaturation index is seen following surgery with an associated increase in sleep efficiency. These parameters were all improved after bariatric surgery. When looking specifically at BMI

Table 5 Development of POSA following bariatric surgery

	POSA post-BS (%)		
POSA pre-BS (%)	Yes	No	McNemar test exact sig. (2-tailed)
Yes	11 (18.6)	3 (5.1)	
No	26 (44.1)	19 (32.2)	<0.001

after surgery, 88 patients had a decrease of at least 1 point in their BMI, 2 patients had no change, and 1 patient had an increase in BMI. Regression analysis showed that only a low AHI was a significant independent predictor for POSA ($p=0.001$). The Hosmer and Lemeshow Goodness-of-Fit test confirmed the model to be a good fit.

Of the 91 patients included in this cohort, 35.2 % (32 patients) no longer had OSA after surgery. The remaining 64.8 % (59 patients) had either OSA or POSA. Table 5 shows that of these 59 patients, 44.1 % who were originally diagnosed with OSA before surgery developed POSA after surgery. These patients had all significantly lost weight after surgery ($p<0.001$). From the patients who started with POSA, 5.1 % subsequently developed non-positional OSA after surgery and 18.6 % remained positional. The remaining 32 % were initially diagnosed with non-positional OSA and remained non-positional after surgery. A McNemar test showed a significant development of POSA following surgery ($p<0.001$).

Discussion

Prevalence of POSA

The prevalence of POSA was first reported in a large retrospective study by Oksenberg et al. where data from 574 patients were analyzed and 56 % of these patients were found to have POSA [6]. Since then, other studies looking at the prevalence of POSA in the general population have found similar results ranging from 53 % to 60 % [3, 5, 11–13]. In these studies, patients with a higher BMI and AHI were less likely to be positional. We therefore hypothesized that the prevalence of POSA in an obese population would be lower than those reported in the general population above. The prevalence of POSA found in our obese population undergoing bariatric surgery was 34 %. This is significantly lower than the prevalence reported in the general population (53–60 %).

Predictors for POSA

Mador et al. conducted a retrospective chart review in 326 patients and found that POSA was significantly more common in patients with a lower AHI. They also found neck circumference to be significantly smaller in the positional group when compared with the non-positional group. No significant differences were seen in

BMI or age [4]. Teerapraipuk et al. specifically studied an Asian population and also found significantly smaller neck sizes and less severe OSA [measured as respiratory disturbance index (RDI)] in patients with POSA, with no differences seen in age, gender, or BMI [7]. Conflicting data, however, does exist. Oksenberg et al. reported that not only did POSA patients have both a significantly lower BMI and AHI but were significantly younger as well [6]. Sunnergren et al. analyzed data collected from 189 patients with OSA and also found that positional patients had both a significantly lower BMI and AHI than their non-positional counterparts. Neck circumference, however, was not analyzed in this study [5]. In our study, significant differences were seen in neck circumference, BMI, and AHI when comparing our POSA patients with those who were non-positional. Patients with POSA had smaller neck circumferences, lower BMI, and milder OSA (lower AHI). There were no differences, however, noted in age between both groups. Although varying results are seen when looking at the role of age, BMI, and neck circumference in POSA patients, it has been consistently noted that patients with POSA have a lower AHI than non-positional patients. Our study also supports this finding. A logistic regression analysis was performed looking at AHI, age, BMI, and neck circumference as potential predictors for POSA. Only AHI was found to be a significant negative predictor for POSA. The lower the AHI, the more likely that a patient would have POSA.

The Effect of Weight Change on POSA

A retrospective study performed by Oksenberg et al. looked at the relationship between weight change and body posture dominance during sleep in a general population of patients with untreated OSA. Patient data comprised two PSG evaluations that were carried out over a 6.2-year interval. The authors reported that patients who were originally diagnosed with POSA, who then became non-positional over time, had a significant increase in weight and total AHI. Conversely, patients who were originally diagnosed with non-positional OSA that subsequently became positional over time had a decrease in weight and total AHI, but these changes were to a lesser degree when compared with changes seen in patients who had become non-positional. Patients who either remained positional or non-positional over time had minimal changes in weight and AHI [8]. In our study, a significant number of obese patients undergoing bariatric surgery, who were originally diagnosed with non-positional OSA, had a significant decrease in AHI and became positional once surgery was performed and weight was lost.

Considerations

Studies looking at the prevalence of and predictors for POSA provide data for early intervention of this disease. As discussed in other chapters of this volume, positional therapy has been shown to be effective in reducing the AHI, and with the development of newer positional therapy devices, compliance rates have improved significantly over time [9]. Early intervention not only has significant clinical implications for preventing long-term negative cardiovascular outcomes in these patients but may also be cost-effective when comparing positional therapy to treatment options such as continuous positive airway pressure (CPAP), oral devices, and surgery for patients with positional OSA. The main limitation to this study was the loss to patient follow-up, where patients either chose not to return for follow-up or had their polysomnograms performed elsewhere.

Conclusion

The prevalence of POSA in the obese population of patients undergoing bariatric surgery is significantly lower than the prevalence noted in the general population. Although lower BMI, smaller neck circumference, and lower AHI were all found to be significant in the POSA population, a low AHI was the only significant predictor for the presence of POSA. The outcomes of this study can play a very important role in guiding future prospective studies looking at appropriate patient selection criteria for positional therapy.

References

1. Young T, Peppard PE, Taheri S. Excess weight and sleep-disordered breathing. J Appl Physiol. 2005;99(4):1592–9.
2. Ravesloot MJ, van Maanen JP, Hilgevoord AA, van Wagensveld BA, de Vries N. Obstructive sleep apnea is underrecognized and underdiagnosed in patients undergoing bariatric surgery. Eur Arch Otorhinolaryngol. 2012;269(7):1865–71.
3. Cartwright RD. Effect of sleep position on sleep apnea severity. Sleep. 1984;7(2):110–4.
4. Mador MJ, Kufel TJ, Magalang UJ, Rajesh SK, Watwe V, Grant BJ. Prevalence of positional sleep apnea in patients undergoing polysomnography. Chest. 2005;128(4):2130–7.
5. Sunnergren O, Brostrom A, Svanborg E. Positional sensitivity as a confounder in diagnosis of severity of obstructive sleep apnea. Sleep Breath. 2013;17(1):173–9.
6. Oksenberg A, Silverberg DS, Arons E, Radwan H. Positional vs nonpositional obstructive sleep apnea patients: anthropomorphic, nocturnal polysomnographic, and multiple sleep latency test data. Chest. 1997;112(3):629–39.
7. Teerapraipruk B, Chirakalwasan N, Simon R, Hirunwiwatkul P, Jaimchariyatam N, Desudchit T, Charakorn N, Wanlapakorn C. Clinical and polysomnographic data of positional sleep apnea and its predictors. Sleep Breath. 2012;16(4):1167–72.
8. Oksenberg A, Dynia A, Nasser K, Gadoth N. Obstructive sleep apnoea in adults: body postures and weight changes interactions. J Sleep Res. 2012;21(4):402–9.
9. van Maanen JP, Meester KA, Dun LN, Koutsourelakis I, Witte BI, Laman DM, Hilgevoord AA, de Vries N. The sleep position trainer: a new treatment for positional obstructive sleep apnoea. Sleep Breath. 2013;17(2):771–9.
10. Epstein LJ, Kristo D, Strollo Jr PJ, Friedman N, Malhotra A, Patil SP, Ramar K, Rogers R, Schwab RJ, Weaver EM, Weinstein MD, Adult obstructive sleep apnea task force of the

American academy of sleep M. Clinical guideline for the evaluation, management and long-term care of obstructive sleep apnea in adults. J Clin Sleep Med. 2009;5(3):263–76.
11. Akita Y, Kawakatsu K, Hattori C, Hattori H, Suzuki K, Nishimura T. Posture of patients with sleep apnea during sleep. Acta Otolaryngol Suppl. 2003;550:41–5.
12. Pevernagie DA, Shepard Jr JW. Relations between sleep stage, posture and effective nasal CPAP levels in OSA. Sleep. 1992;15(2):162–7.
13. Richard W, Kox D, den Herder C, Laman M, van Tinteren H, de Vries N. The role of sleep position in obstructive sleep apnea syndrome. Eur Arch Otorhinolaryngol. 2006;263(10): 946–50.

The Impact of Body Weight Changes on Body Posture Dominance in Adult Obstructive Sleep Apnea Patients

Arie Oksenberg, Aida Dynia, Khitam Nasser, Vlada Goizman, Edith Eitan, and Natan Gadoth

Introduction

One of the unique phenotypes of obstructive sleep apnea (OSA) patients is related to body posture during sleep.

OSA patients could be divided into *positional patients (PP)*, i.e., OSA patients who have more than twice the number of breathing abnormalities in the supine posture compared with the lateral (right or left) posture, and *non-positional patients (NPP)*, i.e., OSA patients who have a similar amount of breathing disorders in the supine and lateral postures or less than twice apneas and hypopnea in the supine, compared to the lateral position.

In the first large study on this topic on seeking treatment for adult OSA patients, it was found that 55.9 % of all 574 consecutive such patients diagnosed by conventional polysomnography (PSG) were positional [1]. This work was the first to clearly show that the majority of OSA patients have much more breathing abnormalities while sleeping on their back compared to the lateral postures.

In a larger population of 2,077 adult OSA patients evaluated by the same group, it was shown that 54 % were positional. When using a more clinical-oriented definition of OSA, i.e., an apnea-hypopnea index (AHI) > 5 and not AHI > 10, the percentage of PP among the whole cohort of OSA patients was similar (53.8 %) [2]. In this study, 60.4 % and 56.2 % were PP in mild (AHI = 5–15) and moderate (AHI > 15–30) OSA, respectively, compared to 44.9 % in severe (AHI > 30) OSA. Similar findings were also reported by other groups [3, 4].

A. Oksenberg, Ph.D. (✉) • K. Nasser, P.S.G.T. • V. Goizman • E. Eitan • N. Gadoth, M.D.
Sleep Disorders Unit, Loewenstein Hospital – Rehabilitation Center, POB 3, Raanana, Israel
e-mail: arieo@clalit.org.il

A. Dynia, M.A.
Fleischman Unit for the Study of Disability, Loewenstein Hospital – Rehabilitation Center, Raanana, Israel

N. de Vries et al. (eds.), *Positional Therapy in Obstructive Sleep Apnea*,
DOI 10.1007/978-3-319-09626-1_18

In patients with mild to moderate OSA, the prevalence of PP is consistently higher than in severe OSA [1, 2], and since such patients are the prevailing group of subjects with OSA [5], those with positional OSA comprise the vast majority of all OSA patients [1, 6].

Moreover, in an Asian study of 1,170 OSA patients who underwent PSG [7], nearly 75 % were PP, while in mild and moderate OSA, 87 % and 84.2 % were PP. In another Asian study on 263 OSA patients [8], the prevalence of PP reached almost 70 %, and in a study evaluating the effect of positional dependency on outcomes of treatment with mandibular advancement device (MAD) in 100 Korean OSA patients, 80 showed positional dependency [9]. Thus, similar to non-Asians, the majority of Asian OSA patients are positional, and the vast majority of mild OSA patients are also positional.

From all the above, it can be concluded that positional or supine-related OSA is the most dominant phenotype of adult sleep apnea.

The high prevalence of positional OSA in the less severe forms of OSA is of concern since mild OSA patients, especially those with milder or having fewer symptoms, are less likely to use CPAP treatment and comply with it [10]. Therefore, they may be good candidates for positional therapy, i.e., the avoidance of the supine posture during sleep.

Obesity is the most commonly identified but modifiable risk factor for OSA.

The crucial role of weight gain in the progression of snoring and OSA among patients seeking treatment was recently reported [11]. The results of this study were similar to most of the previous studies that have investigated the evolution of snoring and OSA in the general population. Studies on populations such as the Wisconsin Sleep Cohort [12], the Cleveland Family Study [13], and the Sleep Heart Health Study [14] showed that weight gain is a crucial predictor of longitudinal changes in the incidence and severity of sleep-disordered breathing. Although the association between increase in weight and worsening of sleep-disordered breathing is also related to sex, age, race, and ethnic origin, it is clear that weight excess is a critical contributor to the incidence and progression of sleep-related breathing disorder (SRBD), i.e., weight gain has a worsening effect and weight loss a positive effect [12, 14, 15]. Similarly, it seems that weight modulates the body posture effect on SRBD. Indeed, we have described several years ago three obese OSA patients, who refused continuous positive airway pressure (CPAP) treatment but successfully lost weight and were converted from NPP to PP [1]. It seems logical that the opposite can also occur, i.e., weight gain will convert PP into NPP. Unfortunately, there are no data concerning the dynamic changes in positional dominance over time in OSA patients.

As a result of time-related changes, four different groups of OSA patients could be characterized: (1) NPP who remained NPP, (2) PP who remained PP, (3) PP who became NPP, and (4) NPP who became PP.

1. NPP ⟹ NPP
2. PP ⟹ PP
3. PP ⟹ NPP
4. NPP ⟹ PP

This categorization will be used in the present study.

The aim of the present work was to study the relationship between changes in body posture dominance and body weight changes over time in OSA patients. For this purpose we have assessed the demographic and polysomnographic data of non-treated OSA patients who had two complete PSG evaluations during a period of approximately 6 years.

Methods

Participants

This was a retrospective study of 638 patients who underwent two complete PSG evaluations at our sleep disorders unit between April 1998 and March 2010.

Following the first PSG, 72 patients were diagnosed as primary snorers and 566 as OSA patients. The majority of patients received the PSG results during a summary meeting with a sleep specialist during which they were informed about the available therapeutic modalities for their problem. Only few preferred and received the PSG results by mail. Before the second PSG, only 189 (33.4 %) OSA patients received treatment, while 377 (66.6 %) were not treated.

Most of the OSA patients have chosen not to get treatment for the time being, and a few of them decided that treatment was not strictly necessary.

Untreated patients were referred for a reevaluation for various reasons such as to verify objectively their subjective sense of worsening or improvement of symptoms or to reevaluate their condition after several years (without a clear subjective sense of change of symptoms). It should be mentioned that polysomnography is included in our medical services free of charge.

The inclusion criteria for the present research group included adult (≥18 years old) nontreated OSA patients who underwent two complete PSG evaluations separated by at least 6 months who slept at least 30 min in the supine and lateral position during each PSG evaluations. After applying the inclusion criteria and excluding patients with insufficient sleep data and/or missing data, the conduction of a randomized selection of OSA patients with completed data, resulted in a sample of 112 nontreated OSA patients (the research group) (Fig. 1). Twelve (10.7 %) of these patients participated also in our previous study [11]. The entire research group was divided into four subgroups according to the positional dominance change which occurred during the time interval between PSG 1 and PSG 2: NPP who remained NPP; PP who remained PP; patients who became worse, i.e., PP who became NPP; and patients who improved, i.e., NPP at PSG 1 who became PP at PSG 2.

To learn more about the effect of weight changes on positional dominance, the patient's sample was divided into three groups according to the weight changes which occurred between PSG 1 and PSG 2. Patients were assigned to the "weight gain group" if their weight increased more than 3 kg. The "weight loss group"

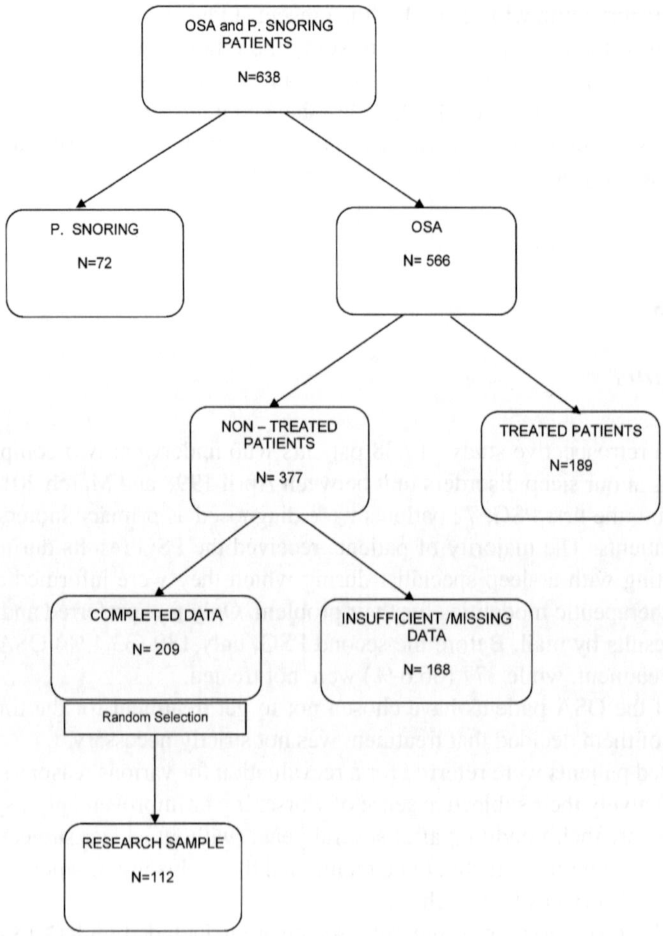

Fig. 1 Flow chart describing the patient's population

consisted of patients who lost more than 3 kg, and patients who had a weight change of 3 kg or less were assigned to the "same weight group." The 3 kg cutoff was based on our clinical experience that even a small increase or decrease in weight could worsen or improve the severity of OSA.

Overnight Polysomnographic Evaluation

Polysomnographic (PSG) recordings were performed with the Rembrandt Manager System (Medcare, Amsterdam, The Netherlands) and included conventional parameters [1]. Sleep stages were scored manually according to the standard criteria [16], by the same polysomnographic technicians during the entire study period.

Apnea was defined as an episode of complete breathing cessation of 10 s or longer, and hypopnea as a reduction in oral/nasal airflow lasting 10 s or longer, accompanied by arousal or by a drop of at least 3 % in SaO_2. The number of apnea + hypopnea events per hours of sleep (apnea-hypopnea index, AHI) [17] was calculated, and severity of OSA was defined as mild for AHI 5–15, moderate for AHI 15–30, and severe for AHI > 30. The Epworth Sleepiness Scale (ESS) [18] was used for the subjective estimation of daytime sleepiness.

The ethical committee of the Loewenstein Hospital Rehabilitation Center approved the study.

Statistical Analysis

Initially, a comparison of the demographic and polysomnographic variables between the four subgroups of OSA patients according to positional dominance at the time of the first and second PSG was performed. Subsequently the same variables were compared in OSA patients who gained weight, who lost weight, and whose weight did not change. For all mentioned parameters, one-way analysis of variance (ANOVA) and Bonferroni adjustment were applied for multiple comparisons. For variables that did not show normal distribution, the nonparametric Kruskal–Wallis one-way analysis of variance was applied. Mann–Whitney U test was used to further explore the difference between groups when the assumption of normality was violated.

The significance level was set at $p \leq 0.05$. Data analysis was performed with the SPSS for Windows, version 15.0. Results are expressed as mean ± SD.

Results

Of the entire research group of OSA patients, 18.8 % were women. The average age was 51.8 ± 10.3 years, the average body mass index (BMI) was 29.9 ± 4.6, and the average AHI was 27.0 ± 19.7. The OSA patient population was first assessed according to body posture dominance.

During an average of 6.2 years of interval between the first and second PSG evaluations, a similar portion of NPP became PP (20, 17.9 %) and PP became NPP (23, 20.5 %). However, the greater portions of the patients were and remained PP (58, 51.8 %) and relatively few were and remained NPP (11, 9.8 %).

Table 1 summarizes the main demographic and polysomnographic characteristics of the four subgroups of OSA patients according to body position dominance at the time of PSG 1.

There was no age difference between the four subgroups of OSA patients. As can be seen in Table 1, patients who were NPP and remained NPP were found initially to be significantly more severely affected than the other three subgroups of OSA patients. Most of those patients had a significant higher body weight, BMI, AHI,

Table 1 Main demographic and polysomnographic (PSG) variables at PSG1 of the four groups of obstructive sleep apnea (OSA) according to changes in body position dominance

	(1) Remained NPP, $n=11$	(2) Remained PP, $n=58$	(3) Became NPP, (worse) $n=23$	(4) Became PP (improved), $n=20$	p^a	Group differences
Age, years	52.9±6.5	52.1±11.2	52.6±7.5	49.2±11.8	N.S.	
Weight, kg	104.4±18.2	82.4±13.3	85.2±14.0	89.6±17.2	0.0001	1≠2* 1≠3* 1≠4*
BMI, kg/m²	34.9±6.2	28.6±3.1	29.5±4.1	31.6±5.8	0.0001	1≠2* 1≠3* 2≠4*
AHI, events per hours of sleep	47.2±28.1	23.5±14.9	22.9±12.2	30.4±26.5	0.012	1≠2** 1≠3** 1≠4**
AHI sup, events per hours of sleep	56.1±35.8	48.6±25.7	49.6±25.5	35.6±27.0	N.S.	
AHI lat, events per hours of sleep	46.1±24.6	9.5±9.6	10.1±7.9	28.1±27.7	0.0001	1≠2** 1≠3** 1≠4** 2≠4** 3≠4**
Snore supine, dB	70.5±7.8	66.0±7.6	69.6±7.5	65.5±7.1 $n=18$	N.S.	
Snore left, dB	63.9±7.6 $n=9$	56.5±10.8 $n=49$	60.6±9.2 $n=20$	60.2±10.4 $n=17$	N.S.	
Snore right, dB	68.4±6.6 $n=10$	58.1±10.8 $n=54$	62.9±8.1 $n=22$	61.3±6.5 $n=16$	0.009	1≠2*
ESS, units	9.8±4.2 $n=4$	10.3±4.8 $n=37$	7.4±4.7 $n=17$	12.7±6.1 $n=14$	0.041	3≠4*
Min SaO_2 REM, %	75.1±8.8	84.7±9.4	84.0±7.1	79.3±14.4	0.013	1≠2** 1≠3**
Min SaO_2 NREM, %	82.8±3.9	85.5±7.0	87.5±5.3	86.6±7.6	0.041	1≠2** 1≠3** 1≠4**

PP—positional patients (OSA patients with more than twice of breathing abnormalities during sleep in the supine posture compared to the lateral posture). NPP—non-positional patients (OSA patients with less than twice the numbers of breathing abnormalities during sleep in the supine compared to the lateral posture). Snore supine, dB—maximum snore loudness at the supine posture. ESS—Epworth Sleepiness Scale [(quite alert) 0–24 (very sleepy)]. Min SaO_2 REM—minimum SaO_2 value during REM sleep. Min SaO_2 NREM—minimum SaO_2 value during NREM sleep. Values are mean±SD

N.S. not significant

*One-way ANOVA post hoc, at $p \leq 0.05$

**Mann–Whitney, at $p \leq 0.05$

[a]Values of $p \leq 0.05$ are from one-way ANOVA post hoc, or Kruskal–Wallis

and lateral AHI (AHI lat) and lower minimum SaO_2 both during REM and NREM sleep, compared to the other subgroups. Although the supine AHI (AHI sup) was also higher in these patients compared to the other groups, the differences did not reach statistical significance.

Although patients who were NPP and remained NPP had a higher maximal snoring loudness in the different body postures than the other three groups, the only significant difference was observed in the right posture compared to PP who remained PP.

Not surprisingly, NPP who improved and became PP had initially a significantly higher Epworth Sleepiness Scale (ESS) value (more sleepy) than PP who became worse and were converted to NPP.

The changes (between PSG 1 and PSG 2) in AHI (total, supine, and lateral) which occurred following the interval between the two PSGs in the four subgroups of OSA patients according to positional dominance are shown in Fig. 2a.

OSA patients who were PP and became NPP showed a major increase in AHI which was significantly different from the other three groups of patients ($p \leq 0.05$). The increased change in AHI of these patients was of 33.1 ± 20.9 events per hours of sleep as compared to a decrease in AHI of only 6.8 ± 24.8 events per hours of sleep in patients who were NPP and became PP. There was no difference in the supine AHI between the four subgroups of OSA patients. This is in contrary to the lateral AHI which was significantly different between the groups ($p \leq 0.05$); PP whose condition worsened and became NPP showed a marked increase in lateral AHI (43.9 ± 19.5) compared to a decrease of 17.2 ± 25.9 in NPP who showed an improvement and became PP.

The weight gain of PP who became NPP was significantly different from the other three groups ($p \leq 0.05$) and more substantial than the weight loss of patients who were NPP and became PP. In patients who remained PP or remained NPP, weight changes were minimal (see Fig. 2b).

Interestingly, the changes in the minimum SaO_2 values during REM sleep were significantly different between the groups ($p \leq 0.05$) (see Fig. 2c). The clearest change occurred in PP who became NPP and had a significant decrease in the minimum SaO_2 value (−11.2 ± 11.9) compared to the relatively small changes present in the other three groups.

Based on these and previous results, and with the aim of learning more about the modulatory effect of weight changes on positional dominance, a similar analysis was performed on three groups of patients, i.e., those who gained weight, lost weight, and maintained a similar weight across time.

Demographic and polysomnographic data obtained at the time of the first PSG study (PSG1), for those three groups of OSA patients according to changes in body weight, are summarized in Table 2.

As shown in the table, patients who lost weight had initially a disease that was significantly more severe in terms of AHI and lateral AHI and a lower minimum SaO_2 value during NREM sleep, than the disease of patients who gained weight and that of the patients with stable weight across time. Although the supine AHI was also higher in the first group compared to the others, the differences did not reach statistical significance.

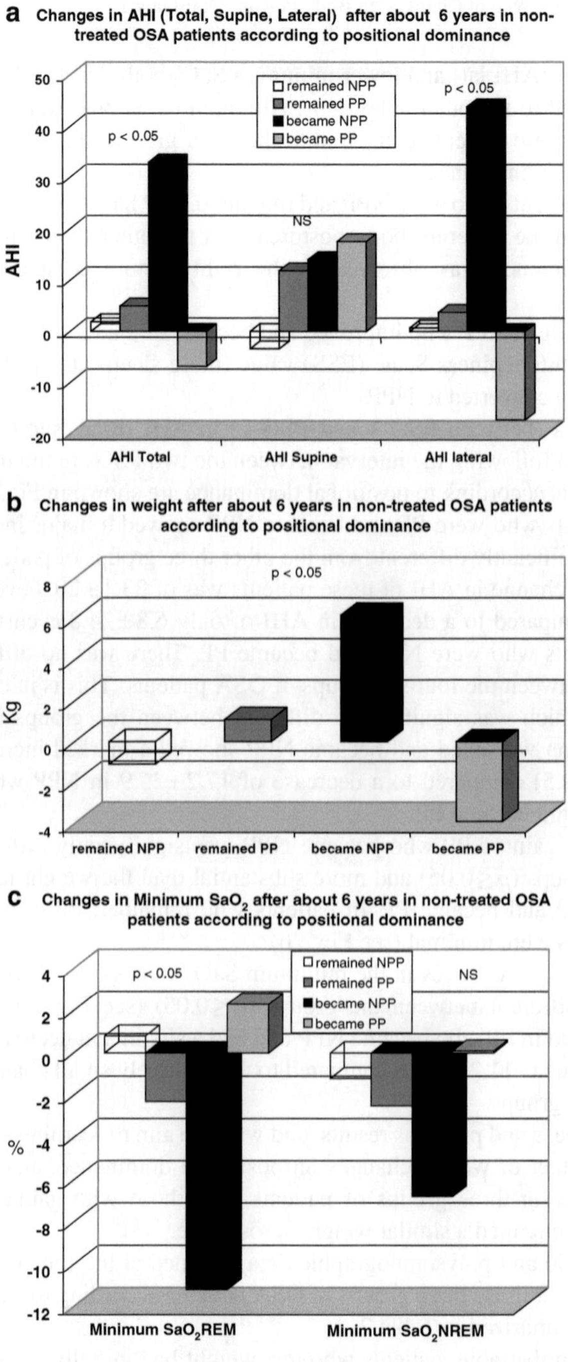

Fig. 2 Changes over time in (**a**) AHI, (**b**) body weight, and (**c**) minimum SaO_2. According to changes in positional dominance in four groups of nontreated OSA patients who had two PSG evaluations about 6 years apart. PP—positional patients; NPP—non-positional patients. Remained NPP (1); remained PP (2); became NPP (3); became PP (4). (**a**) AHI total: $p \leq 0.05$ (1)≠(3); (2)≠(3); (3)≠(4). AHI lateral $p \leq 0.05$ (1)≠(3); (2)≠(3); (2)≠(4); (3)≠(4). (**b**) Body weight: $p \leq 0.05$ (1)≠(3); (2)≠(3); (2)≠(4); (3)≠(4). (**c**) Minimum SaO_2 REM: $p \leq 0.05$ (1)≠(2); (1)≠(3); (2)≠(3); (3)≠(4)

Table 2 Main demographic and PSG variables at PSG 1 of the three groups of OSA patients according to changes in body weight

	(1) Weight gain, $n=42$	(2) Same weight, $n=46$	(3) Weight loss, $n=24$	p^a	Group differences
Age, years	49.4±8.9	52.2±10.3	55.2±11.6	N.S.	
Weight, kg	89.4±15.4	81.3±14.0	90.9±18.1	0.016	1≠2* 2≠3*
BMI, kg/m²	30.2±4.1	29.0±4.0	31.3±6.2	N.S.	
AHI, events per hours of sleep	24.5±18.0	23.6±18.7	37.7±21.2	0.001	1≠3** 2≠3**
AHI sup, events per hours of sleep	46.3±28.1	45.1±28.8	52.7±22.7	N.S.	
AHI lat, events per hours of sleep	12.3±16.1	15.5±18.2	26.1±25.4	0.004	1≠3** 2≠3**
Snore supine, dB	69.4±6.7 $n=41$	64.7±8.3 $n=45$	67.6±6.8	0.014	1≠2*
Snore left, dB	61.0±11.5 $n=36$	56.3±8.9 $n=40$	59.6±10.1 $n=19$	N.S.	
Snore right, dB	61.0±10.9 $n=39$	59.1±9.3 $n=41$	62.9±8.6 $n=22$	N.S.	
ESS, units	9.3±4.8 $n=25$	9.8±5.9 $n=32$	11.8±4.4 $n=15$	N.S.	
Min SaO_2 REM, %	84.9±7.8	82.9±11.2	78.3±11.7	N.S.	
Min SaO_2 NREM, %	86.5±6.0	86.9±6.4	82.7±7.1	0.011	1≠3** 2≠3**

Values are mean±SD. See explanation for abbreviations in the legend of Table 1
N.S. not significant
*One-way ANOVA post hoc, at $p \leq 0.05$
**Mann–Whitney, at $p \leq 0.05$
[a]Values of $p \leq 0.05$ are from one-way ANOVA post hoc, or Kruskal–Wallis

There were no significant age differences between the three groups of patients, but the initial body weight of the three groups of patients was significantly different. Patients who gained weight and those who lost weight had similar body weight that was significantly higher than the body weight of patients who kept a stable weight. However, the BMI comparison did not reveal significant differences between the groups.

The ESS and the maximal snoring intensity were not significantly different in the three groups, except for a higher mean snoring intensity in the supine posture in the patients who gained weight than that of patients with a stable weight.

Although OSA patients who succeed to lose weight showed at the time of the first PSG a lower minimum SaO_2 values during REM sleep compared to the other two groups of patients, the differences between the groups reached statistical significance only for the differences in minimum SaO_2 values during NREM sleep.

Figure 3a shows the changes (between PSG 1 and PSG 2) of AHI (total, supine, and lateral) which occurred during the interval between the two evaluations for the three groups of OSA patients according to changes in body weight.

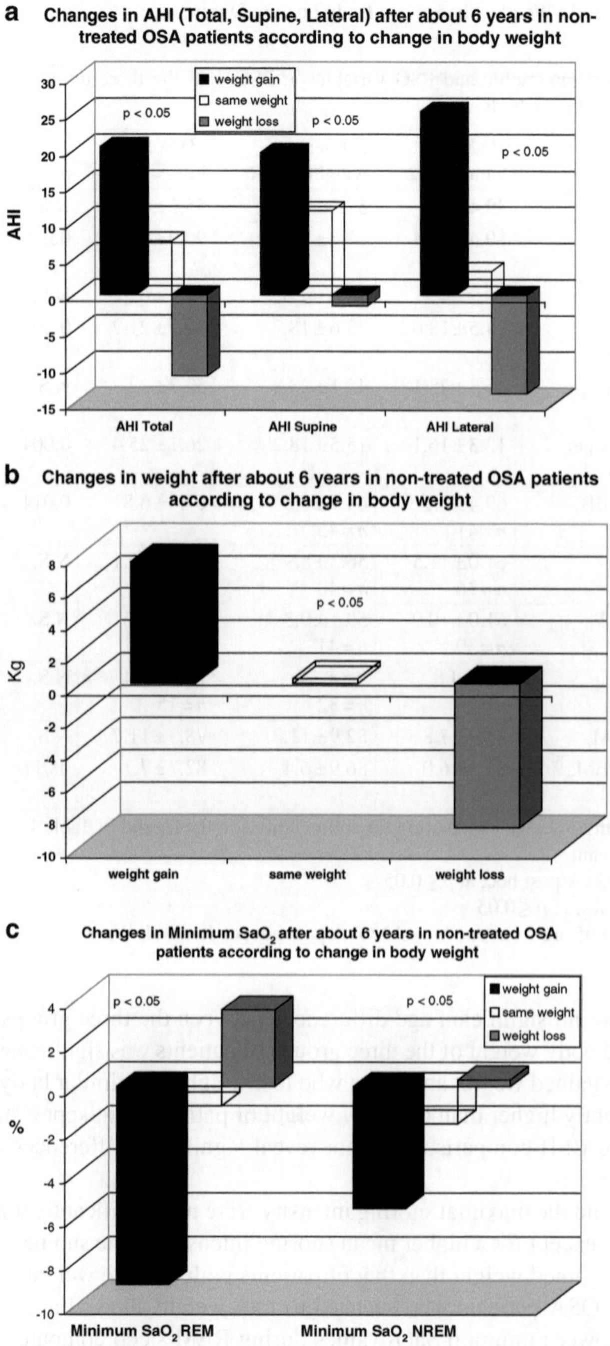

Fig. 3 Changes over time in (**a**) AHI, (**b**) body weight, and (**c**) minimum SaO_2. According to changes in body weight in three groups of nontreated OSA patients who had two PSG evaluations about 6 years apart. Weight gain (1); same weight (2); weight loss (3). (**a**) AHI total: $p \leq 0.05$ (1) ≠ (2); (1) ≠ (3); (2) ≠ (3). AHI supine: $p \leq 0.05$ (1) ≠ (3). AHI lateral: $p \leq 0.05$ (1) ≠ (2); (1) ≠ (3); (2) ≠ (3). (**b**) Body weight: $p \leq 0.05$ (1) ≠ (2); (1) ≠ (3); (2) ≠ (3). (**c**) Minimum SaO_2 REM: $p \leq 0.05$ (1) ≠ (2); (1) ≠ (3). (**c**) Minimum SaO_2 NREM: $p \leq 0.05$ (1) ≠ (2); (1) ≠ (3)

The severity of the disease as expressed by AHI increased in patients who gained weight (+20.5 ± 21.5 units) and decreased in patients who succeeded to lose weight (−11.2 ± 19.4 units) ($p \leq 0.05$). In addition, weight gain was associated with an increase in both supine and lateral AHI, while weight loss was associated with a decrease in lateral AHI ($p \leq 0.05$), but only a minor decrease in supine AHI.

After an average interval of about 6 years, patients who gained weight had an average increase of 7.5 ± 3.9 kg, while patients who lost weight had an average decrease of 8.9 ± 5.5 kg (see Fig. 3b). Weight gain was also associated with a decrease in the oxygen saturation during both REM and NREM sleep in comparison to the two other groups ($p \leq 0.05$). Again, the worsening effect of weight gain in terms of minimum SaO_2 during REM and NREM sleep was more prominent than the improvement effect of weight loss on these parameters (see Fig. 3c).

Thus, consistent with previous published data, weight gain was associated with a more striking increase in disease severity than the improvement of the disease associated with weight loss [14].

It is important to mention that OSA patients who did not show a change in body weight at the second PSG evaluation had only a small increase in disease severity, as expressed by the increased AHI, especially the supine AHI. This result is perhaps related to the passage of time as a risk factor for OSA worsening [11].

There were no significant differences in the supine total sleep time and in the percentage of supine total sleep time between the four subgroups of OSA which were formed according to body position dominance as well as between the three subgroups formed according to body weight changes (data not showed).

Discussion

The main findings of this study are related to the interaction between changes in body weight and their association with changes in positional dominance in non-treated OSA patients. To the best of our knowledge, this issue has not been previously reported. Moreover, the analysis of four groups of OSA patients, according to changes related to positional dominance, is an innovative approach to document and further understand the interactions between body posture and weight changes.

Positional patients (PP) who became non-positional patients (NPP) had a significant gain in weight and a significant increase in AHI, mainly in lateral AHI. On the contrary, NPP who became PP had a significant decrease in weight (but less than the increase in weight of PP who became NPP) and showed a significant improvement in AHI, mainly in the lateral AHI. The NPP who became PP had initially a less severe disease in terms of AHI, lateral AHI, and minimum SaO_2 during NREM sleep and were less obese than NPP who remained NPP. NPP who remained NPP had initially a more severe disease showing higher AHI and lateral AHI and lower minimum SaO_2 in both REM and NREM sleep than the rest of the OSA patients. Weight and BMI were also significantly higher in this particular group. After several years these patients showed only minor insignificant changes in body weight and in distinct parameters of OSA severity such as AHI, lateral and supine AHI, and minimum SaO_2 during NREM and REM sleep.

These data suggest that in adult OSA patients changes in body weight appear to modulate the body posture effect on breathing abnormalities during sleep, affecting several breathing parameters mainly the lateral AHI.

Clinical Implications

This study highlights at least two important clinical implications for OSA patients:

1. NPP who suffered from a severe disease and cannot adhere to CPAP may become PP after losing weight. Initiation and maintenance of positional therapy (i.e., the avoidance of the supine posture during sleep) may result in major improvement in their sleep quality as well as quality of life and general health.
2. On the contrary, PP who gain weight may become NPP. Therefore, for them CPAP is the treatment of choice since positional therapy is insufficient to overcome their OSA severity. These results indicate that PP who have a tendency to gain weight should be encouraged to watch their weight carefully, and this should be followed up by their personal physician.

If a PP who is using successfully positional therapy is beginning to feel sleepier during daytime hours, it is possible that he/she gained weight and now is having also breathing abnormalities while sleeping in the lateral position. A new PSG evaluation is necessary, and if this is the case, CPAP treatment should be suggested.

The effect of weight gain and weight loss on the progression and regression of sleep-disordered breathing (SDB) was previously assessed in a large multiethnic cohort of middle-aged and older men and women, across the United States—the Sleep Heart Health Study [14]. These individuals had two portable sleep assessments about 5 years apart. It was found that weight loss was associated with less regression of SDB than the association of weight gain with progression of SDB, mainly in women but also in men.

Similarly, in the present study, we have found that weight loss was associated with a relatively small decrease in AHI and lateral AHI but with almost no change in supine AHI. On the contrary, weight gain of only a few kilograms was associated with a large increase in AHI and both lateral and supine AHI. The parameter that appeared to be more sensitive to the changes in body weight in OSA patients was the lateral AHI.

What could be the possible mechanism responsible for the modulatory effect of weight on body position in patients with sleep-related breathing abnormalities?

The precise mechanism by which weight gain and weight loss affect the positional dominance in OSA patients is still unknown. A possible explanation which may provide some insight into this issue could be the differences in volume of the soft tissue and the three-dimensional size of the craniofacial structures of the pharyngeal airway between positional and non-positional OSA patients. Indeed,

Saigusa et al. [19] showed that the dominant determinant for positional dependency was the volume of the lateral pharyngeal wall, in positional and non-positional OSA patients matched for BMI, age, and AHI. They also found that positional OSA patients in general had a smaller volume of the lateral pharyngeal wall soft tissues.

Thus, based on these results, it may be suggested that an increase or a decrease in the volume or thickness of the lateral pharyngeal wall, due to changes in the amount of fat tissue, is most probably one of the main mechanisms responsible for the conversion of a PP into a NPP and vice versa (see Fig. 4, from Saigusa et al. 2009, with permission).

It has already been shown that OSA patients have abnormally thick lateral pharyngeal wall compromising the pharyngeal lumen during sleep [20]. Therefore, when an OSA patient sleeps in the lateral posture, it is the width of the lateral pharyngeal wall (which fluctuates according to changes in the amount of the surrounding fat tissue) that will determine if the gravitational forces acting on the pharyngeal lumen are sufficient, as it occurs in positional patients, or insufficient, as it occurs in non-positional patients, to prevent the collapse of the pharyngeal space during sleep.

There is a possibility that the quality of sleep has an impact on body posture during sleep and weight change interactions. The deterioration of sleep quality in OSA patients is characterized by a typical pattern of severe sleep fragmentation and ultimately sleep deprivation. This condition may affect the regulation of leptin and ghrelin levels and lead to an increase in hunger and appetite resulting in an increase in caloric intake and consequent increased body weight [21]. Thus, OSA by itself, through a complex metabolic dysregulation, may predispose the worsening of obesity. This fact indicates that the relationship between OSA and obesity is apparently multifaceted and bidirectional [22].

NPP who remained NPP after about 5 years are those patients with the worst sleep quality due to a high amount of breathing abnormalities, but also due to a high degree of obesity which by itself could worsen the nocturnal sleep quality and lead to daytime sleepiness independent of breathing abnormalities [23]. On the other hand, PP enjoy a much better sleep quality (they sleep well in the lateral postures) [1, 2], and this perhaps contributed to the fact that most of the PP remained PP.

What could be the reason that some NPP were unable to improve their condition and remained NPP?

It is possible that the high degree of obesity, and the very poor quality of sleep caused by sleep fragmentation related to severe OSA, produces a condition of chronic physiologic and emotional stress leading to a depression-like state, with lower than required mental and physical energies sufficient to deal with the difficult task of weight loss. In our opinion, those are the OSA patients that should be encouraged to consider seriously the option of bariatric surgery as a good alternative (and perhaps, the only one) for obesity treatment, which will in many cases noticeably improve, although not always resolve, OSA syndrome [24].

Several limitations of this study should be mentioned. The number of patients studied was relatively small, and thus, a corroboration of the present results is necessary by studying a larger population. Also, due to the small number of patients in

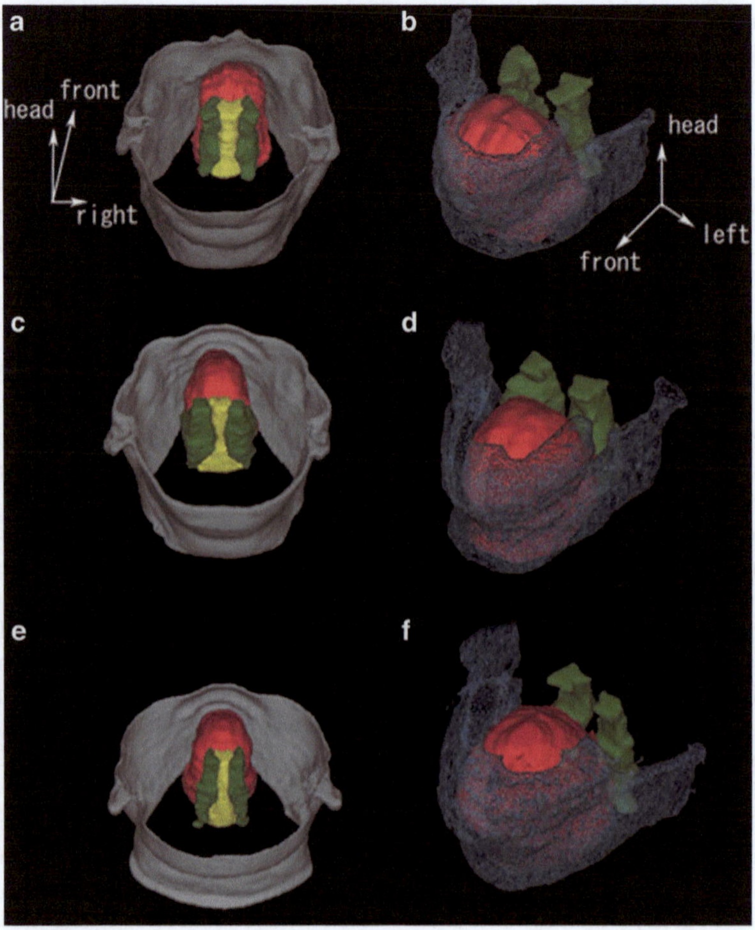

Fig. 4 Three-dimensional magnetic resonance imaging reconstructions of subjects with (**a**, **b**) positional obstructive sleep apnea syndrome (OSAS), (**c**, **d**) non-positional OSAS, and (**e**, **f**) control subjects. (**a**, **c**, **e**) Lateral pharyngeal wall, tongue, and pharyngeal airway with outline of the face, posterosuperior view; (**b**, **d**, **f**) lateral pharyngeal wall, tongue, and craniofacial structures (mandible and lower part of maxilla), anterosuperior left oblique view. *Green*, lateral pharyngeal wall; *red*, tongue; *yellow*, upper airway space; and *blue web*, craniofacial structures. Note that positional OSAS had relatively small volume of the lateral pharyngeal wall and smallest craniofacial volume; non-positional OSAS had relatively large craniofacial volume and largest volume of the lateral pharyngeal wall; the control subjects had the largest craniofacial volume and the smallest volume of the lateral pharyngeal wall. (From Saigusa et al. 2009, with permission)

each group, it was not possible to assess adequately the effect of age and gender on the results. Moreover, it should be stressed that the interaction described between changes in body weight and changes in body posture dominance preclude defining causality between these two parameters. In order to find out the direction of causality between these parameters, it is imperative to carry out a large, prospective, longitudinal study.

In conclusion, the present findings indicate that there is a dynamic interaction between changes in body weight and changes in body posture dominance in OSA patients. Improvement in OSA severity of non-positional patients (NPP) who converted to positional patients (PP) was associated with a decrease in body weight. In contrast, PP conversion into NPP was associated with an increase in body weight and a worsening of OSA. It appears that weight changes have a modulatory effect on positional dominance and that the lateral AHI appears to be a sensitive parameter of these changes.

References

1. Oksenberg A, Silverberg DS, Arons E, Radwan H. Positional vs nonpositional obstructive sleep apnea patients. Anthropomorphic, nocturnal polysomnographic and multiple sleep latency test data. Chest. 1997;112:629–39.
2. Oksenberg A, Arons E, Greenberg-Dotan S, Nasser K, Radwan H. The significance of body posture on breathing abnormalities during sleep: data analysis of 2077 obstructive sleep apnea patients. Harefuah. 2009;148:157–62 (Article in Hebrew).
3. Mador MJ, Kufel TJ, Magalang UJ, Rajesh SK, Watwe V, Grant JB. Prevalence of Positional sleep apnea in patients undergoing polysomnography. Chest. 2005;128:2130–7.
4. Richard W, Kox D, den Herder C, Laman M, van Tinteren H, de Vries N. The role of sleep position in obstructive sleep apnea syndrome. Eur Arch Otorhinolaryngol. 2006;263:946–50.
5. Young T, Palta M, Dempsey J, Skatrud J, Weber S, Badr S. The occurrence of sleep disordered breathing among middle-aged adults. N Engl J Med. 1993;328:1230–5.
6. Oksenberg A, Silverberg DS. Avoiding the supine posture during sleep for patients with mild obstructive sleep apnea. Am J Respir Crit Care Med. 2009;180:101. (letter); author reply 101–2.
7. Mo JH, Lee CH, Rhee CS, Yoon IY, Kim JW. Positional dependency in Asian patients with obstructive sleep apnea and its implication for hypertension. Arch Otolaryngol Head Neck Surg. 2011;137:786–90.
8. Teerapraipruk B, Chirakalwasan N, Simon R, Hirunwiwatkul P, Jaimchariyatam N, Desudchit T, et al. Clinical and polysomnographic data of positional sleep apnea and its predictors. Sleep Breath. 2012;16:1167–72.
9. Lee CH, Jung HJ, Lee WH, Rhee CS, Yoon IY, Yun PY, et al. The effect of positional dependency on outcomes of treatment with a mandibular advancement device. Arch Otolaryngol Head Neck Surg. 2012;138:479–83.
10. Rosenthal L, Gerhardstein R, Lumley A, Guido P, Day R, Syron ML, et al. CPAP therapy in patients with mild OSA: implementation and treatment outcome. Sleep Med. 2000;1:215–20.
11. Berger G, Berger R, Oksenberg A. Progression of snoring and obstructive sleep apnea: the role of increasing weight and time. Eur Respir J. 2009;33:338–45.
12. Peppard PE, Young T, Palta M, Dempsey J, Skatrud J. Longitudinal study of moderate weight changes and sleep disordered breathing. JAMA. 2000;284:3015–21.
13. Redline S, Schluchter MD, Larkin EK, Tishler PV. Predictors of longitudinal change in sleep-disordered breathing in a non-clinic population. Sleep. 2003;26:703–9.
14. Newman AB, Foster G, Givelber R, Nieto FJ, Redline S, Young T. Progression and regression of sleep-disordered breathing with changes in weight: the Sleep Heart Health Study. Arch Intern Med. 2005;165:2408–13.
15. Randerath WJ, Verbraecken J, Andreas S, Bettega G, Boudewyns A, Hamans E, et al. Non CPAP therapies in obstructive sleep apnea. Eur Respir J. 2011;37:1000–28.

16. Rechtschaffen A, Kales A, editors. A manual of standardized terminology techniques and scoring system for sleep stages of human subjects. Los Angeles, CA: Brain Information Service/Brain Research Institute, University of California at Los Angeles; 1968.
17. Guilleminault C, editor. Sleep and breathing in sleeping and waking disorders: indications and techniques. Menlo Park, CA: Addison-Wesley; 1982. p. 155–82.
18. Johns MW. A new method for measuring daytime sleepiness: the Epworth sleepiness scale. Sleep. 1991;14:540–5.
19. Saigusa H, Suzuki M, Higurashi N, Kodera K. Three-dimensional morphological analyses of positional dependence in patients with obstructive sleep apnea syndrome. Anesthesiology. 2009;110:885–90.
20. Schwab RJ, Pasirstein M, Pierson R, Mackley A, Hachadoorian R, Arens R, et al. Identification of upper airway anatomic risk factors for obstructive sleep apnea with volumetric magnetic resonance imaging. Am J Respir Crit Care Med. 2003;168:522–30.
21. Spiegel K, Tasali E, Penev P, Van Cauter E. Sleep curtailment in healthy young men is associated with decreased leptin levels, elevated ghrelin levels, and increased hunger and appetite. Ann Intern Med. 2004;141:846–56.
22. Pillar G, Shehadeh N. Abdominal fat and sleep Apnea. The chicken or the egg? Diabetes Care. 2008;31 Suppl 2:S303–9.
23. Vgontzas AN, Bixler EO, Tan TL, Kantner D, Martin LF, Kales A. Obesity without sleep apnea is associated with daytime sleepiness. Arch Intern Med. 1998;158:1333–7.
24. Greenburg DL, Lettieri CJ, Eliasson AH. Effects of surgical weight loss on measures of obstructive sleep apnea: a meta-analysis. Am J Med. 2009;122:535–42.

Positional Central Sleep Apnea

Hennie Janssen, Johan A. Verbraecken, Dirk Pevernagie, and Sebastiaan Overeem

Introduction

As illustrated in this book, the effect of body position in mild to moderately severe obstructive sleep apnea is well known. Much less known—although not less interesting—is the possible positional dependency of central sleep apnea.

Positional dependency in central sleep apnea has not been extensively studied, and research is complicated by the fact that multiple phenotypes of central sleep apnea exist. In the third edition of the International Classification of Sleep Disorders (ICSD-3) [1], eight types of central sleep apnea are listed (Table 1). Although the pathophysiology is heterogeneous, these eight types of central sleep apnea can be divided into two groups, i.e. hypocapnic and hypercapnic forms, or due to hyperventilation or hypoventilation, respectively. Central sleep apnea due to hypoventilation is found in neuromuscular or chest wall disease, in opioid use and in central sleep apnea in infancy. These forms are often mixed with an obstructive component of sleep-disordered breathing, and underlying mechanisms of positional dependency are difficult to unravel. In this chapter we will therefore focus on the role of body position in central sleep apnea due to hyperventilation.

H. Janssen, M.D., Ph.D. (✉) • D. Pevernagie, M.D., Ph.D. • S. Overeem, M.D., Ph.D.
Sleep Medicine Centre, Kempenhaeghe, Heeze, PO Box 61, 5590 AB, The Netherlands
e-mail: janssenhe@kempenhaeghe.nl

J.A. Verbraecken, M.D., Ph.D.
Department of Pulmonary Medicine, Antwerp University Hospital, Edegem, Antwerp, Belgium

Multidisciplinary Sleep Disorders Centre, Antwerp University Hospital, Edegem, Antwerp, Belgium

N. de Vries et al. (eds.), *Positional Therapy in Obstructive Sleep Apnea*,
DOI 10.1007/978-3-319-09626-1_19

Table 1 Central sleep apnea as defined in the international classification of sleep disorders (ICSD-3)

• Central sleep apnea with Cheyne-Stokes breathing
• Central apnea due to a medical disorder without Cheyne-Stokes breathing
• Central sleep apnea due to high altitude periodic breathing
• Central sleep apnea due to a medication or substance
• Primary central sleep apnea
• Primary central sleep apnea of infancy
• Primary central sleep apnea of prematurity
• Treatment-emergent central sleep apnea

Positional Dependency in Central Sleep Apnea Due to Hyperventilation Not Related to Chronic Heart Failure

Clinical Presentation

In CSA due to hyperventilation not related to chronic heart failure, positional dependency has been reported in only a few cases.

Zaharna et al. [2] recently described a 29-year-old male with severe idiopathic central sleep apnea with an apnea-hypopnea index (AHI) of 49.3 per hour and a central apnea-hypopnea index (CAHI) of 42.7 per hour. Positional dependency was present with a supine CAHI of 101.6 per hour in contrast to a right lateral CAHI of 7.1 per hour and left lateral CAHI of 39 per hour. The patient denied any symptoms of an underlying cardiac, renal or neurological condition, and no further diagnostic tests were performed. He was successfully treated with CPAP and he declined positional therapy.

Another case of positional CSA was presented by DelRosso et al. [3]. A 66-year-old man with hypertension complained of excessive daytime sleepiness, dyspnoea upon exertion, episodes of dream-enacting behaviour and tongue biting when sleeping in the right lateral decubitus position. Polysomnography (PSG) revealed severe positional CSA, with predominance in the supine position (187 events) and right lateral decubitus position (35 events), and only 2 events in the left lateral decubitus position. Obstructive events were minimal (6 events). MRI scan of the brain revealed a calcified left vertebral artery that caused compression of the pre-Bötzinger complex in the left anterolateral medulla and patient was treated with BIPAP-ST.

Oksenberg et al. [4] presented a 57-year-old female with both obstructive and central sleep apnea after an ischemic cerebrovascular accident. In this patient the first PSG was performed 2 months post-stroke and revealed severe CSA/CSB in non-REM and a severe OSA pattern during REM sleep, independent of body position (RDI supine 85.2 per hour and lateral 95.4 per hour). After 3 months and overall clinical improvement, a second PSG showed a complete disappearance of breathing abnormalities in the lateral position for both CSB and OSA (RDI 0 per hour) but only a small improvement in supine position (supine RDI 73.2 per hour), with the

CSA/CSB characterized mainly by central hypopneas. Finally, Yaegashi et al. [5] reported a statistically significantly higher total CAHI in supine position during NREM sleep in complex sleep apnea syndrome during the baseline polysomnography, but these data can hardly be considered clinically relevant (2.5 ± 3.1 vs. 0.9 ± 2.3).

Possible Mechanisms of Positional Central Sleep Apnea Due to Hyperventilation Not Related to Chronic Heart Failure

Development of central sleep apnea in the supine position, although unexpected, can be explained by a considerable overlap in the pathogenesis and pathophysiology of central and obstructive apneas [6–8]. The behaviour of the upper airway in the case of obstruction may not be uniform. Badr et al. [9] described the occurrence of gradual progressive pharyngeal narrowing during induced hypocapnic central apnea and frequent complete pharyngeal occlusion in 146 of 160 investigated cases. Resumption of inspiratory effort was associated with persistent narrowing or complete occlusion unless electroencephalographic arousal was noted. They concluded that subatmospheric intraluminal pressure is not required for pharyngeal occlusion to occur and may be due to passive collapse or active constriction. Vanderveken et al. [10] reported that during central apnea, respiratory impedance was highly variable ranging from a wide open pharynx to complete upper airway closure. In 20 % of analysed central events, a definite closure of the upper airway occurred as demonstrated by Zrs values of 35–57 hPa/l/s. In 10 % an increase by >200 % Zrs was observed, reaching a value of 22–23 hPa/l/s. In 70 %, only a partial occlusion or no change at all in airway patency occurred with Zrs < 17 hPa/l/s. Pepin et al. [11] reported on a case of central apnea with upper airway collapse visualized by somnofluoroscopy. In this patient, the pharyngeal collapse occurred at the end of the central events. On the other hand, Guilleminault et al. [12] did not find evidence for complete upper airway collapse during central apnea in an EMG study. Another argument for upper airway closure during central events is the effectiveness of CPAP for the treatment of central apnea, with a role for the upper airway factor in the pathogenesis of central sleep apnea [13, 14].

Altogether, the aforementioned obstructive component reported in central apnea could explain the occurrence of supine dependency in some patients. It is however in contradiction with the traditional paradigm that central apnea is characterized by recurrent apnoeic episodes in the absence of upper airway obstruction during sleep, according to the guidelines of the AASM [15].

Airway obstruction, especially in the supine position, can mimic central apnea, and nearly 30 % of obstructive events appeared phenomenologically as central apneas in a study by Luo et al. [16]. On the other hand, central hypocapnic hypopnea may exhibit obstructive features [8]. Boudewyns et al. [17] pointed at methodological issues in the assessment of central apnea, with an overestimation of central apneas based on strain gauges in patients with obstructive sleep apnea syndrome. In this perspective, supine dependency in misclassified obstructive events is obvious.

Positional Dependency in Central Sleep Apnea Due to Hyperventilation, Type CSA/CSB Related to Chronic Heart Failure

CSA/CSB in Heart Failure Patients: Clinical Picture and Pathophysiology

CSA/CSB is common in chronic heart failure patients with reported prevalences of 30–40 % [18, 19] and is also observed in stroke patients and in patients with renal failure. CSA/CSB is characterized by a typical waxing and waning breathing pattern, with a relatively long cycle length of about 60 s (Fig. 1). The pathophysiology underlying this typical breathing pattern is complex, and detailed discussion is beyond the scope of this section (please refer to Yumino and Bradley [20] for further reading). Briefly, CSA/CSB results from activation of pulmonary stretch receptors due to pulmonary congestion and enhanced sensitivity of the peripheral and central chemoreceptors leading to hyperventilation and intermittent ventilatory overshooting. This mechanism cyclically drives the $PaCO_2$ below the CO_2 apnoeic threshold, and the ventilatory instability is further enhanced by increased circulation time in heart failure, hypoxaemia, arousals causing sleep stage shifts and sleep state instability with further aggravation of CSA/CSB [21], metabolic alkalosis and upper airway narrowing (Fig. 2).

CSA/CSB is present predominantly in sleep stages N1 and N2, much less in slow wave sleep and usually absent in REM sleep [22], supposedly because the atonia of REM sleep is 'protective' against the hyperventilation in CSA/CSB and the absence of the CO_2 threshold in REM sleep. Moreover, it is more predominant at the end of the night. This may be due to the prevalence in sleep stages N1 and N2 on the one hand but on the other hand also may reflect a gradual fluid shift from the extravascular peripheral space rostrally to the lungs, thereby worsening pulmonary congestion [23]. Orthopnoea is one of the nocturnal signs of heart failure, and patients report relief when sleeping with their upper body in an elevated angle.

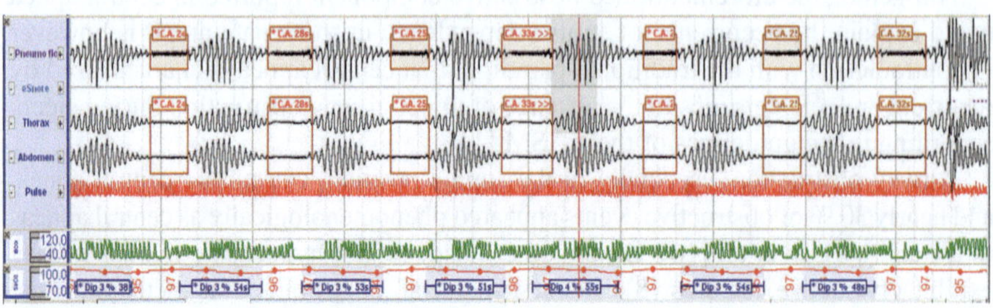

Fig. 1 PSG recording of central sleep apnea type Cheyne-Stokes breathing

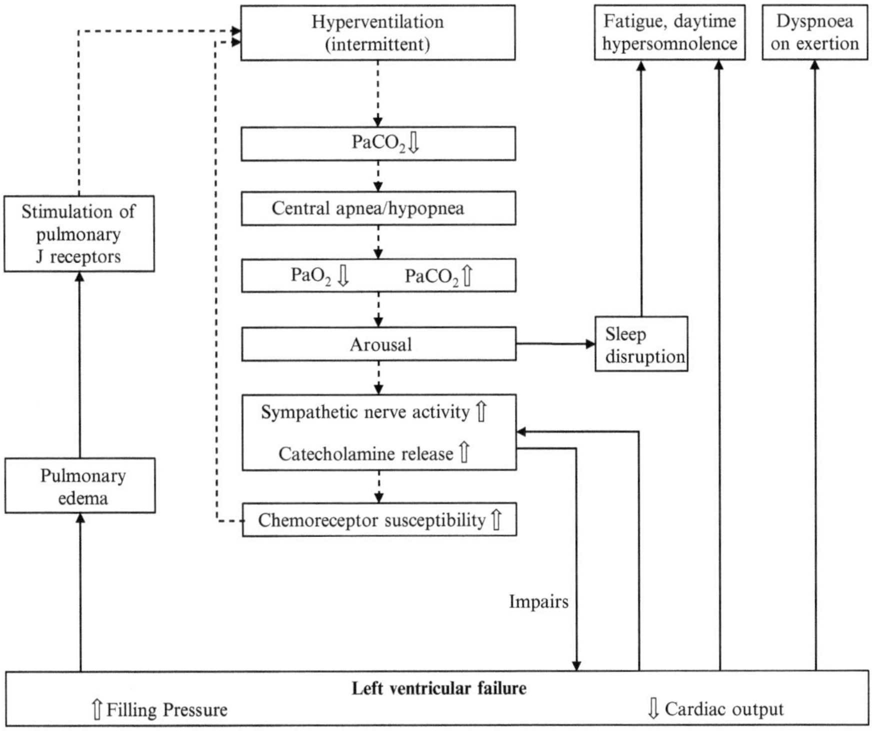

Fig. 2 Mechanisms involved in the pathophysiology of central sleep apnea type Cheyne-Stokes breathing. Reprinted with permission from the Neth Heart J. 2010 May;18(5):260-3

Positional CSA/CSB: Prevalence, Severity and Clinical Determinants

We performed a literature search using PubMed as well as Web of Science, using the keywords 'central sleep apnea', 'CSA', 'Cheyne Stokes breathing' and 'CSB', combined with 'position dependent', 'position', 'positionality', 'lateral' or 'supine'. Only studies reporting on systematically obtained, original data were included.

Sahlin et al. [22] reported on 20 consecutive patients with CSA/CSB of which 18 had congestive heart failure (NYHA classes II–III) and 2 had atrial fibrillation and experienced a stroke before. The mean central AHI (CAHI) was 31 ± 9 per hour, and the obstructive AHI was 2 ± 2 per hour. The average BMI was 27 ± 3 kg/m^2 and only two subjects reported snoring. The CAHI was higher in supine as compared with the non-supine position in 17 out of 20 patients (mean supine CAHI 41 ± 13 and non-supine CAHI 26 ± 12, $p < 0.001$), and BMI did not correlate with the postural effect of central sleep apnea.

Szollosi et al. [24] also reported on 20 patients (age 59.9 ± 2.3 years) with stable heart failure (mean left ventricular ejection fraction 26.5 ± 2.2 %) and CSA/CSB

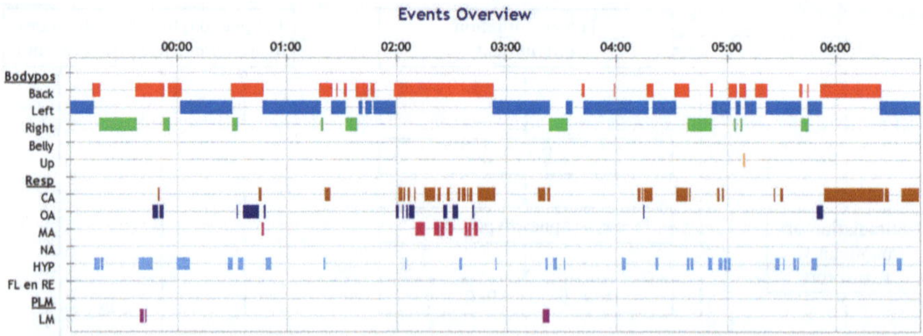

Fig. 3 Positional CSA/CSB. *Red bar*: supine position; *green bar*: right lateral decubitus position; *blue*: left lateral decubitus position. *CA* central apnea, *OA* obstructive apnea, *MA* mixed apnea. Central apneas were of Cheyne-Stokes breathing type. Most central events cluster with the supine body position

with an average BMI of 26.5 ± 0.8 kg/m². Total AHI was 26.4 ± 3 per hour, with 21.2 ± 2.7 central, 3.3 ± 1.6 mixed and 2.1 ± 0.4 obstructive events per hour. The lateral body position was associated with a significant reduction in AHI in all sleep stages: stage N1 54.7 ± 4.2 per hour vs. 27.2 ± 4.1 per hour, stage N2 43.3 ± 6.1 per hour vs. 14.4 ± 3.6 per hour, SWS 15.9 ± 6.4 per hour vs. 5.4 ± 2.9 per hour and REM 38.7 ± 7.3 per hour vs. 11.0 ± 3.0 per hour (p for all <0.01). In addition, the lateral position was associated with reduced AHI-related hypoxemia during sleep stages 1 and 2, during which most events occurred, but event duration was not influenced by sleep stage nor sleeping position.

Joho et al. [25] found that 12 (48 %) of 25 patients with stable heart failure (left ventricular ejection fraction <0.45, a mean AHI 28 ± 8 per hour and CAHI 21 ± 10 per hour) had positional CSA. Overall, subjects with positional CSA/CSB had a lower AHI, a lower NYHA score and better physical activity; used β-blockers; had a lower BNP (brain natriuretic peptide); and a better LVEF. When eight patients with non-positional CSA/CSB were intensively treated to improve cardiac function, non-positional CSA/CSB changed to positional CSA/CSB in all eight patients.

In our own sleep laboratory in a tertiary referral centre, we looked at 28 consecutive patients with CSA/CSB (27 males, mean age 66.3 ± 10 years , mean BMI 30.1 ± 5.1 kg/m², mean AHI 42 ± 19.7, with ≥30 min in either supine and non-supine sleeping position, and >50 % central events type CSB). Nineteen patients used PAP therapy during the sleep registration. Mean AHI in non-supine position was 34.5 ± 20.3 vs. AHI supine 55.0 ± 23.9 (p < 0.001). In 25 patients AHI supine was higher than AHI non-supine. Positional CSA, defined as an AHI ratio non-supine/supine ≤0.5, was seen in 11 out of 28 patients (39 %). See Fig. 3 for an example of positional CSA/CSB in a young male patient with atrial fibrillation. In positional CSA average, AHI was 29 ± 16.7, while in non-positional CSA, average AHI was 50.4 ± 16.9 (p = 0.003). If positional CSA was present, average AHI non-supine was 15.9 ± 11.8 as compared with AHI supine 49.3 ± 24.3 (p = 0.003; unpublished data).

We found one study by Soll et al. [26] in which the effect of a semi/recumbent body position (the head of the bed tilted at a certain angle) on the severity of CSA/CSB was determined. They studied 25 subjects (mean age 64 ± 12 years) with stable heart failure and mean BMI of 28 ± 5.5 kg/m^2. Six had complaints of habitual snoring. 17 of the 25 patients had CSA/CSB (68 %), and an additional 6 patients had central hypopneas but no central apneas. Patients underwent overnight polysomnography starting at their sleeping angle of comfort. During the night they spent 60–90 min at different sleeping angles, namely, 0°, 15°, 30° and 45°, in a random order. The non-supine CAHI was lower than the supine CAHI (25.4 ± 42.9 vs. 34.4 ± 27.8) but did not reach statistical significance, probably due to small numbers and a wide standard deviation. In the supine position, increasing the sleeping angle decreased the CAHI significantly, from 34.4 ± 27.8 at 0° to 8.2 ± 13.8 at 45° ($p < 0.001$). In the non-supine sleeping position, increasing the sleeping angle did not change the CAHI, partly because of the small numbers. Hypopneas did not respond to sleeping angle. Left ventricular haemodynamics and thoracic fluid content index (TFCI: thoracic fluid content/body surface area) as determined by impedance cardiography remained constant despite changes in sleeping angle.

Positional CSA/CSB: Possible Mechanisms

Pathophysiologically, the ventilatory instability of CSA/CSB in heart failure patients is the result of activation of pulmonary stretch receptors due to pulmonary congestion and enhanced chemosensitivity leading to intermittent ventilatory overshooting. This ventilatory instability is further enhanced by increased circulation time in heart failure, hypoxaemia, arousals and upper airway narrowing. The effect that sleeping body position has on each of these mechanisms might explain positional CSA/CSB.

Body position during sleep affects cardiac function. Chronic heart failure patients preferred the right lateral decubitus position above the left lateral decubitus and the supine position during sleep [27, 28], with a twofold longer time in right lateral decubitus position as compared to the other sleeping positions. This was accompanied by a better parasympathetic to sympathetic balance and lower norepinephrine concentration in the right lateral decubitus position. In the right lateral decubitus position, the position of the heart is higher with decreased venous return and reduced pulmonary congestion. This observation is in accordance with the findings of Pump et al. [29] who found an increase in left atrial diameter and a simultaneous decrease in mean arterial pressure in the left lateral decubitus position, possibly by causing stimulation of low-pressure receptors and reduced compression of the inferior caval vein.

Another explanation is an effect of the supine body position on the pulmonary system. Heart failure patients may have reduced lung volumes due to pulmonary congestion and an enlarged heart, with reduced buffer capacity to store oxygen and carbon dioxide. In favor of this theory is the finding by Szollosi et al. [24], who found that a reduction in AHI in the lateral sleeping position was accompanied by attenuated hypoxemia, while the event duration was not influenced. Together, these findings might suggest postural changes in lung volumes responsible for the ventilator instability and hence lower oxygen storage capacity.

The fact that a change in sleeping position immediately influenced central apnea frequency [22, 26] suggests a more rapid mechanism than a change in pulmonary congestion or a change in cardiac function [30]. Instability of the upper airway in CSA/CSB might be an alternative explanation for the rapid change in the central apnea frequency observed. This is supported by the fact that in the supine position, tilting the head improved CAHI, in contrast to the non-supine position and in wake, in which sleeping angle did not influence CAHI [26]. Furthermore, in nine males with compensated heart failure and CSA/CSB (mean age 66.3 ± 3.4 years, mean AHI 46.1 ± 4.4 per hour, with 66.3 ± 3.6 % central events and mean BMI 29.5 ± 2.7 kg/m^2), forced oscillation technique (FOT) was used to determine upper airway patency during predominantly central events [31]. Upper airway narrowing (defined as an impedance value of twice the baseline value during tidal breathing) occurred during 50 ± 12 % of central apneas, with immediate airway reopening associated with the onset of inspiratory effort. This indicates a passive airway narrowing during a central event and might contribute on the one hand to ventilatory instability and on the other hand may make a patient more prone to obstructive events.

To determine the effect of upper airway collapse on the positional dependency of CSA/CSB, Szollosi et al. [24] determined the ratio mixed events/central events in supine versus non-supine position. The supine position was associated with a higher total apnea index compared with the lateral position (19.0 ± 4.9 per hour vs. 7.0 ± 2.9 per hour, $p < 0.001$), due an increase in both central and mixed events, and the proportion of mixed versus central was similar in both sleeping positions. This would indicate that in these subjects upper airway narrowing did not play a role in the supine dependency or in any case did not result in an obstructive component.

Implications for Clinical Practice

The available studies show that body position during sleep is important in about 40–50 % of patients with CSA/CSB. If position dependency is present in CSA/CSB, this indicates a less severe underlying disease and CSA, which is similar to obstructive sleep-disordered breathing, where position dependency is mostly found in mild to moderately severe OSA. In idiopathic central sleep apnea, it can be estimated that only a minority will have benefit from position therapy, since less than 20 % of central events are associated with upper airway closure.

In clinical practice, when considering treatment of CSA/CSB in chronic heart failure, it is important to discuss with the patient to what extent symptoms may be attributed to the breathing disorder, such as frequent arousals at night and daytime sleepiness, in contrast with symptoms related to the underlying disorder, such as fatigue and dyspnoea on exertion. Nocturnal oxygen saturation in CSA/CSB is usually above 90 %, because of the baseline SaO_2 and interapnoeic hyperventilation, which is the main feature of this breathing disorder. Therefore, hypoxaemia is often not a therapeutic issue, and treatment of CSA/CSB should be aimed at improving nocturnal and daytime symptoms in the first place.

By optimizing cardiac treatment and improving cardiac function, position-independent CSA/CSB became position dependent [25]. This underlines the importance in clinical practice to optimize cardiac function as a first-line treatment of CSA/CSB.

Besides optimizing cardiac treatment, continuous positive airway pressure is the first-line treatment modality in CSA/CSB, although therapeutic results are not always satisfactory, with an overall reduction in apnea-hypopnea index after 3 months of about 50 % [32]. Acetazolamide [33] or oxygen [34] can be added, with varying results and side effects, and compliance is a problem. Adaptive servo ventilation (ASV) seems to be the optimal therapy in CSA/CSB [35], but reimbursement is not available in all countries.

Therefore, a stepped-care approach to treating CSA/CSB may be recommended. Next to enhancement of cardiac function, management of positional dependency is to be considered. Particularly in patients with CPAP intolerance, this might be an important intermediate step and may obviate the need to prescribing acetazolamide and oxygen. However, this approach obviously will need validation in prospective studies.

References

1. American Academy of Sleep Medicine. International classification of sleep disorders, 3rd ed. Darien, IL: American Academy of Sleep Medicine, 2014.
2. Zaharna M, Rama A, Chan R, Kushida C. A case of positional central sleep apnea. J Clin Sleep Med. 2013;9:265–8.
3. DelRosso L, Gonzalez-Toledo E, Chesson Jr AL, Hoque R. Positional central sleep apnea and vascular medullary compression. Neurology. 2012;79:2156–7.
4. Oksenberg A, Arons E, Snir D, Radwan H, Soroker N. Cheyne-Stokes respiration during sleep: a possible effect of body position. Med Sci Monit. 2002;8:CS61–5.
5. Yaegashi H, Fujimoto K, Abe H, Orii K, Eda S, Kubo K. Characteristics of Japanese patients with complex sleep apnea syndrome: a retrospective comparison with obstructive sleep apnea syndrome. Intern Med. 2009;48:427–32.
6. Verbraecken J, De Backer W. Upper airway mechanics. Respiration. 2009;78:121–33.
7. Eckert DJ, Jordan AS, Merchia P, Malhotra A. Central sleep apnea: pathophysiology and treatment. Chest. 2007;131:595–607.
8. Sankri-Tarbichi AG, Rowley JA, Badr MS. Expiratory pharyngeal narrowing during central hypocapnic hypopnea. Am J Respir Crit Care Med. 2009;179:313–9.
9. Badr MS, Toiber F, Skatrud JB, Dempsey J. Pharyngeal narrowing/occlusion during central sleep apnea. J Appl Physiol. 1995;78:1806–15.
10. Vanderveken OM, Oostveen E, Boudewyns AN, Verbraecken JA, Van de Heyning PH, De Backer WA. Quantification of pharyngeal patency in patients with sleep-disordered breathing. ORL. 2005;67:168–79.

11. Pepin JL, Pajon A, Veale D, Ferretti G, Levy P. Central sleep apnoea syndrome with upper airway collapse. Eur Respir J. 1993;6:592–5.
12. Guilleminault C, Hill MH, Simmons FB, Powell N, Riley R, Stoohs R. Passive constriction of the upper airway during central apneas: fiberoptic and EMG investigations. Respir Physiol. 1997;108:11–22.
13. Verbraecken J, Willemen M, Wittesaele W, Van de Heyning PH, De Backer W. Short-term CPAP does not influence the increased CO_2 drive in idiopathic central sleep apnea. Monaldi Arch Chest Dis. 2002;57:10–8.
14. Hoffstein V, Slutsky AS. Central sleep apnea reversed by continuous positive airway pressure. Am Rev Respir Dis. 1987;135:1210–2.
15. Report of the American Academy of Sleep Medicine Task Force. Sleep-related breathing disorders in adults. Recommendations for syndrome definition and measurement techniques in clinical research. Sleep 1999;22:667–89.
16. Luo YM, Tang J, Jolley C, et al. Distinguishing obstructive from central sleep apnea events. Diaphragm electromyogram and esophageal pressure compared. Chest. 2009;135:1133–41.
17. Boudewyns A, Willemen M, Wagemans M, DeCock W, Van de Heyning PH, DeBacker W. Assessment of respiratory effort by means of strain gauges and esophageal pressure swings: a comparative study. Sleep. 1997;20:168–70.
18. Javaheri S, Parker TJ, Liming JD, et al. Sleep apnea in 81 ambulatory male patients with stable heart failure. Circulation. 1998;97:2154–9.
19. Macdonald M, Fang J, Pittman SD, White DP, Malhotra A. The current prevalence of sleep disordered breathing in congestive heart failure patients treated with beta-blockers. J Clin Sleep Med. 2008;4:38–42.
20. Yumino D, Bradley TD. Central sleep apnea and Cheyne-Stokes respiration. Proc Am Thorac Soc. 2008;5:226–36.
21. Pinna GD, Maestri R, Robbi E, La Rovere MT. Periodic breathing and state instability during supine laboratory recordings in chronic heart failure patients. Conf Proc IEEE Eng Med Biol Soc 2008;2008:5398–401.
22. Sahlin C, Svanborg E, Stenlund H, Franklin KA. Cheyne-Stokes respiration and supine dependency. Eur Respir J. 2005;25:829–33.
23. Kasai T, Motwani SS, Yumino D, et al. Contrasting effects of lower body positive pressure on upper airway resistance and partial pressure of carbon dioxide in men with heart failure and obstructive or central sleep apnea. J Am Coll Cardiol. 2013;61:1157–66.
24. Szollosi I, Roebuck T, Thompson B, Naughton MT. Lateral sleeping position reduces severity of central sleep apnea/Cheyne-Stokes respiration. Sleep. 2006;29:1045–51.
25. Joho S, Oda Y, Hirai T, Inoue H. Impact of sleeping position on central sleep apnea/Cheyne-Stokes respiration in patients with heart failure. Sleep Med. 2010;11:143–8.
26. Soll BAG, Yeo KK, Davis JW, et al. The effect of posture on Cheyne-Stokes respirations and hemodynamics in patients with heart failure. Sleep. 2009;32:1499–506.
27. Fujita M, Miyamoto S, Sekiguchi H, Eiho S, Sasayama S. Effects of posture on sympathetic nervous modulation in patients with chronic heart failure. Lancet. 2000;356:1822–3.
28. Miyamoto S, Fujita M, Sekiguchi H, et al. Effects of posture on cardiac autonomic nervous activity in patients with congestive heart failure. J Am Coll Cardiol. 2001;37:1788–93.
29. Pump B, Talleruphuus U, Christensen NJ, Warberg J, Norsk P. Effects of supine, prone, and lateral positions on cardiovascular and renal variables in humans. Am J Physiol Regul Intergr Comp Physiol. 2002;283:R174–80.
30. Hanly PJ. Impact of sleeping angle on the upper airway and pathogenesis of Cheyne Stokes respiration. Sleep. 2009;32:1412–3.
31. Jobin V, Rigau J, Beauregard J, et al. Evaluation of upper airway patency during Cheyne-Stokes breathing in heart failure patients. Eur Respir J. 2012;40:1523–30.
32. Bradley TD, Logan AG, Kimoff RJ, et al. Continuous positive airway pressure for central sleep apnea and heart failure. N Engl J Med. 2005;353:2025–33.

33. Javaheri S. Acetazolamide improves central sleep apnea in heart failure: a double-blind, prospective study. Am J Respir Crit Care Med. 2006;173:234–7.
34. Andreas S, Weidel K, Hagenah G, Heindl S. Treatment of Cheyne-Stokes respiration with nasal oxygen and carbon dioxide. Eur Respir J. 1998;12(2):414–9.
35. Teschler H, Dohring J, Wang YM, Berthon-Jones M. Adaptive pressure support servo-ventilation: a novel treatment for Cheyne-Stokes respiration in heart failure. Am J Respir Crit Care Med. 2001;164:614–9.

Part VI
Treatment of Positional OSA

History of Positional Therapy: Transition from Tennis Balls to New Devices

Madeline Ravesloot, Arjan van der Star, and Eline C. Vrijland van Beest

History of Obstructive Sleep Apnea

OSA is a relatively new disease entity, much remains to be discovered and improved, and many areas of the field remain controversial or unproven, especially concerning treatment of OSA patients [1]. An exponential increase has taken place in peer-reviewed publications on OSA. A search in the electronic bibliographical database PubMed leads to more than 1,600 research publications on OSA which were published in the year 2012, whilst in 1992, there were just over 200 [2].

The clinical picture of OSA has long been recognized as a character trait, without understanding of the pathophysiology, especially in obese people. The word "apnea" derives from the Greek word *a-pnoia*, which means "without breath". Obesity was frequently associated with daytime sleepiness and sleep-disordered breathing.

Features of sleep apnea were described in antiquity. Dionysus, a tyrant of Heraclea, was an "unusually fat man" as reported in *Varia Historia* written by *Claudio Aelianus* (235–170 BC) [3]. Aelianus wrote: "I am informed that Dionysius the Heracleote, son of Clearchus the tyrant, through daily gluttony and intemperance, increased to an extraordinary degree of Corpulency and Fatness, by reason whereof he had much adoe to take breath" [4]. It is thought that his difficulties in breathing also took place during sleep. Athenaeus describes that because of his obesity, Dionysus was afflicted with shortness of breath and fits of choking. He describes a curious method to keep him awake: "So the physicians prescribed that he should get some fine needles, exceedingly long, which they thrust through his

M. Ravesloot, M.D., Ph.D. (✉)
Department of Otorhinolaryngology, Sint Lucas Andreas Ziekenhuis,
Jan Tooropstraat 164, 1061 AE Amsterdam, The Netherlands
e-mail: m.ravesloot@slaz.nl

A. van der Star, M.Sc. • E.C.V. van Beest, M.Sc., M.B.I.
NightBalance B.V., Delft, The Netherlands

N. de Vries et al. (eds.), *Positional Therapy in Obstructive Sleep Apnea*,
DOI 10.1007/978-3-319-09626-1_20

ribs and belly whenever he happened to fall into a deep sleep" [5]. It is said that "At last, however, he was choked by his own fat".

Other prominent historical figures suspected to have suffered from sleep-disordered breathing included Henry VIII, Napoleon Bonaparte, Queen Victoria, Johannes Brahms, Winston Churchill, Grover Cleveland, Franklin and Theodore Roosevelt and William Taft [6–14].

Features of obstructive sleep apnea were often used in fictional literature. In *Henry IV*, by William Shakespeare, the character Sir John Falstaff was well known for his corpulence and tendency for napping and was occasionally found "fast asleep behind the arras, and snoring like a horse" [15]. But Charles Dickens is most famous for the first detailed description of an obese patient with obstructive sleep apnea. The supporting character Joe, from the *Pickwick Papers*, is described as "a wonderfully fat boy" who falls asleep easily and against his will [3, 15].

Dickens' description was so stereotypical that the term "Pickwickian syndrome" was later used to describe obese and sleepy patients [16].

The first scientific description of what we term today as "obstructive sleep apnea" was not published until 1877, when W.H. Broadbent, a physician from St. Mary's Hospital in London, described a strange case of sleep-disordered breathing that was "similar to Cheyne–Stokes breathing" [17].

"When a person, especially if he is advanced in years, is sleeping on his back in deepest sleep, and snoring loudly, it occurs very often that a total silence for two, three or four breaths is produced, in which for breathing the chest doesn't open finally the air enters with a loud snort, accompanied by a sharp snort, after which occurs several deep breaths to compensate the loss of air. After a while, breathing returns to normal rhythm. In the case that I mean, well described, there is the cessation of snoring at regular intervals and the respiratory pause stretched enough to attract attention, and sometimes becoming worrisome."

Interestingly, even though Broadbent concluded his article that "All theories that have attempted to explain this phenomenon are inadequate and I have none of my own", he recognized the role of sleep position.

In the 1950s various articles were published analysing sleepy, obese individuals, and in the 1960s, researchers began to understand that the symptoms also presented themselves in nonobese patients and started to unravel the pathogenesis [3]. It wasn't until 1976 when pioneers Guilleminault and Dement recognized that obstructive sleep apnea did not solely occur in patients with obesity and provided the first clinical description as well as coining the term obstructive sleep apnea [18].

The management of OSA was revolutionized with the introduction of continuous airway pressure (CPAP), by Sullivan [19].

History of Positional Sleep Apnea

Obesity wasn't the only exogenous factor appreciated in the ancient worlds as a risk factor for snoring or sleep-disordered breathing; the causal relationship between snoring and the patient's body position was recognized: "It also befalls those who are inadequately positioned" [20]. In 1581 Levinus, a Dutch physician and author, reported that mouth breathing in supine position causes restless sleep [21]. In medical scientific literature, the supine sleeping position was first mentioned as "a common cause of snoring" by Robin in 1948 [22]. He reasoned, "by changing the position of the head the tongue will be prevented from falling back". Harper and Sauerland suggested, "when sleep apnea patients sleep in supine position, the tongue tends to fall backward against the pharyngeal wall, due to gravity" [23].

History of Positional Therapy

Tennis Ball Therapy

To our best knowledge, first historical mention of positional therapy can be found in military documentation. During the American War of Independence (1775–1783) and later during World War I (1914–1918), soldiers were advised to wear their rucksacks (filled with a bulky mass) whilst sleeping, or a small cannonball would be sewn into the back of a soldier's uniform by the regimental tailor to prevent the soldier from adopting a supine position and reduce snoring, as to avoid making their location known to the enemy [24].

The first patent for positional therapy dates back to 1872: "Apparatus for preventing a person while asleep from turning on his back" [25]. This device consisted of a bulky mass, strapped and worn on the user's back.

Since then, a variety of inventions have been patented over the years, depicted in Fig. 1 in chronological order.

In 1900, L.E. Wilson, from Nebraska, filed a patent for a "Shoulder brace and antisnoring attachment" [26]. The device consisted of a metal "prodding device", kept in place by adjustable, washable and ventilated straps. Not only did the device block the patient from adopting the supine position, the device also forced the patient to roll over to a lateral position. The first patent for a device for medical application was filed by T. Thomas in 1907: "A belt and shield to be worn at night to give support to the wearer, prevent his sleeping on his back, to prevent dreaming and snoring…" [27].

In 1908, two patents were filed, both titled "Antisnoring device" by C.F. Rohwer and L.F. Liebhardt. These devices aimed to "provide a simple and easily applied device, which will effectively prevent snoring, sleep talking, bad dreams and other disagreeable features with which many persons contend when sleeping on their backs", by securing a hollow ball composed of compressible material, such as rubber on the wearer's back [28, 29].

E.R. Boots invented a new sleeping garment, for which a patent was filed in 1941 [30]. This garment consisted of a pocket sewn onto the back panel of a nightshirt or pyjama, sized to retain a so-called "anti-snore medium such as a sponge rubber ball". This ball served as an obstacle for the wearer to sleep in supine position.

Under a decade later, the journal CHEST published a letter written by a patient's wife [31]. She had cured her husband's sleep apnea snoring problem by "having

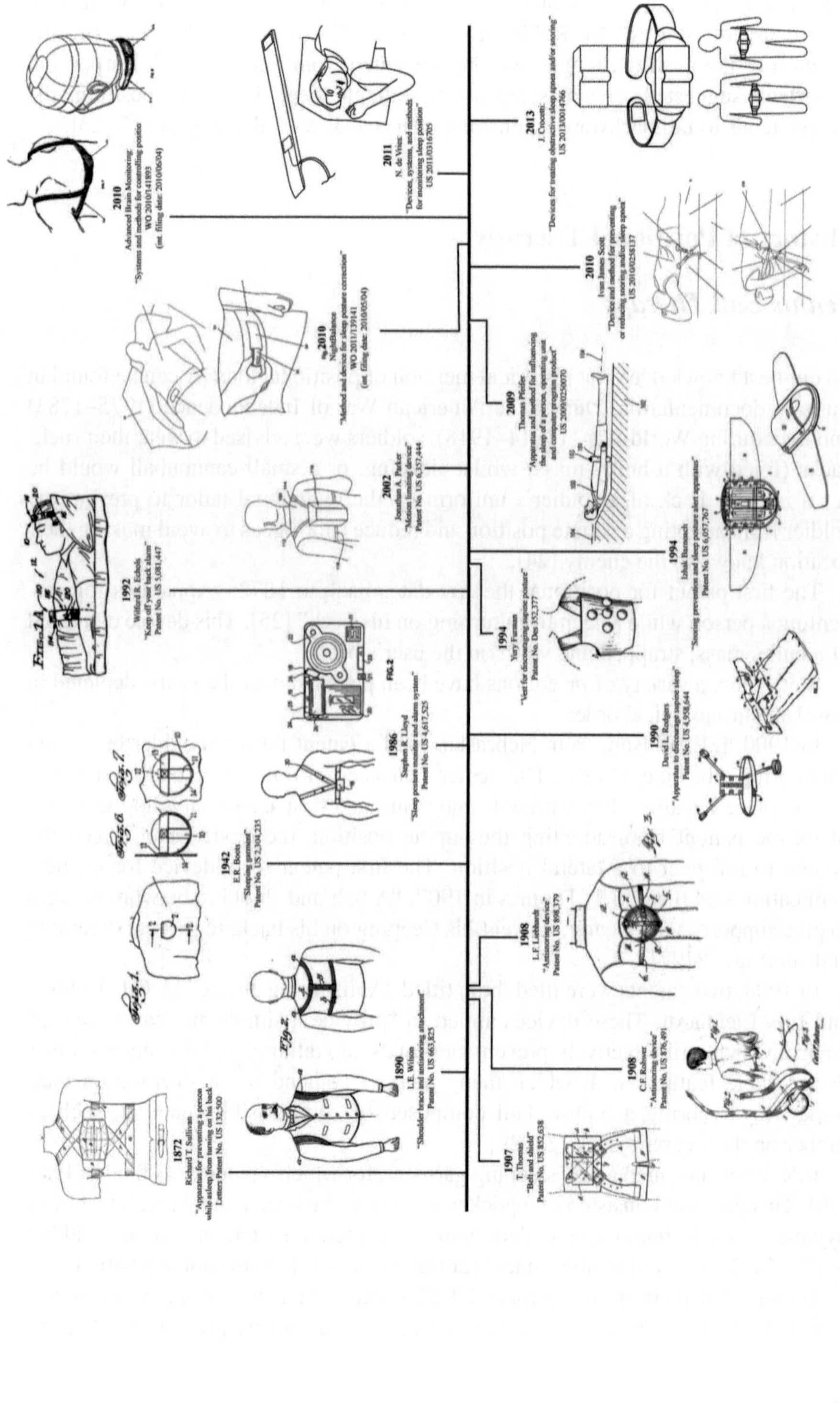

Fig. 1 Patents in positional therapy

sewn a pocket into the back of a T-shirt and having inserted a hollow, lightweight plastic ball, to prevent her husband sleeping on his back". To our best knowledge, this is the first publication of "positional therapy" in medical literature.

It was not until the mid-1980s that the first scientific studies on positional therapy were published.

Kavey published the results of two patients who had been instructed to attach a ball in a sock to the back of their nightshirt in such a way as to make the supine position uncomfortable [32]. Henceforth, variations of the tennis ball techniques have been described in the literature varying from vests, "shark fins" or special pillows, as shown in Table 1. After running a thorough search strategy in the MEDLINE and Embase databases, 24 relevant articles were found. Seven studies were excluded from the overview. Two studies did not provide information on the effect of PT on OSA parameters and were omitted from the overview. Five studies evaluated the effect on OSA of an array of devices resulting in an elevated posture and head extension. As these devices did not prevent the patient from assuming the supine position, the studies were not included in the overview. All studies report positive effect of positional therapy on the AHI [24–33, 40, 43, 44, 48, 49, 55, 56, 58].

Nevertheless, ineffectiveness, backache, discomfort and no improvement in sleep quality or daytime alertness have been responsible for poor compliance and subsequent disappointing long-term results of positional therapy. As prime example, in 1990, D. L. Rodgers filed a patent named "Apparatus to discourage supine sleep" [41]. This device was invented to cause "a supine sleeper to shift to a non-supine position, or to cause sufficient, preferably non-awakening, arousal to maintain respiration and/or to avoid snoring". An apparatus containing a plurality of prods is attached to the back of the patient. The sharpness of the prods, as felt by the sleeper, is adjustable, such as by adjusting the surface area, thickness or compressibility of material surrounding the prods or modifying or coating the prod points.

Yury Furman introduced the "Snorr Ball", a "vest for discouraging supine posture", in 1994 [42]. It consists of a vest with balls attached to the back to discourage a supine sleeping position.

In 1999, Jokic et al. studied the effect of positional therapy compared to CPAP in a randomized crossover study setup. The researchers included 13 patients who were randomized to 2 weeks of treatment with nCPAP or positional therapy (backpack with softball) followed by a crossover to the other modality [43]. They found "positional therapy to be highly effective in reducing time spent in a supine position". And although both treatment modalities were found to improve OSA severity, nCPAP was found to be more effective in reducing the AHI (17.9–3.4 on nCPAP, to 9.5 with positional therapy).

After the paper by the group of Jokic in 1999, Skinner et al. included 20 patients in a randomized crossover comparing the efficacy of a thoracic anti-supine band (TASB) with nasal CPAP (nCPAP) in 2009 [44]. Subjects were randomly assigned to receive the TASB or nCPAP for the first month followed by a 1-week washout before commencing the alternative treatment. The baseline AHI was 22.7 and decreased to 12.0 with TASB and 4.9 with nCPAP. A successful treatment outcome was defined as an AHI < 10, which was achieved in 13 of 18 subjects when using

Table 1 Overview literature on positional therapy

	Year	Design	LoE	No.	BMI (kg/m²)	PT method	Mean AHI without PT	Mean AHI with PT	Mean TST in supine position without PT (%)	Mean TST in supine position with PT (%)	AHI in supine position without PT	AHI in supine position with PT	AHI in non-supine position without PT	AHI in non-supine position with PT	Sleep efficiency without PT (%)	Sleep efficiency with PT (%)	Follow-up
Cartwright [48]	1985	Case series	4	10	30.6	Positional alarm	54.7	21.4	51.4	2.1	72.0	11.0	19.3	21.6	ND	ND	–
Kavey [32]	1985	Case series	4	2/4	24.5	Ball in sock on back	9.2[b,c]	3.8[b,c]	40.4[c]	8.8[c]	13.7[b,c]	5.1[b,c]	ND	ND	ND	ND	4–12 months
Kavey [32]	1985	Case series	4	2/4	26.5	Verbal instructions	40.8[b,c]	2.8[b,c]	92.1[c]	11.2[c]	42.4[b,c]	6.9[b,c]	ND	ND	ND	ND	3–4 months
Cartwright [49]	1991	Case series	4	15/60	ND	Positional alarm	33.3	20.8	141.1[f]	3.4[f]	62.5	32.9	9.7	21.7	ND	ND	8 weeks
Cartwright [49]	1991	Case series	4	15/60	ND	Verbal instructions	26.7	7.7	101.3[f]	16.5[f]	87.3	26.8	7.7	4.6	ND	ND	8 weeks
Braver [33]	1994	Randomized crossover trial	2b	20	36	Foam wedges	17.5	14.1	68	ND	ND	ND	ND	ND	ND	ND	–
Jokic [43]	1999	RCT	2b	13	30	Backpack with softball inside	17.9	9.5	25.6	1.	63.8	ND	4.9	ND	ND	82	–
Maurer [34]	2003	Case series	4	12	26.5	Vest with semirigid foam on dorsal part	26.7	7.6	300[f]	63[f]	39.3	ND	5.5	ND	81	83	–
Zuberi [35]	2004	Case series	4	22	23–48[a]	Triangular pillow	23.5	11.1	ND	ND	ND	ND	ND	ND	ND	ND	–
Oksenberg [36]	2006	Case series	4	28825	28.1	Tennis ball technique	46.5	17.5	79	12.3	57.0	44.4	11.6	13.8	80.9	78.9	2 months
Wenzel [37]	2007	Case series	4	12	28.1	Vest with semirigid foam on dorsal part	31.3	13.8	72.2	2.1	ND	ND	ND	ND	86.3	78.9	-

Loord [38]	2007	Case series	4	18/23	ND	Soft vest attached to a board with pillow	21.8	14.3	ND	ND	50.4	ND	ND	ND	ND	ND	3 months
Skinner [44]	2009	Randomized crossover trial	2b	20	30.7	Thoracic anti-supine band (TASB)	22.7	12.0	34.4	6.3	59.6	37.8	4.7	10.3	ND	ND	1 month
Permut [60]	2010	Randomized crossover trial	2b	38	31	Vest with semirigid foam on dorsal part	11^{d}	2^{d}	40^{d}	0^{d}	31^{d}	ND	2^{d}	ND	89^{d}	88^{d}	–
Choi [39]	2011	Case series	4	17	ND	Vest with inflatable chambers	7.7	4.8	67.1	25	ND	ND	ND	ND	89.8	87.6	
Svatikova [40]	2011	Randomized, controlled, crossover trial	2b	18	29	Triangular pillow	39^{d}	27^{d}	39	8	49^{d}	51^{d}	27^{d}	27^{d}	ND	ND	–
Bignold [56]	2011	Randomized crossover trial	2b	15	28.8	Position monitoring and supine alarm device	24.1	$–^{e}$	36.4	ND	51.3	ND	9.7	ND	81.4	ND	–
Maanen [55]	2012	Randomized controlled single-blind, crossover trial	2b	30	27.7	Neck-worn vibrating apparatus	27.7	12.8	40	19	59.7	12.5	6.7	11.2	91.9	88.3	–
Maanen [58]	2013	Case series	4	31	27	Sleep position trainer	16.4^{d}	5.2^{d}	49.9^{d}	0.0^{d}	35.7^{d}	0.0^{d}	3.2^{d}	4.3^{d}	89.1^{d}	89.4^{d}	1 month

AHI apnea–hypopnea index, *BMI* body mass index, *LoE* level of evidence, *ND* not described, *PT* positional therapy, *TST* total sleep time

[a]Range

[b]AI

[c]Initial diagnosis based on 2 consecutive PSGs. After initial diagnosis, patients studied for an additional one or two nights between 4 months and 3 years later during which time they avoided sleeping in the supine position

[d]Median

[e]AHI reduction in the order of 45 % with active treatment estimated from nasal cannula/oximetry from home-sleep studies

[f]In minutes

TASB and in 16 of 18 subjects when using nCPAP. Once again they found the self-reported compliance was significantly better with TASB than with nCPAP. Nineteen of 20 patients reported a 7-h nightly use of the TASB, whilst only 9/20 patients managed to use their nCPAP at least 4 h per night.

In 2002, another patent called "Motion limiting device" was filed by J.A. Parker [45]. The device positioned on one's back limits body motion through a pad, shaped to prevent the patient from rolling over the pad.

Ivan James Scott invented a new device for positional therapy and filed his patent in 2010, named "Device and method for preventing or reducing snoring and/or sleep apnea" [46]. The user wears a vest, which through straps attached to the vest and bed prevents the users from rolling to a supine sleeping position.

Even today, patents for variations of the tennis ball technique continue to be filed. In 2013, J. Crocetti filed a patent for this so-called "Devices for treating obstructive sleep apnea and/or snoring" [47]. This device passively controls the sleeping position by preventing the user to sleep in supine position through the use of a bulky mass. This wedge-shaped object is attached to a strap around the torso, which is secured with a Velcro closure anteriorly.

Positional Alarm Devices

The pioneer of research on positional sleep apnea and its therapy is Dr. Rosalind Cartwright. She was the first to define positional therapy as well as the first to publish scientific reports studying the efficacy various techniques aimed to assist the patient in avoiding the supine sleeping position. Ten male patients with OSA associated with the supine sleep position were trained for one night to avoid the supine sleep position by wearing a gravity-activated position monitor/alarm on the chest. This device emitted an auditory signal if the patient remained supine for more than 15 s. The number of apneic events was significantly reduced, as was the number of episodes of significant O_2 desaturation. While wearing the alarm, the apnea index of seven patients remained within or near normal limits. On a follow-up night, with only instructions to maintain the lateral decubitus posture, five patients remained significantly improved [48].

After Cartwright et al. referred to sleep position training in 1985, they coined the term *positional therapy* in 1991, defined as "preventing patients to sleep in the worst sleeping position". The worst sleeping position is usually, but not always the supine position [49].

In 1986, a patent for this type of device was filed by S. R. Lloyd titled "Sleep posture monitor and alarm system" [50]. The patent was for "A device for awakening a sleeping person when the sleeping person attempts to sleep in a particular sleep posture includes a sensor, a time-delay circuit, and an alarm or other device for generating a stimulus for awakening the person. The time-delay circuit is designed such that it activates the alarm only when the sensor indicates the person is in the particular sleep posture for a predetermined period of time and also stops the alarm when the person stops sleeping in the particular sleep posture. The device can also be used for monitoring the sleeping person's sleep posture for diagnostic purposes."

W. R. Echols published a patent for a positional alarm in 1992 [51]. This was the first patented device that was not designated to be worn on one's back, since it uses a gravity-activated sensor to measure the supine sleeping position. Patients could either attach the apparatus to the head or to the body. After a time delay, this so-called "Keep off your back alarm" sounds an alarm to inform the patient when he/she is resting on his/her back, thereby enticing the person to sleep on one side or the other and not on his back.

During the same year, T. Pfeifer filed another patent for the innovation called "Apparatus and method for influencing the sleep of a person, operating unit and computer program product" [52]. This device comprises a sensor that detects positions of the user's body. Furthermore, based on one's *prohibited* position, a predetermined stimulus pattern is given based on a procedural mechanism from embedded software.

Vibrational Alarm Devices

The devices for positional therapy further developed when Barnoach filed a patent for his "Snoring prevention and sleep posture alert apparatus" in the year 2000 [53]. The device, especially designed for infants, is worn on the chest. It uses a time-delay period after detecting the supine sleeping position of its user measured with a gravity-actuated sensor. After the supine position is detected for a longer time than the predetermined time slot, a vibrator is activated "to alert the user without awaking".

In an attempt to decrease discomfort and improve compliance, the group of van Maanen et al. developed a new treatment concept in 2011: a small neck-worn vibrating device, which prevents patients from applying a supine sleeping position. When wearing the device, adopting a supine position triggers a vibration that increases in intensity until a new position is adopted, without significantly reducing total sleep time or disrupting sleep. The patent for this new device was filed as part of a patent application "Devices, systems, and methods for monitoring sleep position" in 2011 by a researcher from this group, N. de Vries and others [54]. This device uses a gravity-activated sensor to measure the undesired sleeping position. Thirty patients with positional sleep apnea were included in a pilot study [55]. No side effects were reported in 2012. The mean AHI dropped from 27.7 ± 2.4 to 12.8 ± 2.2. Seven patients developed an overall AHI below 5 when using the device in ON modus. Although the results are encouraging, several items remain to be addressed with this device and there is room for improvement. The long-term effect remains to be studied.

In 2011, Bignold et al. evaluated the efficacy of a similar device in 15 patients fulfilling the following criteria: overall AHI ≥ 15 per hour, supine AHI $\geq$ twice or greater than the non-supine AHI and ≥20 min of sleep in supine and non-supine postures and non-supine AHI < 15 [56]. Subjects were assigned to receive the active positional therapy or the inactive positional therapy in a random order for a week followed by a 1-week washout before commencing the alternative treatment. The mean baseline AHI (24.1) was reduced in the order of 45 % with active treatment. The device consists of a position monitoring and supine alarm device fastened to the chest, which vibrates after a user-selected delay when the supine position is detected. Furthermore, it also comes with a dedicated computer program, which is designed to enable overnight sleep position monitoring.

In 2010, the patent for a sleep posture alerting apparatus invented by NightBalance was filed [57]. When the device detects that the body sleeping posture is within a predetermined range, the wearer is alerted by the device to change position. The device uses a predefined sleep-in time period to enable the wearer to fall asleep in every preferred position. Furthermore, it introduces a training programme to gradually train patients not to sleep in supine position after two diagnosis nights, in which no feedback is given. The level of the feedback is adapted to the threshold of the user in order to be able to provide vibrotactile feedback effectively without being too disturbing. Moreover, a software program is added to provide users with feedback on night-to-night progress and their sleeping behaviour.

Van Maanen et al. researched the effect of this Sleep Position Trainer (SPT) in patients with POSA later in 2013, the median percentage of supine sleeping time decreased from 49.9 % [20.4–77.3 %] to 0.0 % [range: 0.0–48.7 %] ($p < 0.001$) [58]. The median AHI decreased from 16.4 per hour [6.6–29.9] to 5.2 per hour [0.5–46.5] ($p < 0.001$). Fifteen patients developed an overall AHI below 5 per hour. Sleep efficiency did not change significantly, the Epworth Sleepiness Scale decreased significantly and Functional Outcomes of Sleep Questionnaire increased significantly. Compliance after 1 month was found to be 92.7 % [62.0–100.0 %].

Levendowski patented its device named "Systems and methods for controlling position" in 2010 [59]. This device is designed to measure the body position and store this information in order to estimate sleep quality. Furthermore, the device can be configured to a specific undesired sleeping position; to be worn around the neck, chest or head; and to customize the level of feedback given to the wearer.

Future Perspectives

Currently, various devices are available on the market, but the efficacy of these modalities has not been studied in clinical trials or been patented. Different other cushion types are commercially available which claim to help its user to sleep in a latent sleeping position. Other options are comparable alternatives to the aforementioned attached straps with bulky masses to prevent the wearer from sleeping in supine position. Slightly more advantaged modern methods use active instead of passive feedback and have self-detecting mechanisms to assess changing body posture rather than passively using buttons to determine an already adapted supine sleeping position. The last generation of positional therapy devices employs a combined arsenal of innovations in order to improve comfort and compliance. Although no long-term results are available yet, researchers expect these devices to be very effective in the application of positional therapy in POSA patients.

The most recent development has been the introduction of software applications for mobile operating systems (i.e. iOS and Android), attempting to provoke a change in the body sleeping position with sound or vibrations. To our best knowledge, no scientific studies have been performed studying the efficacy of these applications. Currently none of these applications are medically certified, whereas as of 2013, new laws require all these applications to have a medical CE mark.

References

1. McNicholas WT, Bonsignore MR, editors. Sleep apnoea, European respiratory society monograph. Sheffield, UK: European Respiratory Society; 2010.
2. http://www.ncbi.nlm.nih.gov/pubmed?term=obstructive%20sleep%20apnoea. 12-1-2013.
3. Kryger MH. From the needles of Dionysius to continuous positive airway pressure. Arch Intern Med. 1983;143:2301–3.
4. Aelianus C. Various history: Book IX. London: Thomas Dung; 1666. p. 177. Chap 13.
5. Gulick CB (trans.) Athenaeus: the deipnosophist. Vol 5. Cambridge, MA: Harvard University Press; 1863. p 491, 497.
6. Margolis ML. Brahms' lullaby revisited: did the composer have obstructive sleep apnoea? Chest. 2000;118:210–3.
7. Campbell J. Winston Churchill's afternoon nap. New York: Simon and Schuster; 1986.
8. Brodsky A. Grover Cleveland: a study in character. New York: St. Martin's Press; 2000. p. 4, 312.
9. Dugan H. Bedlam in the boudoir. Colliers. 1947; Feb. 22. Cited by: Fairbanks DNF. Snoring: an overview with historical perspectives. In: Fairbanks DNF, Fujita S, editors. Snoring and obstructive sleep apnoea. 2nd ed. New York: Raven, 1994. p. 1–16.
10. Boller Jr PF. Presidential anecdotes. New York: Oxford University Press; 1981. p. 178.
11. Brewer C. The death of kings: a medical history of the kings and queens of England. London: Abson; 2000.
12. Ferrell RH. The dying president: Franklin D. Roosevelt 1944-1945. Columbia, MO: University of Missouri Press; 1998.
13. Boulware MH. Snoring: new answers to an old problem. Rockaway, NJ: American Faculty Press; 1974. Cited by: Fairbanks DNF. Snoring: an overview with historical perspectives. In: Fairbanks, DNF, Fujita S, editors. Snoring and obstructive sleep apnoea. 2nd ed. New York: Raven; 1994. p. 1–16.
14. Hoover IH (Ike). 42 years in the White House. Boston, MA: Houghton Mifflin; 1934. p. 270.
15. Zupancic M, Lavie P. History. In: Kushida CA, editor. Obstructive sleep apnoea, pathophysiology, comorbidities and consequences: pathophysiology, comorbidities, and consequences (sleep disorders). 1st ed. Boca Raton, FL: CRC; 2007.
16. Burwell CS, Robin ED, Whaley RD, et al. Extreme obesity associated with alveolar hypoventilation; a Pickwickian syndrome. Am J Med. 1956;21(5):811–8.
17. Broadbent WH. Cheyne Stokes respiration in cerebral hemorrhage. Lancet. 1877;3:307–9.
18. Guilleminault C, Tilkiam A, Dement WC. The sleep apnoea syndromes. Annu Rev Med. 1976;27:465–84.
19. Sullivan CE, Issa FG, Berthon-Jones M, Eves L. Reversal of obstructive sleep apnoea by continuous positive airway pressure applied through the nares. Lancet. 1981;1:862–5.
20. Pirsig W. Snoring in the ancient World. Sleep Breath. 2002;6:29–39.

21. Levinus Lemnious. The touchstone of complexions. London; 1581.
22. Robin IG. Snoring. Proc R Soc Med. 1948;41(3):151–3.
23. Harper R, Sauerland E. The role of the tongue in sleep apnoea. In: Guilleminault C, Dement W, editors. Sleep apnoea syndromes. New York: Alan R Liss; 1978. p. 219–34.
24. Ravesloot MJL, van Maanen JP, Dun L, de Vries N. The undervalued potential of positional therapy in position-dependent snoring and obstructive sleep apnoea—a review of the literature. Sleep Breath. 2013;17(1):39–49.
25. Sullivan RT. U.S. Patent No. 132,500. Washington, DC: U.S. Patent and Trademark Office; 1872.
26. Wilson LE. U.S. Patent No. 663,825. Washington, DC: U.S. Patent and Trademark Office; 1900.
27. Thomas T. U.S. Patent No. 852,638. Washington, DC: U.S. Patent and Trademark Office; 1907.
28. Rohwer CF. U.S. Patent No. 876,491. Washington, DC: U.S. Patent and Trademark Office; 1908.
29. Liebhardt LF. U.S. Patent No. 898,379. Washington, DC: U.S. Patent and Trademark Office; 1908.
30. Boots ER. U.S. Patent No. 2,304,235. Washington, DC: U.S. Patent and Trademark Office; 1942.
31. Editor's note. Patient's wife cures his snoring. Chest. 1984;85(4):582.
32. Kavey NB, Blitzer A, Gidro-Frank S, Korstanje K. Sleeping position and sleep apnoea syndrome. Am J Otolaryngol. 1985;6(5):373–7.
33. Braver HM, Block AJ. Effect of nasal spray, positional therapy, and the combination thereof in the asymptomatic snorer. Sleep. 1994;17(6):516–21.
34. Maurer JT, Stuck BA, Hein G, Verse T, Hörmann K. Schlafapnoetherapie mit einer neuartigen rückenlage-verhinderungs-weste. DMW-Deutsche Medizinische Wochenschrift. 2003; 128(03):71–5.
35. Zuberi NA, Rekab K, Nguyen HV. Sleep apnoea avoidance pillow effects on obstructive sleep apnoea syndrome and snoring. Sleep Breath. 2004;8(4):201–7.
36. Oksenberg A, Silverberg D, Offenbach D, Arons E. Positional therapy for obstructive sleep apnoea patients: a 6 month follow up study. Laryngoscope. 2006;16(11):1995–2000.
37. Wenzel S, Smith E, Leiacker R, Fischer Y. Efficacy and long-term compliance of the vest preventing the supine position in patients with obstructive sleep apnoea. Laryngorhinootologie. 2007;86(8):579–83.
38. Loord H, Hultcrantz E. Positioner—a method for preventing sleep apnoea. Acta Otolaryngol. 2007;127(8):861–8.
39. Choi JH, Park YH, Hong JH, Kim SJ, Park DS, Miyazaki S, Lee SH, Shin C, Lee J. Efficacy study of a vest-type device for positional therapy in position dependent snorers. Sleep Biol Rhythms. 2009;7(3):181–7.
40. Svatikova A, Chervin RD, Wing JJ, Sanchez BN, Migda EM, Brown DL. Positional therapy in ischemic stroke patients with obstructive sleep apnoea. Sleep Med. 2011;12(3):262–6.
41. Rodgers DL. U.S. Patent No. 4,958,644. Washington, DC: U.S. Patent and Trademark Office; 1990.
42. Furman Y. U.S. Patent No. D352,377. Washington, DC: U.S. Patent and Trademark Office; 1994.
43. Jokic R, Klimaszewski A, Crossley M, Sridhar G, Fitzpatrick MF. Positional treatment vs continuous positive airway pressure in patients with positional obstructive sleep apnoea syndrome. Chest J. 1999;115(3):771–81.
44. Skinner MA, Kingshott RN, Filsell S, Taylor DR. Efficacy of the 'tennis ball technique' versus nCPAP in the management of position-dependent obstructive sleep apnoea syndrome. Respirology. 2009;13(5):708–15.
45. Parker JA. U.S. Patent No. 6,357,444. Washington, DC: U.S. Patent and Trademark Office; 2002.
46. Scott IJ. (2010). U.S. Patent Application 12/755,653.
47. Crocetti J. U.S. Patent No. 20,130,014,766. Washington, DC: U.S. Patent and Trademark Office; 2013.
48. Cartwright RD, Lloyd S, Lilie J, Kravitz H. Sleep position training as treatment for sleep apnoea syndrome: a preliminary study. Sleep. 1985;8(2):87–94.

49. Cartwright RD, Diaz F, Lloyd S. The effects of sleep posture and sleep stage on apnoea frequency. Sleep. 1991;14(4):351–3.
50. Lloyd SR. U.S. Patent No. 4,617,525. Washington, DC: U.S. Patent and Trademark Office; 1986.
51. Echols WR. U.S. Patent No.5,081,447. Washington, DC: U.S. Patent and Trademark Office; 1992.
52. Pfeifer T. (2009). U.S. Patent Application 12/416,613.
53. Barnoach I. U.S. Patent No. 6,057,767. Washington, DC: U.S. Patent and Trademark Office; 2000.
54. De Vries N, Boucher RP, Doelling EN. U.S. Patent No. 20,110,316,705. Washington, DC: U.S. Patent and Trademark Office; 2011.
55. Van Maanen JP, Richard W, Van Kesteren ER, Ravesloot MJL, Laman DM, Hilgevoord AAJ, de Vries N. Evaluation of a new simple treatment for positional sleep apnoea patients. J Sleep Res. 2012;21(3):322–9.
56. Bignold JJ, Mercer JD, Antic NA, McEvoy RD, Catcheside PG. Accurate position monitoring and improved supine-dependent obstructive sleep apnoea with a new position recording and supine avoidance device. J Clin Sleep Med. 2011;7(4):376–83.
57. Van Beest E. WIPO Patent No. 2011139141. Geneva: World Intellectual Property Organization; 2011.
58. Van Maanen JP, Meester KA, Dun LN, Koutsourelakis I, Witte BI, Laman DM, Hilgevoord AAJ, de Vries N. The sleep position trainer: a new treatment for positional obstructive sleep apnoea. Sleep Breath. 2013;17(2):771–9.
59. Levendowski DJ, Zavora T, Westbrook PR, Mitrovic M, Veljkovic B, Berka C, Trejo J. WIPO Patent No. 2010141893. Geneva: World Intellectual Property Organization; 2010.
60. Permut I, Diaz-Abad M, Chatila W, Crocetti J, Gaughan JP, D'Alonzo GE, Krachman SL. Comparison of positional therapy to CPAP in patients with positional obstructive sleep apnoea. J Clin Sleep Med. 2012;6(3):238–43.

Long-Term Results and Compliance of a Special Vest Preventing the Supine Position

Joachim T. Maurer

Introduction

Sleeping in the supine position has been linked to snoring since long. Upper airway obstruction has been shown to worsen during sleep when lying on the back. In some patients obstructive events exclusively occur in this body position, which is called positional obstructive sleep apnea (POSA). Avoiding the supine position is therefore considered a viable treatment option for more than three decades in POSA.

In general, there are two possibilities to reduce or even completely eliminate the time sleeping supine: using any kind of obstacle placed in the back such as a tennis ball, a backpack, or a vest, making it impossible to lay on it on one side, and any kind of training to learn not to sleep on the back on the other side. Historical reports and patents from the last more than hundred years mainly focus on applying the first principle in snoring treatment. Kavey et al. [1] evaluated first the efficacy of the tennis ball technique (TBT) in four OSA patients and found a reduction of time spent supine as well as respiratory events. However, patients, relatives, or health-care personnel mainly manufacture the TBT themselves. Furthermore, sleeping supine was not eliminated entirely having possibly a negative effect on treatment efficacy. Some people consider the tennis ball to be too small and its fixation too loose and slippery around the patient's body. Hence, some patients are still able to sleep supine part of the night when using the TBT. Therefore, we tested a vest specifically designed and well fit hoping to reliably eliminate supine sleep and improve efficacy. Furthermore, this chapter reviews available data on efficacy and long-term compliance of supine prevention vests.

J.T. Maurer, M.D. (✉)
Department of Otorhinolaryngology, Head & Neck Surgery, Sleep Disorders Center, University Hospital Mannheim, Theodor-Kutzer-Ufer 1-3, 68167 Mannheim, Germany
e-mail: joachim.maurer@umm.de

N. de Vries et al. (eds.), *Positional Therapy in Obstructive Sleep Apnea*,
DOI 10.1007/978-3-319-09626-1_21

Description of the Supine Prevention Vest

The vest consists of strong linen tissue and contains a half-cylindrical piece of hard foam in its dorsal part (Fig. 1). It can be closed tight fit by adhesive strips. There are several sizes available according to body height, chest, and waist circumference. If necessary it can also be made custom fit. When wearing the vest, it is impossible to sleep completely on the back, but an intermediate position between lateral and supine can occur.

Variations of the vest in size of the rigid foam sold by different manufacturers exist in the international market.

Existing Data

In our case study [2], we examined 12 patients with POSA as defined by an overall AHI > 10, a supine AHI > twice non-supine AHI and at least 1 h of sleep supine and non-supine, respectively. All patients received a baseline polysomnography according to standard criteria followed by fitting the vest (Fig. 1) and getting used to it during the day and a second polysomnography at night while wearing the vest.

We could show that the vest eliminated supine posture effectively. AHI was reduced in every single patient with only one patient showing a drop in AHI of less than 50 %. The average AHI dropped from 26.7 ± 11.9 to 7.6 ± 5.1. So was time spent with oxygen saturation below 90 % (from 11.7 ± 11.3 to 1.5 ± 2.1). However, snoring was not reduced to the same extent (from 180 ± 125 to 110 ± 52 min) with

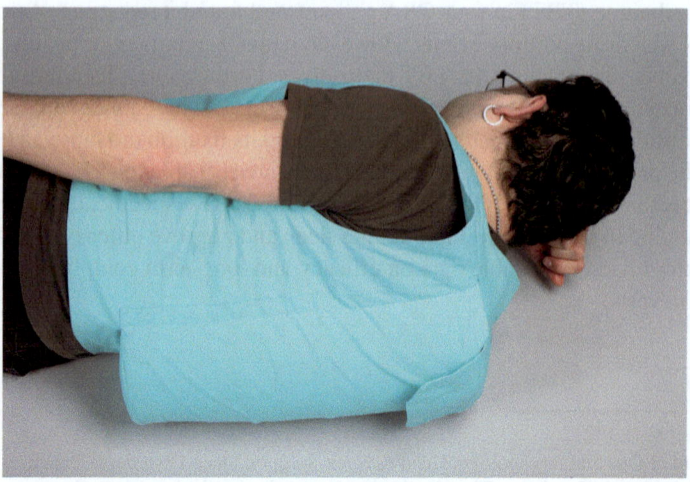

Fig. 1 Supine prevention vest (RLV-Weste, Fa. Fanderl, Neumarkt, Germany) as worn by the patient

an increase of snoring time in 30 % of the cases. Sleep parameters such as sleep efficiency, the amount of sleep stages S1 and S2, slow wave sleep and REM sleep, as well as arousal index remained unchanged. All patients could sleep with the vest but two patients deemed it necessary getting used to. In summary, the supine prevention vest was able to show its efficacy during the first night of use.

However, until today there is only one study comparing a supine prevention vest with CPAP. Permut et al. [3] tested 38 patients with POSA as assessed by a baseline polysomnogram (AHI 13 ± 5) in a randomized crossover design for two consecutive nights. PT as well as CPAP reduced the AHI below 5 in 92 % vs. 97 %. Again there was a between-group difference of the treatment AHI in favor of CPAP (2 vs. 0), which may be considered clinically meaningless. Sleep parameters as well as oxygenation were comparable.

Both studies clearly show that upper airway obstruction and consecutive impaired breathing can be normalized effectively with vests preventing the supine position. Results are even comparable to CPAP treatment. Unfortunately, long-term data was not assessed in either of the studies.

Wenzel and co-workers [4] presented similar short-term results with the same type of vest in 14 patients. In addition, they conducted a structured telephone interview 13.7 ± 15.9 months after the initial fitting of the vest. Only four patients (29 %) continued using the vest daily after the sleep specialist had recommended it. Two among them were initial nonresponders, one a partial responder and one a complete responder. The latter was using the vest for 5 years at the time of the interview. All long-term users experienced a relevant subjective benefit regarding daytime sleepiness with a significant reduction of Epworth Sleepiness Scale from 8.5 ± 6.5. Patients who refused using the vest complained about the uncomfortable posture due to the rigid foam in the back (ten of ten), sleep interruptions (nine of ten), inability to sleep supine being the preferred sleep position (seven of ten), sweating (four of ten), feeling of tightness and hence the lack of subjective benefit. Of this group, three patients each decided to undergo surgery or weight reduction instead. Four patients followed rules of sleep hygiene more consequently as their own decision. Objective long-term data were not collected.

Similarly low subjective adherence rates have been reported with the TBT Oksenberg [5] reported that 19 of 50 (38 %) patients were still using the TBT after 6 months and Bignold [6] found only four long-term users of 67 (6 %) patients responding to a mail-based questionnaire after a follow-up of 2.5 ± 1.0 years. Reasons for interrupting positional treatment in both studies were again uncomfortable and disturbed sleep, back pain, or ineffectivity. Measuring objective compliance as done with CPAP is therefore of major importance when using positional therapy, too.

Taking this problem into account, the Swiss group of Heinzer [7] inserted and fixed an actigraph into another type of supine prevention vest and prospectively assessed objective compliance in 16 patients with POSA over a 3-month period. One patient stopped using the vest due to back pain, a second one after a car accident. The remaining 14 patients used the vest for an average of 73.7 ± 29.3 % of the nights during 8.0 ± 2.0 h per night. Respiratory parameters were significantly improved with the positional device during the first as well as during the follow-up night but did not significantly differ between each other. Sleep parameters or other outcome measures such as daytime vigilance or cardiovascular parameters were not assessed. Possible reasons for the far better compliance in this study are the following: The device used might be more comfortable as there was only a plastic hump at the scapula of each side but no long and stiff half cylinder along the whole back, follow-up was only 3 months, and patients were aware that compliance was monitored objectively.

Other important outcome measures have been evaluated for the TBT in controlled trials. TBT had a similar effect on quality of life, mood, daytime performance [8], and blood pressure [9] as CPAP even though respiratory parameters during PSG were still slightly inferior to CPAP. There is no such data regarding supine prevention vests so far.

Conclusion

Specifically designed vests effectively eliminate supine position and eliminate POSA as effectively as CPAP. However, compliance cannot be measured in commercially available vests, and long-term treatment adherence is very low in clinical use due to the discomfort while wearing the vests. If vests become more comfortable and treatment compliance as well as adherence can be monitored objectively, then it probably will become a first-line alternative to CPAP or Auto-CPAP in POSA patients.

References

1. Kavey NB, Blitzer A, Gidro-Frank S, Korstanje K. Sleeping position and sleep apnea syndrome. Am J Otolaryngol. 1985;6:373–7.
2. Maurer JT, Stuck BA, Hein G, Verse T, Hörmann K. Treatment of obstructive sleep apnea with a new vest preventing the supine position. Dtsch Med Wochenschr. 2003;128:71–5.
3. Permut I, Diaz-Abad M, Chatila W, Crocetti J, Gaughan JP, D'Alonzo GE, Krachman SL. Comparison of positional therapy to CPAP in patients with positional obstructive sleep apnea. J Clin Sleep Med. 2010;6:238–43.
4. Wenzel S, Smith E, Leiacker R, Fischer Y. [Efficacy and longterm compliance of the vest preventing the supine position in patients with obstructive sleep apnea]. Laryngorhinootologie. 2007;86:579–83.
5. Oksenberg A, Silverberg D, Offenbach D, Arons E. Positional therapy for obstructive sleep apnea patients: a 6-month follow-up study. Laryngoscope. 2006;116:1995–2000.
6. Bignold JJ, Deans-Costi G, Goldsworthy MR, Robertson CA, McEvoy D, Catcheside PG, Mercer JD. Poor long-term patient compliance with the tennis ball technique for treating positional obstructive sleep apnea. J Clin Sleep Med. 2009;5:428–30.
7. Heinzer RC, Pellaton C, Rey V, Rossetti AO, Lecciso G, Haba-Rubio J, Tafti M, Lavigne G. Positional therapy for obstructive sleep apnea: an objective measurement of patients' usage and efficacy at home. Sleep Med. 2012;13:425–8.

8. Jokic R, Klimaszewski A, Crossley M, Sridhar G, Fitzpatrick MF. Positional treatment vs continuous positive airway pressure in patients with positional obstructive sleep apnea syndrome. Chest. 1999;115:771–81.
9. Berger M, Oksenberg A, Silverberg DS, Arons E, Radwan H, Iaina A. Avoiding the supine position during sleep lowers 24 h blood pressure in obstructive sleep apnea (OSA) patients. J Hum Hypertens. 1997;11:657–64.

Results of a First-Generation New Device for Positional Therapy

J. Peter van Maanen, Wietske Richard, Ellen R. van Kesteren, Madeline Ravesloot, D. Martin Laman, Antonius J. Hilgevoord, and Nico de Vries

Introduction

More than half of OSA patients appear to have position-dependent obstructive sleep apnea (POSA), defined as an apnea–hypopnoea index (AHI) during sleep in supine position that is at least twice as high as the AHI during sleep in other positions [1, 2].

The therapeutic armamentarium for obstructive sleep apnea (OSA) comprises several treatment options. Continuous positive airway pressure (CPAP) is often regarded as the gold standard in the treatment of moderate and severe cases. Oral

J.P. van Maanen, M.D. (✉)
Department of Otolaryngology, Sint Lucas Andreas Ziekenhuis, Amsterdam, The Netherlands
e-mail: p.vanmaanen@slaz.nl

W. Richard, M.D., Ph.D.
Department of Otolaryngology/Head and Neck Surgery, Sint Lucas Andreas Hospita, Jan Tooropstraat 164, 1061 AE Amsterdam, The Netherlands

E.R. van Kesteren, B.Sc. • A.A.J. Hilgevoord, M.D., Ph.D.
Department of Neurology and Clinical Neurophysiology, St. Lucas Andreas Hospital, Amsterdam, The Netherlands

M. Ravesloot, M.D., Ph.D.
Department of Otorhinolaryngology, Sint Lucas Andreas Ziekenhuis, Amsterdam, The Netherlands

D.M. Laman, M.D., Ph.D.
Department of Clinical Neurophysiology, St. Lucas Andreas Hospital, Amsterdam, The Netherlands

N. de Vries, M.D., Ph.D.
Department of Otolaryngology, Sint Lucas Andreas Ziekenhuis, Amsterdam, The Netherlands

Department of Otolaryngology, University Hospital Antwerp, Antwerp, Belgium

N. de Vries et al. (eds.), *Positional Therapy in Obstructive Sleep Apnea*,
DOI 10.1007/978-3-319-09626-1_22

appliances and upper airway surgery are both used in mild and moderate cases or in reserve of CPAP failure. In all patients with OSA, conservative approaches including abstinence of alcohol and sedatives, weight reduction, cessation of smoking and avoidance of the supine sleeping position in POSA should be considered [3]. The role of positional therapy as a minimally invasive treatment modality in patients with positional OSA looks promising [4]. The discomfort and disruption of sleep architecture however have been responsible for poor compliance and subsequent disappointing results of these interventions in the past. In this chapter a new neck-worn device that influences sleep position whilst getting around the problem of sleep quality disruption will be presented.

Methods

Design

Consecutive patients, aged >18 years, who were diagnosed, using full overnight in-hospital polysomnography, with positional sleep apnea (AHI > 5, AHI supine ≥ 2 × AHI other positions, percentage of total sleep time in supine position ≥10 % and ≤90 %) were requested to participate in this study. In addition to the first baseline polysomnography, patients underwent two more in-hospital polysomnographies after they had given written informed consent. These two test recordings were scheduled with at least 1 week and no more than 2 weeks in between, so that possible sleep deprivation resulting from the first would not influence the second recording. During the test recordings, patients wore the electronic device attached to their neck. Randomly, in one of the two polysomnographies, the device was active (ON); in the other, it was inactive (OFF). Patients were blinded for the chosen activity state of the device. The study was approved by the local human research ethics review board.

Device

The device consisted of a small vibrating apparatus (3 × 3 × 1 cm, powered by three small batteries; see Fig. 1a) similar to the silent alarm device used in mobile phones. This silent, vibrating alarm was triggered by a position sensor. The position sensor started the trigger with a delay of 10 s after the supine position was detected, causing the device to vibrate with gradually incremental strength for as long as it took the position sensor to detect another position, in which case the vibrations ceased immediately. The small device was worn secured to the skin of the neck with hypoallergenic adhesive tape (Fig. 1b) and connected to the polysomnography system.

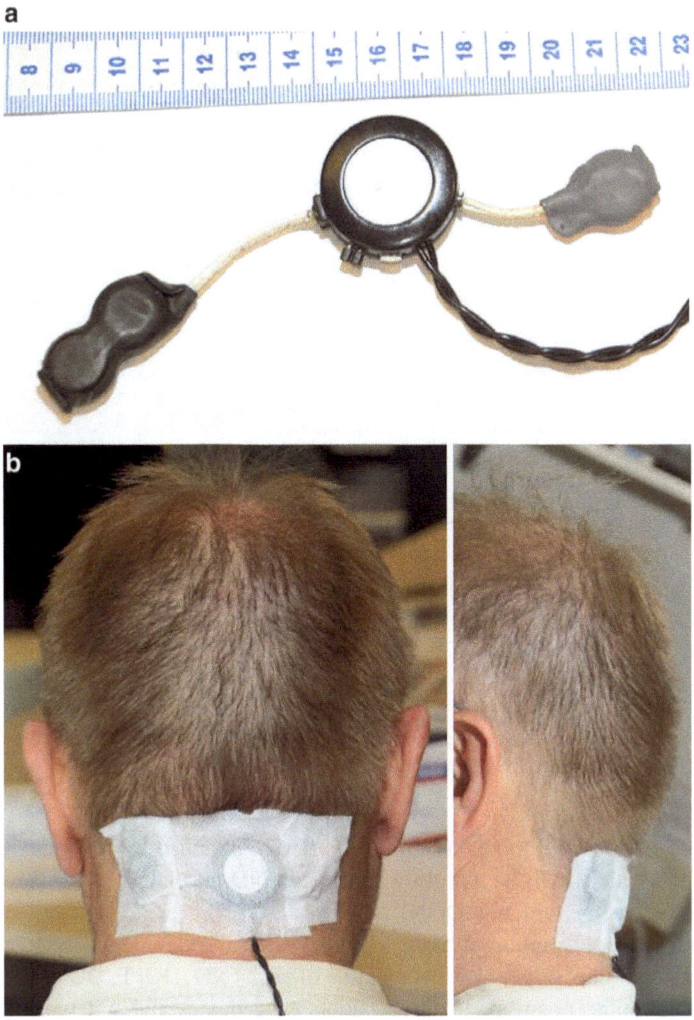

Fig. 1 (**a**, **b**) The middle part (ring structure) of the apparatus shown consists of a small vibrating motor (like the one used in cell phones) and a position sensor. Three small round batteries (two positioned on the *left*, one on the *right*) are connected via the white cables. The braided black cables connect the device to the polysomnograph system

Results

During a study period of 18 months, 30 patients were included. In these patients the third PSG was performed 1 week to 3 months, median 1.5 months, after the first PSG (Table 1). Individual body mass indices over time did not differ more than 0.2 kg/m^2. Polysomnography results were divided into three groups: no device (ND),

Table 1 Baseline characteristics of all patients ($n=30$)

Patient characteristics	
Age (years)	48.0±9.5
Body mass index (kg/m²)	27.7±3.6
Male:female ratio	6:1
Median months from PSG 1–3	1.5

Age and body mass index are shown as mean ± standard deviation

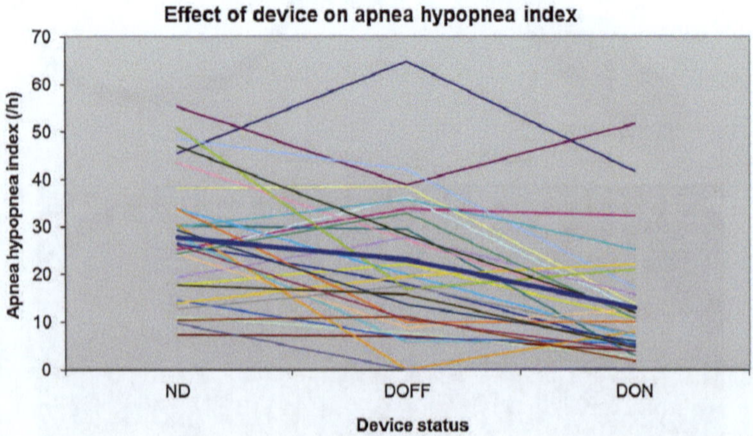

Fig. 2 The *thickened line* depicts the mean value. *ND* no device, *DOFF* device attached in OFF modus, *DON* device attached in ON modus

device attached in OFF modus (DOFF) and device attached in ON modus (DON). Display of *p*-values will be as follows: between ND and DOFF, between ND and DON and between DOFF and DON.

Analysis of polysomnography data showed that the device worked well in 27 patients. All patients slept at least some time of each (ND, DOFF, DON) of the three nights in a supine position. In three patients the device did not work properly. According to the position sensor in these patients, despite an episode of supine position, the device did not vibrate. The analysis was performed on intention-to-treat basis, and therefore, these patients were not excluded from analysis. No side effects were reported.

The effect of the device on mean sleep parameters ± standard error of the mean is shown in Fig. 4. Highlighted values indicate significance.

In Fig. 2 the effect of the device on apnea–hypopnoea index for each individual patient is shown. The thicker line shows the mean value for all patients. Although wearing the device in OFF modus already had a significant effect on the AHI, the decrease in AHI was much larger when the device was worn in ON modus. Differences in AHI between ND and DOFF and between DOFF and DON were not affected by sleeping the first or the second night with the device attached in ON modus (data not shown here).

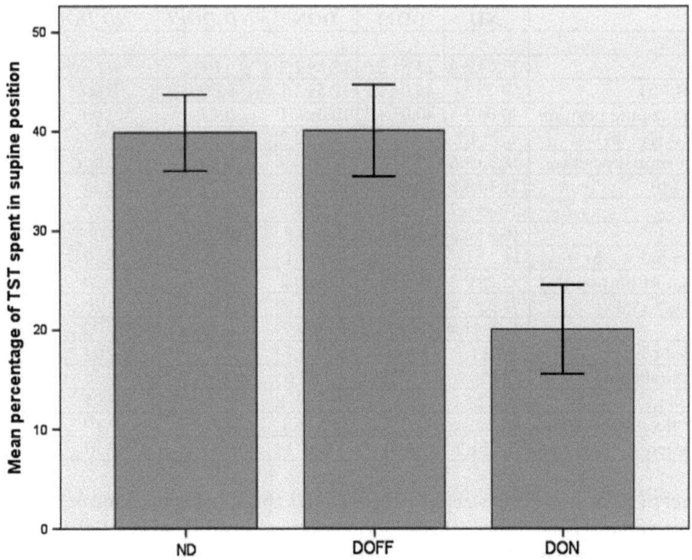

Fig. 3 Effect of device on percentage of TST in supine position. *TST* total sleep time, *ND* no device, *DOFF* device attached in OFF modus, *DON* device attached in ON modus. The *y error bars* depict the standard error of the mean

The average percentage of total sleep time spent in supine position significantly decreased from 40.0 (ND) and 40.0 (DOFF) to 19.0 % (DON) when the device was worn in ON modus ($p=0.93$, 0.00, 0.00) (Fig. 3). Individuals who wore the device in ON modus the first night did not seem to avoid the supine position more effectively the second night (without vibration) compared to those who wore the device off in the first night (data not shown). This could be due to the time (1–2 weeks) in between the two recordings.

The device attached in OFF modus did not have a significant effect on the desaturation index when compared to no device. The device in ON modus did have a significant effect on the desaturation index when compared to no device and in OFF modus (Fig. 4).

Mean total sleep times were 436 (ND), 417 (DOFF) and 393 (DON) minutes ($p=0.14$, 0.00, 0.13), showing that the device in ON modus leads to a significant reduction in total sleep time when compared to no device attached.

Arousal index was found to be 9.0 (ND), 9.9 (DOFF) and 6.8 (DON) ($p=0.77$, 0.04, 0.01). The arousal index was significantly lower in the group with the device in ON modus when compared to the no device group and the group with the device in OFF modus.

The effect of the device and its status on mean oxygen saturation, sleep efficiency, percentage of deep sleep and number of awakenings was insignificant. Sleep efficiency was found to be 91.9 % (ND), 89.9 % (DOFF) and 88.3 % (DON) ($p=0.21$, 0.10, 0.59); percentage of deep sleep was 19.8 (ND), 18.5 (DOFF) and 19.7 (DON) ($p=0.73$, 0.95, 0.84). Mean number of awakenings was 3.4 (ND), 3.9 (DOFF) and 4.1 (DON) ($p=0.74$, 0.36, 0.76).

	ND	DOFF	DON	*p ND DOFF*	*p ND DON*	*p DOFF DON*
AHI (/h)	27.7±2.4	23.5±2.6	12.8±2.2	*0.04*	*0.00*	*0.00*
Supine AHI (/h)	59.7±3.6	45.0±4.8	12.5±3.1	*0.00*	*0.00*	*0.00*
% of TST in supine position	40.0±3.5	40.0±4.5	19.0±4.1	*0.93*	*0.00*	*0.00*
Nonsupine AHI (/h)	6.7±1.2	13.4±2.7	11.2±2.2	*0.02*	*0.03*	*0.49*
% TST non supine position	58.5±3.6	55.5±4.9	78.5±4.0	*0.63*	*0.00*	*0.00*
AHI REM (/h)	21.1±4.2	24.6±4.9	16.2±4.3	*0.25*	*0.35*	*0.29*
% REM	21.7±1.2	18.3±1.5	19.2±1.5	*0.11*	*0.27*	*0.67*
AI (/h)	16.3±2.3	11.5±1.6	3.4±0.8	*0.01*	*0.00*	*0.00*
desaturation index (/h)	11.5±1.7	9.7±1.8	4.6±1.1	*0.26*	*0.00*	*0.01*
mean oxygen saturation (%)	95.2±0.3	95.2±0.3	95.6±0.2	*0.24*	*0.20*	*0.34*
sleep efficiency (%)	91.9±1.4	89.9±1.6	88.3±1.8	*0.21*	*0.10*	*0.59*
TST (min)	436±11.4	417±10.6	393±9.7	*0.14*	*0.00*	*0.13*
arousal index (/h)	9.0±1.1	9.9±1.0	6.8±0.7	*0.77*	*0.04*	*0.01*
number of awakenings	3.4±0.6	3.9±0.9	4.1±0.6	*0.74*	*0.36*	*0.76*
% of deep sleep	19.8±1.6	18.5±1.5	19.7±1.4	*0.73*	*0.95*	*0.84*
Wake after sleep onset (min)	40.7±9.5	42.2±7.6	39.5±6.1	*0.81*	*0.40*	*0.77*
% Stage 1 sleep	5.3±1.2	5.3±0.9	5.6±1.1	*0.86*	*0.76*	*0.64*

Fig. 4 Effect of device on mean sleep parameters. *AHI* apnea-hypopnoea index, *AI* apnea index, *TST* total sleep time, *ND* no device, *DOFF* device attached in OFF modus, *DON* device attached in ON modus. *Shaded* are *p*-values <0.05. Standard error of the means is shown

Discussion

Fifty-six percent of sleep apnea patients suffer from position-dependent OSA (POSA), with position dependency defined as an at least two times higher AHI in supine position than the mean AHI in the other positions and a percentage of total sleep time in supine position ≥10 % and ≤90 % [1, 2]. Positional therapy can be defined as preventing patients to sleep in the worst sleeping position. The worst sleeping position is usually but not always the supine position. Previous attempts by strapping an object on the back (tennis balls, squash balls, special vests [5–8], "shark fins", etc.) were unsuccessful due to arousals whilst turning from one position to the other, thereby disturbing sleep architecture and sleep quality. This leads to serious lack of compliance. Tennis ball therapy, for example, has a long-term compliance of less than 10 %, mainly because of its effect on sleep quality and comfort complaints [7].

The present device gets around this problem, since this small, light and comfortable to wear device did not seem to cause any discomfort during position change.

Permut et al. recently showed that positional therapy with a bulky mass strapped to the back was equal to CPAP in normalizing the AHI in patients with mild to moderate POSA [9]. However, patient selection criteria and thus definition of POSA were not the same as in our study. In their proposal for an alternative definition of POSA, patients should have a non-supine AHI of <5. We believe this definition of POSA to be too restrictive, because a significant number of patients with position-dependent obstructive sleep apnea would be excluded, whilst using positional therapy in these patients could lead to a clinical significant lowering of the AHI. So unlike the group of Permut, we did include patients suffering from severe POSA with AHI > 5 in lateral sleeping position. This explains that our mean AHI was 12.8 and not below 5.

When Sher's AHI definition of surgical success (AHI < 20 and >50 % reduction of AHI) is used, a 60.0 % (18/30) success rate is achieved [10]. This success rate would have been even higher (66.6 %) if the three patients in which the device did not work properly due to technical failure were not taken into account. In 7 out of 30 (23 %) patients, the overall AHI dropped below 5 when using the device in ON modus, whereas using the device in OFF modus did not cause the AHI to drop below 5.

Wearing the device in ON modus had a significant effect on AHI when compared to wearing no device ($p=0.00$). When worn in OFF modus, however, the device also had a significant effect on AHI when compared to wearing no device ($p=0.04$). This could be because subjects felt the device in their neck, shifting the preferred position of the head without leading to clear changes in other sleep parameters.

Apnea–hypopnoea index, apnea index and desaturation index usually increase during REM sleep. So longer periods of REM sleep would lead to higher index values. However, no significant differences in REM sleep percentages of total sleep time nor AHI during REM sleep were found between ND, DOFF and DON group.

The effect of wearing or not wearing the device and its status on sleep efficiency, percentage of deep sleep and number of awakenings was insignificant. There was, however, a significant shortening of the mean total sleep time in the DON modus compared to the ND. Other sleep quality items were not different between groups, except for the arousal index. This was significantly reduced in the DON, implying that the arousals evoked by the device outweigh the arousals caused by the otherwise occurring apneas and hypopnoeas. Since validated post-PSG quality of sleep questionnaires do not exist, we did not investigate this any further; therefore, interpretation of the sleep time shortening in the DON modus is difficult.

Since overnight AHI and sleep quality were our primary end points of the study, we did not further analyse how often stimulator activity led to position change and either an arousal or awakening. Another limitation of this study is the lack of subjective data. The initial set-up of this study was to have patients fill in Epworth Sleepiness Scales following each night in hospital and ask them about their experiences with the device and their subjective sleep quality. Unfortunately, at the end of the study period, we noticed that a considerable number of patients had not received the questionnaire.

The average percentage of total sleep time spent in supine position significantly changed from 40 to 19 %. The data analysis was performed on intention-to-treat basis. The relatively high residual percentage of supine sleeping position is mostly due to the three patients in whom the device did not work properly. The median percentage supine sleeping position was found to be 5 % (data not shown). This indicates that with technical improvements in the next generation of such a device, it is realistic to believe that a much lower mean percentage supine sleeping position can be achieved. The second reason it did not decrease to 0 % could be because of a discrepancy between the two separate position recording sensors. The position sensor in the device was in the neck, and the PSG position sensor was attached to the midline of the abdominal wall. In some subjects obstructive episodes might be alleviated through mere rotation of the head sideways whilst the trunk remained in the supine position. The finding that the occurrence of obstructive sleep apnea not solely depends on position of the trunk but also depends on the position of the head has been discussed in more detail elsewhere [11]. Also, the extent to which participants respond to the stimulus to change their body position might be different, depending on their response threshold. That is to say, the higher their response threshold, the longer the TST in supine position, indicating our stimulus might have been too weak for some of the patients. Future research in our hospital is ongoing and concentrating on collecting subjective results and offering different stimuli to be able to decrease the percentage of total sleep time spent in supine position and thereby the overall AHI.

The results of treating POSA patients with this device are convincing, and the impact on future treatment of sleep apnea could be enormous. In approximately 80 % of patients, sleeping position plays a role (56 % with a factor 2 difference in AHI, the rest with less than factor 2). Positional therapy with a device like the one presented in this chapter can be applied as single treatment in many patients with mild to moderate position-dependent obstructive sleep apnea, whilst in patients with a more severe obstructive sleep apnea syndrome, such a device could be used in combination with other treatment modalities. Also many patients with central sleep apnea syndrome might benefit from this simple, cheap and successful treatment [12, 13]. Further research should focus on long-term compliance and direct comparison to other treatment modalities.

References

1. Oksenberg A, Silverberg DS, Arons E, Radwan H. Positional vs nonpositional obstructive sleep apnea patients. Chest. 1997;112:629–39.
2. Richard W, Kox D, den Herder C, Laman M, van Tinteren H, de Vries N. The role of sleeping position in obstructive sleep apnea. Eur Arch Otorhinolaryngol. 2006;263:946–50.
3. Randerath WJ, Verbraecken J, Andreas S, Bettega G, Boudewyns A, Hamans E, et al. European Respiratory Society task force on non-CPAP therapies in sleep apnoea. Non-CPAP therapies in obstructive sleep apnoea. Eur Respir J. 2011;37:1000–28.
4. Ravesloot MJL, van Maanen JP, Dun L, de Vries N. The undervalued potential of positional therapy in position dependent snoring and obstructive sleep apnea – a review of the literature. Sleep Breath. 2013;17:39–49.
5. Maurer JT, Stuck BA, Hein G, Verse T, Hörmann K. Schlafapnoetherapie mit einer neuartigen rückenlage-verhinderungs-weste. Dtsch Med Wochenschr. 2003;128:71–5.
6. Wenzel S, Smith E, Leiacker R, Fischer Y. Efficacy and longterm compliance of the vest preventing the supine position in patients with obstructive sleep apnea. Laryngorhinootologie. 2007;86:579–83.
7. Bignold JJ, Deans-Costi G, Goldsworthy MR, Robertson CA, McEvoy D, Catcheside PG, Mercer JD. Poor long-term patient compliance with the tennis ball technique for treating positional obstructive sleep apnea. J Clin Sleep Med. 2009;5:428–30.
8. Oksenberg A, Silverberg D, Offenbach D, Arons E. Positional therapy for obstructive sleep apnea patients: a 6-month follow-up study. Laryngoscope. 2006;116:1995–2000.

9. Permut I, Diaz-Abad M, Chatila W, Crocetti J, Gaughan JP, D'Alonzo GE, Krachman SL. Comparison of positional therapy to CPAP in patients with positional obstructive sleep apnea. J Clin Sleep Med. 2010;6:238–43.
10. Sher AE, Schechtman KB, Piccirillo JF. The efficacy of surgical modifications of the upper airway in adults with obstructive sleep apnea syndrome. Sleep. 1996;19:156–77.
11. Van Kesteren ER, van Maanen JP, Hilgevoord AAJ, Laman DM, de Vries N. Quantitative effects of trunk and head position on the apnea hypopnea index in obstructive sleep apnea. Sleep. 2011;34:1075–81.
12. Joho S, Oda Y, Hirai T, Inoue H. Impact of sleeping position on central sleep apnea/Cheyne-Stokes respiration in patients with heart failure. Sleep Med. 2010;11:143–8.
13. Szollosi I, Roebuck T, Thompson B, Naughton MT. Lateral sleeping position reduces severity of central sleep apnea/Cheyne-Stokes respiration. Sleep. 2006;29:1045–51.

Short-Term (4 Weeks) Results of the Sleep Position Trainer for Positional Therapy

J. Peter van Maanen, Kristel A.W. Meester, Lideke N. Dun, Ioannis Koutsourelakis, Birgit I. Witte, D. Martin Laman, Antonius A.J. Hilgevoord, and Nico de Vries

Introduction

In three studies from Israel and the Netherlands, a remarkable steady 56 % of patients have positional sleep apnea (POSA), defined as a supine AHI twice or more as compared to the AHI in the other sleeping positions [1–3].

Attempts to decrease the severity of sleep apnea by influencing sleep position have been reported but with limited success [4]. The tennis ball technique, where a tennis ball is placed in the centre of the back, was one of the first described positional therapies and has been shown to be effective in normalizing AHI in positional

J.P. van Maanen, M.D. (✉)
Department of Otolaryngology, Sint Lucas Andreas Ziekenhuis,
Jan Tooropstraat 164, 1061 AE Amsterdam, The Netherlands
e-mail: p.vanmaanen@slaz.nl

K.A.W. Meester, B.Sc. • D.M. Laman, M.D., Ph.D.
Department of Clinical Neurophysiology, St. Lucas Andreas Hospital,
Amsterdam, The Netherlands

L.N. Dun, M.Sc. • I. Koutsourelakis, M.D., Ph.D.
Department of Otolaryngology/Head and Neck Surgery, Sint Lucas Andreas Hospital,
Jan Tooropstraat 164, 1061 AE Amsterdam, The Netherlands

B.I. Witte, M.Sc., Ph.D.
Department of Epidemiology and Biostatistics, VU University Medical Centre,
Amsterdam, The Netherlands

A.A.J. Hilgevoord, M.D., Ph.D.
Department of Neurology and Clinical Neurophysiology, St. Lucas Andreas Hospital,
Amsterdam, The Netherlands

N. de Vries, M.D., Ph.D.
Department of Otolaryngology, Sint Lucas Andreas Ziekenhuis,
Amsterdam, The Netherlands

Department of Otolaryngology, University Hospital Antwerp, Antwerp, Belgium

N. de Vries et al. (eds.), *Positional Therapy in Obstructive Sleep Apnea*,
DOI 10.1007/978-3-319-09626-1_23

OSA patients. Several variations of the tennis ball technique (positional alarms, verbal instructions, vests, special pillows) have also been tested with similarly good results [5–18]. However, the clinical significance of positional therapy is so far hampered by a very low compliance rate which ranges from 40 %, short term, to 10 %, long term [8, 12, 13]. These results show the need for a positional therapy system that is able to ensure high compliance and little discomfort and disruption of the sleep architecture, both being the reason for the poor compliance rates seen in the past. A simple small neck-worn vibrating device that corrects patients when sleeping in supine position has shown to be effective in significantly reducing the AHI without disrupting sleep quality [18]. In line with this technology and its encouraging results, a new medical device appropriate for wide clinical use was developed, the sleep position trainer (SPT). In this chapter short-term subjective and objective effects of using the SPT will be evaluated in POSA patients.

Methods

Design

All patients underwent two full night in-hospital polysomnographic assessments. The baseline assessment consisted of an overnight polysomnography (PSG) to confirm the diagnosis of POSA. Within 28 days after the baseline PSG, patients started using the sleep position trainer (SPT) for 29 ± 2 nights. On day one patients filled out the Epworth Sleepiness Scale (ESS) [19] and the Functional Outcomes of Sleep Questionnaire (FOSQ) [20] to assess their daytime sleepiness and quality of life.

Treatment with the SPT was divided into three phases: a diagnostic phase, a training phase and a therapy phase. The first two nights were defined as the diagnostic phase, where the SPT monitored and recorded the sleeping position and in which no active feedback was given to the patient. The following seven nights entailed the training phase, where the SPT began to vibrate in an increasing amount of episodes of supine sleep. From night ten onwards, the therapy phase started in which the SPT vibrated every time a supine sleeping position was detected in order to urge the patient to change his or her sleeping position. To promote continued use, subjects could upload and read-out information about their nightly behaviour (e.g. percentages of different sleeping positions) to their own personal computer at any desired time.

The final assessment took place after 29 ± 2 days and included a PSG whilst using the SPT. Additionally, ESS and FOSQ questionnaires were completed for a second time.

The Sleep Position Trainer Device

The sleep position trainer (SPT) is a small, lightweight device (72 × 35 × 10 mm, 25 g) which is worn around the chest in a neoprene strap (Fig. 1). The neoprene strap comprises a pocket in which the device is placed on the sternum and can be

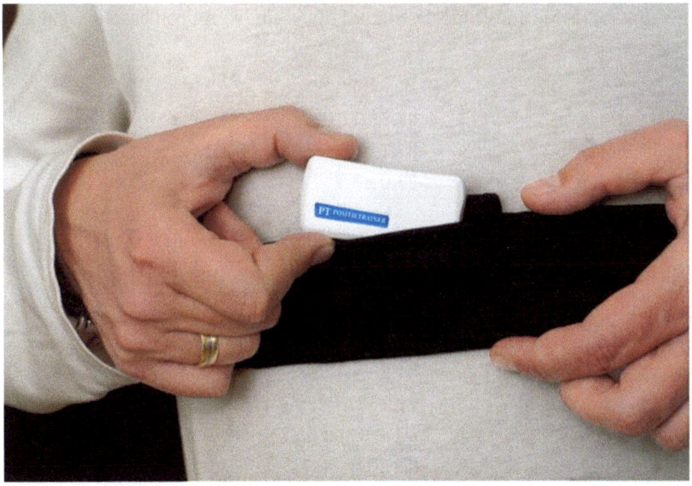

Fig. 1 Subject wearing the sleep position trainer

closed with a Velcro tab. The device measures the orientation using a three-dimensional digital accelerometer. The measurements were used to define the posture of the user: left side, right side, supine, prone or upright. The device responded to supine position with a vibration stimulus to provide feedback to the user. The stimulus started after the supine position was detected, and no turning movement was detected anymore. The device continued with a gradually increasingly strength and stimulus duration, until non-supine position was detected. If the patient did not react to the stimulus, the vibrations would be paused to be reinitiated after 2 min. Furthermore, the SPT provided an internal memory to store the sleeping posture of the user for a period of at least 90 days. The device employs a USB port to communicate data to a personal computer (PC) and to recharge the integrated battery.

Results

Thirty-one patients were enrolled ((27 males); mean age 48.1 ± 11.0 years; mean body mass index 27.0 ± 3.7 kg m^{-2}). The compliance rate was 100 % with a median use of 6.1 h per night (range, 4.1–8.6) over all nights observed. The polysomnographic and clinical characteristics of patients at baseline and after 1 month of SPT are shown in Table 1. As the results show, the total AHI but also the AHI in supine position as well as the percentage of sleep time spent in supine position, desaturation index, apnea index and ESS score presented significant decrease, whereas minimum oxygen desaturation, the percentage of sleep time spent in non-supine position and FOSQ score exhibited significant increase. Sleep efficiency did not change significantly. Individual values of the apnea–hypopnoea index, the percentage of time spent in supine position and ESS and FOSQ scores at baseline and after 1 month of positional therapy are shown in Table 2.

Table 1 Polysomnographic and clinical variables of the study group at baseline and after 1 month of SPT therapy ($n=31$)

	Baseline	After SPT	p-value
Age, years	48.1±11.0		
Male sex, %	87.1		
BMI	27.0±3.7	27.4±4.0	0.387
Compliance rate, %		100.0	
AHI, events/h	16.4 [6.6–29.9]	5.2 [0.5–46.5]	**<0.001**
AHI in supine, events/h	35.7 [9.3–81.0]	0.0 [0.0–100.7]	**<0.001**
AHI in non-supine, events/h	3.2 [0.0–16.2]	4.3 [0.1–48.0]	0.052
Average oxygen saturation, %	95.1±1.4	95.5±1.6	0.101
Minimum oxygen desaturation, %	84.5±4.1	88.4±3.6	**<0.001**
Desaturation index, events/h	11.2 [2.2–22.4]	5.2 [0.9–39.6]	**<0.001**
Apnea index, events/h	10.4 [1.0–26.3]	2.5 [0.0–21.3]	**<0.001**
Arousal index, events/h	6.1 [0.0–28.4]	5.5 [0.0–22.8]	0.289
Number of awakenings	4.0 [0.0–60.0]	3.0 [0.0–10.0]	0.323
Total sleep time, min	456±76	429±87	0.187
N2 sleep/total sleep time, %	52.0±8.7	50.0±12.1	0.322
N3 sleep/total sleep time, %	22.4±9.8	21.7±7.7	0.618
REM sleep/total sleep time, %	19.5±5.6	20.9±6.4	0.364
Sleep efficiency, %	89.1 [61.1–99.7]	89.4 [58.0–98.6]	0.544
Percentage supine	49.9 [20.4–77.3]	0.0 [0.0–48.7]	**<0.001**
Percentage non-supine position	50.1 [22.7–79.6]	100.0 [51.3–100.0]	**<0.001**
ESS score	11 [2–20]	9 [0–19]	**0.004**
FOSQ core	86.0±22.1	93.8±21.7	**0.001**

Data are presented either as mean ± SD or as median [range]
SPT sleep position trainer

Twenty-two patients were considered responders (71.0 %) and 9 nonresponders (29.0 %). The clinical and polysomnographic characteristics of responders and non-responders are presented in Table 3.

AHI, apnea index, desaturation index, supine AHI and Epworth Sleepiness Scale score all significantly decreased in the responder group. Furthermore, average oxygen saturation, minimum oxygen saturation and FOSQ score significantly increased in the responder group. In the nonresponder group, a significant increase was seen in non-supine AHI. In both responders and nonresponders, a significant increase in percentage non-supine position sleeping time and a significant decrease in percentage of supine position sleeping time were seen. Percentage of N3 or deep sleep did not change significantly during SPT therapy. Responders had a significantly lower AHI, desaturation index and apnea index than non-responders after SPT ($p<0.001$, $p=0.004$ and $p=0.001$). Non-responders had a significantly higher non-supine AHI and significantly lower number of awakenings than responders after SPT ($p<0.001$ and $p=0.008$).

Table 2 Individual values of apnea–hypopnoea index, percentage of supine position and Epworth Sleepiness Scale scores of all patients at baseline and after 1 month of SPT therapy

	AHI		% supine position		ESS		FOSQ	
Patient no	Baseline	After SPT	Baseline	After SPT	Baseline	After SPT	Baseline	After SPT
1	6.6	3.3	63.6	12.0	19	19	88	88
2	12.1	5.2	20.5	0.0	16	9	77	78
3	20.2	15.5	65.6	48.7	2	2	85	99
4	16.2	1.8	32.2	0.0	17	18	36	40
5	21.0	10.2	40.0	10.3	14	10	48	72
6	19.0	9.9	28.8	0.1	11	5	90	111
7	20.8	15.4	24.1	2.7	18	19	71	62
8	11.0	10.1	40.5	0.0	12	13	84	92
9	21.0	16.0	56.0	0.0	10	7	101	101
10	11.7	4.3	77.3	0.0	12	12	97	97
11	10.4	0.5	28.7	0.0	17	3	108	118
12	13.4	4.5	70.4	1.3	4	4	111	116
13	24.0	3.5	59.0	0.0	6	3	91	101
14	23.4	9.6	33.5	0.0	15	14	66	74
15	14.5	6.9	21.4	0.0	3	3	119	119
16	16.2	7.6	49.9	7.5	15	13	63	86
17	27.5	4.7	54.5	8.8	5	1	75	80
18	11.8	3.1	20.4	0.0	9	10	73	76
19	18.3	48.4	21.4	4.0	8	4	90	74
20	16.0	19.5	43.8	1.0	7	8	112	120
21	11.9	3.3	57.3	0.0	20	16	82	114
22	29.8	1.9	50.7	0.4	18	9	55	99
23	29.9	8.8	21.2	9.2	12	13	64	75
24	11.1	6.9	71.1	0.0	9	12	59	56
25	6.8	4.9	33.9	0.0	5	0	118	109
26	21.2	2.1	59.5	11.8	11	2	104	120
27	16.6	5.4	68.9	36.3	16	19	105	113
28	11.5	2.0	28.3	10.7	4	1	122	122
29	18.3	1.6	66.5	0.0	8	9	100	108
30	22.9	8.9	55.2	0.0	5	5	70	75
31	10.8	0.7	51.0	0.0	11	4	102	114

Figures 2 and 3 show the effect of SPT on, respectively, the percentage of supine position and AHI. Post hoc analyses showed that the decrease between diagnostic phase and training phase was highly significant ($p<0.001$), as was the case for the decrease between diagnosis phase and therapy phase and between training phase and therapy phase (data not shown here).

Table 3 Anthropometrical data and clinical and polysomnographic variables in responders and non-responders at baseline and after 1 month

	Responders ($n=22$)			Non-responders ($n=9$)			
	Baseline	After SPT	*p*-value[a]	Baseline	After SPT	*p*-value[a]	*p*-value[b]
Age, years	49.8 ± 11.6			44.1 ± 8.6			
Male sex, %	86.4			88.9			
BMI	27.3 ± 3.4			26.3 ± 4.6			
AHI, events/h	16.2 [6.6–29.9]	3.9 [0.5–10.3]	**<0.001**	18.2 [6.7–21.0]	14.1 [4.9–46.5]	0.214	**<0.001**
AHI in supine, events/h	36.5 [9.3–81.0]	0.0 [0.0–37.3]	**<0.001**	34.7 [14.9–63.6]	0.0 [0.0–100.7]	0.173	0.685
AHI in non-supine, events/h	3.2 [0.0–16.2]	3.2 [0.1–9.6]	0.833	3.7 [0.2–9.1]	10.1 [3.5–48.0]	**0.011**	**<0.001**
Average oxygen saturation, %	95.0 ± 1.5	95.5 ± 1.4	**0.004**	95.4 ± 1.0	95.2 ± 2.0	0.681	0.620
Minimum oxygen desaturation, %	84.4 ± 4.5	89.4 ± 2.3	**<0.001**	84.7 ± 3.4	86.0 ± 5.1	0.431	0.087
Desaturation index, events/h	11.2 [2.2–22.4]	4.6 [0.9–13.1]	**<0.001**	11.6 [5.5–19.0]	8.5 [3.4–39.6]	0.213	**0.004**
Apnea index, events/h	11.0 [2.2–26.3]	1.8 [0.0–7.3]	**<0.001**	8.0 [1.0–19.4]	8.3 [1.6–21.3]	0.953	**0.001**
Arousal index, events/h	7.5 [3.0–28.4]	5.2 [0.0–20.5]	**0.027**	0.0 [0.0–18.5]	6.5 [0.0–22.8]	0.176	0.203
Number of awakenings	3.5 [0.0–60.0]	4.0 [1.0–10.0]	0.659	4.0 [0.0–15.0]	1.0 [0.0–9.0]	0.068	**0.008**
Total sleep time, min	466 ± 80	433 ± 94	0.218	432 ± 63	418 ± 68	0.666	0.656
N2 sleep/total sleep time, %	49.8 ± 8.2	47.3 ± 12.2	0.366	57.3 ± 8.0	56.6 ± 9.5	0.700	0.051
N3 sleep/total sleep time, %	24.7 ± 9.3	23.6 ± 7.4	0.518	16.7 ± 8.8	17.1 ± 6.8	0.846	**0.032**
REM sleep/total sleep time, %	19.3 ± 5.9	21.0 ± 7.1	0.348	20.1 ± 5.1	20.6 ± 4.4	0.858	0.891
Sleep efficiency, %	88.6 [61.1–99.7]	86.1 [58.0–98.6]	0.306	89.1 [70.1–96.0]	92.0 [68.9–98.1]	0.594	0.086
Percentage supine	50.9 [20.4–77.3]	0.0 [0.0–36.3]	**<0.001**	40.5 [21.4–71.1]	0.1 [0.0–48.7]	**0.008**	1.000
Percentage non-supine position	49.2 [22.7–79.6]	100.0 [63.7–100.0]	**<0.001**	59.5 [29.0–78.6]	99.9 [51.3–100.0]	**0.008**	0.881
ESS score	12 [3–20]	9 [1–19]	**0.007**	9 [2–18]	7 [0–19]	0.291	0.623
FOSQ core	84.4 ± 23.6	94.8 ± 21.8	**<0.001**	90.0 ± 18.6	91.6 ± 22.6	0.710	0.715

Data are presented either as mean ± SD or as median [range]

SPT sleep position trainer

[a]Comparing baseline values with values after SPT per group responders/non-responders

[b]Comparing responders with non-responders after SPT

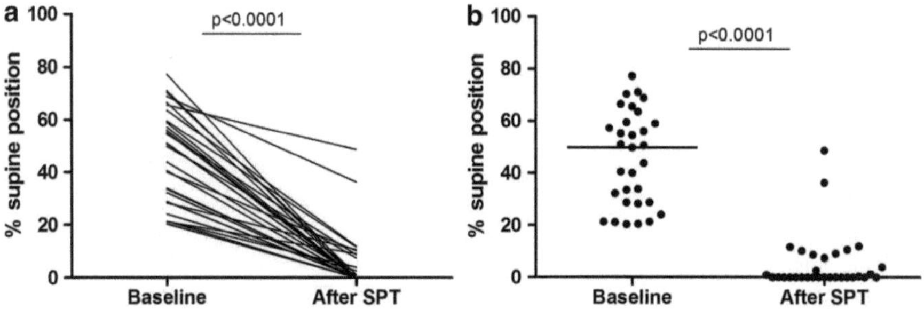

Fig. 2 Effect of SPT therapy on percentage of supine sleeping time. (**a**) *Lines* depict individual changes in percentage of supine sleeping time from baseline to after 1 month of SPT therapy. (**b**) *Dots* depict individual percentages of supine sleeping time. The *horizontal black lines* show the median. *SPT* sleep position trainer

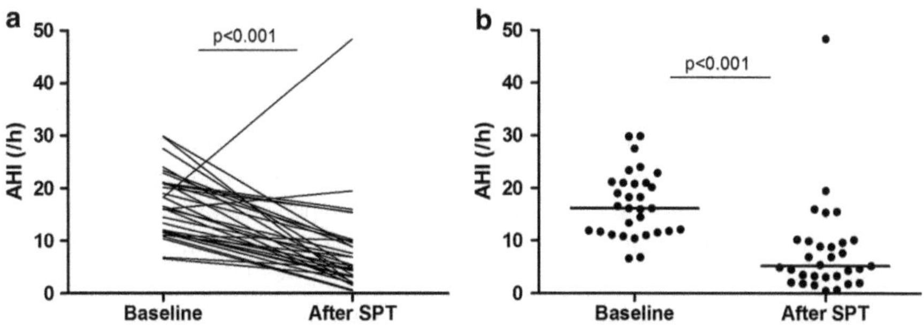

Fig. 3 Effect of SPT therapy on AHI. (**a**) *Lines* depict individual changes in AHI from baseline to after 1 month of SPT therapy. (**b**) *Dots* depict individual AHI values. The *horizontal black lines* show the median. *SPT* sleep position trainer, *AHI* apnea–hypopnoea index

Discussion

If one would set requirements for an ideal (P)OSA treatment, it would be effective and well tolerated, it would not disturb sleep or would even improve it and it would be reversible and would have negligible side effects, at acceptable costs. The analysis of more than 900 sleep nights described in this chapter indicates that the SPT fulfils these six criteria to a high degree.

It shows that the SPT is highly effective in the treatment of POSA. The percentage of time slept in supine position decreased significantly, with a median of 0 %. When Sher's criteria of surgical success [21] were used (i.e. the responder group), a 71.0 % (22/31) success rate was achieved with a median decrease of 61.1 % in AHI value. Six out of nine non-responders had an AHI reduction between 20 and 50 %. With this novel treatment, 15 patients dropped in AHI value below five and had their (P) OSA cured (Table 2). Another study with a neck-worn device [18] showed a 60 % success rate with a decrease of 53.8 % in AHI value. The mean reduction in AHI

Table 4 Comparison of first-generation device versus SPT

	First generation	SPT
Device placement	Neck (taped)	Chest (strapped)
Vibrational stimulus	Yes	Yes
Timing vibrational stimulus	After 30 s	Directly
Varying in frequency	No	Yes
Varying in amplitude	Yes	Yes
Training programme	No	Yes
Start delay	No	Yes
Data viewing feedback system	No	Yes

was similar in both studies. Apparently, the location of the device, neck or chest, and duration of usage do not influence the average reduction in AHI. Table 4 shows the comparison between the first-generation device and the SPT.

Even the most effective medical devices are only successful when used properly. CPAP is used in moderate and severe OSA. Many patients refuse or simply cannot tolerate CPAP; about 25 % of patients quit the probationary period [22]. Others use CPAP for a few hours per night, every night or incidental [23]. Treatment with oral appliances is reasonably effective in mild and moderate OSA and snoring but can have negative side effects such as jaw discomfort, hypersalivation or dry mouth, whilst in the long term, dental occlusion might change. In addition, up to one-third of patients have contraindications for using oral appliances [24].

Compliance was defined as the use of the SPT for at least 4 h per night, seven nights a week, in line with CPAP's compliance definition [25]. The compliance, in a period of 29 ± 2 nights, was 100 %, which is an exceptionally high rate in comparison to CPAP, oral device therapy or other studies which researched compliance in positional therapy. Ineffectiveness, backaches, discomfort and no improvement in sleep quality or daytime alertness have been responsible for poor compliance in positional therapy in the past. Compliance was enhanced by using a very small, comfortably fitting device with optimal physical movement freedom. Increased comfort was further supported by several algorithms like a sleep-in period and a training programme so that patients gradually could get used to sleeping in non-supine positions. In addition, patients were able to check their progress by viewing the data on their nightly behaviour on a personal computer. Improving compliance in PT is a major step forward since the recent study by Permut et al., which showed that positional therapy was equal to CPAP in normalizing the AHI in patients with mild to moderate POSA [17]. Also positive predictions have been made about the learning effect of PT. Cartwright et al. suggested that patients may learn to avoid the supine position following PT and therefore do not need to use PT on a regular basis. Others may need PT either periodically to reinforce training or consistently to ensure non-supine sleep [26].

As discussed briefly in an earlier section, compliance is very likely related to improvement in sleep quality, daytime alertness and treatment comfort. Sleep efficiency was not disrupted by the use of the SPT nor was the percentage of deep sleep.

Arousal index and number of awakenings both showed a non-significant decrease. Subjective parameters like the ESS showed a significant decrease, whereas the FOSQ significantly increased, which means that patients experienced less daytime sleepiness and a higher level of sleep-related quality of life. This finding, the significant effect on ESS and FOSQ scoring, partly might be influenced by the feedback from the device (e.g. a computer read-out of the percentage of supine sleep time) when using the therapy.

Due to the built-in training period of the SPT, patients can gradually get used to the lateral and prone positions. Fortunately, when a patient has no beneficial effects or has side effects of the device, the treatment is reversible without harming the patient, unlike surgery. Another advantage is the acceptable costs for the SPT. It is a one-time purchase, which is expected to be cheaper than CPAP. In case CPAP or PT is ineffective, it presumably can be returned to the distributor. Oral devices however are custom made and in case of failure cannot be returned and used by another patient.

There are some limitations that need to be addressed. First of all, the average percentage of total time spent in supine position changed significantly from 45.6 to 5.3 %, with a median of 0 %; 16 out of 31 patients did not sleep in supine position anymore using the SPT. One of the reasons the average percentage did not reach zero might be the finding that two patients did not respond very well to the stimulus; they were able to sleep in supine position for 48.7 and 36.3 % of total sleep time (Table 2). Sleep position was measured in position sensors placed on the trunk (one for the PSG, one for the SPT). The finding that the occurrence of obstructive sleep apnea depends not solely on the position of the trunk but also on the position of the head has already been discussed earlier by van Kesteren et al. [27]. Also, in patient 19 (Table 2) it would have been interesting to have investigated the position of the head in the polysomnographies as the AHI in lateral position was much higher in the second PSG compared to the first PSG (data not shown here), whilst percentage of supine sleep time significantly decreased.

As described in the literature, long-term results are disappointing in PT because of lack of compliance. The patients described in this chapter used the SPT for 29 ± 2 days; therefore, long-term (>6 months) effects, compliance, side effects and benefits are yet unknown. The data however showed that some people learned to avoid supine position rapidly, whilst others did not seem to have such a therapeutical effect or at least not within the period of 1 month. Further research is ongoing, concentrating on long-term compliance and data collection from a larger group of subjects.

The sleep position trainer applied for 1 month (1) cures (P)OSA in 48 % of patients (15/31), (2) is a well-tolerated treatment for patients with positional OSA with a high compliance (100.0 %), (3) is associated with a response rate of 71.0 % and a median decrease of AHI of 61.1 %, (4) reduces the percentage of total sleeping time spent in supine position to a median of zero, (5) does not negatively affect sleep quality and (6) diminishes subjective sleepiness and improves sleep-related quality of life.

In conclusion, it appears that the SPT applied for 1 month is a highly successful and well-tolerated treatment for patients with positional OSA, which diminishes subjective sleepiness and improves sleep-related quality of life without disrupting sleep quality. Further research, especially on long-term results, is ongoing.

References

1. Oksenberg A, Silverberg DS, Arons E, Radwan H. Positional vs nonpositional obstructive sleep apnea patients. Chest. 1997;112:629–39.
2. Richard W, Kox D, den Herder C, Laman M, van Tinteren H, de Vries N. The role of sleeping position in obstructive sleep apnea. Eur Arch Otorhinolaryngol. 2006;263:946–50.
3. Oksenberg A, Khamaysi I, Silverberg DS, Tarasiuk A. Association of body position with severity of apneic events in patients with severe nonpositional obstructive sleep apnea. Chest. 2000;118:1018–24.
4. Ravesloot MJL, van Maanen JP, Dun L, de Vries N. The undervalued potential of positional therapy in position dependent snoring and obstructive sleep apnea – a review of the literature. Sleep Breath. 2013;17:39–49.
5. Choi JH, Park YH, Hong JH, Kim SJ, Park DS, Miyazaki S, et al. Efficacy study of a vest-type device for positional therapy in position dependent snorers. Sleep Biol Rhythms. 2009;7:181–7.
6. Maurer JT, Stuck BA, Hein G, Verse T, Hörmann K. Schlafapnoetherapie mit einer neuartigen rückenlage-verhinderungs-weste. Dtsch Med Wochenschr. 2003;128:71–5.
7. Zuberi NA, Rekab K, Nguyen HV. Sleep apnea avoidance pillow effects on obstructive sleep apnea syndrome and snoring. Sleep Breath. 2004;8:201–7.
8. Wenzel S, Smith E, Leiacker R, Fischer Y. Efficacy and long-term compliance of the vest preventing the supine position in patients with obstructive sleep apnea. Laryngorhinootologie. 2007;86:579–83.
9. Loord H, Hultcrantz E. Positioner – a method for preventing sleep apnea. Acta Otolaryngol. 2007;127:861–8.
10. Berger M, Oksenberg A, Silverberg DS, Arons E, Radwan H, Iaina A. Avoiding the supine position during sleep lowers 24 h blood pressure in obstructive sleep apnea (OSA) patients. J Hum Hypertens. 1997;11:657–64.
11. Jokic R, Klimaszewski A, Crossley M, Sridhar G, Fitzpatrick MF. Positional treatment vs continuous positive airway pressure in patients with positional obstructive sleep apnea syndrome. Chest. 1999;115:771–81.
12. Oksenberg A, Silverberg D, Offenbach D, Arons E. Positional therapy for obstructive sleep apnea patients: a 6-month follow-up study. Laryngoscope. 2006;116:1995–2000.
13. Bignold JJ, Deans-Costi G, Goldsworthy MR, Robertson CA, McEvoy D, Catcheside PG, et al. Poor long-term patient compliance with the tennis ball technique for treating positional obstructive sleep apnea. J Clin Sleep Med. 2009;5:428–30.
14. Skinner MA, Kingshott RN, Filsell S, Taylor R. Efficacy of the 'tennis ball technique' versus nCPAP in the management of position-dependent obstructive sleep apnoea syndrome. Respirology. 2008;13:708–15.
15. Svatikova A, Chervin RD, Wing JJ, Sanchez BN, Migda EM, Brown DL. Positional therapy in ischemic stroke patients with obstructive sleep apnea. Sleep Med. 2011;12:262–6.
16. Bignold JJ, Mercer JD, Antic NA, McEvoy RD, Catcheside PG. Accurate position monitoring and improved supine-dependent obstructive sleep apnea with a new position recording and supine avoidance device. J Clin Sleep Med. 2011;7:376–83.
17. Permut I, Diaz-Abad M, Chatila W, Crocetti J, Gaughan JP, D'Alonzo GE, et al. Comparison of positional therapy to CPAP in patients with positional obstructive sleep apnea. J Clin Sleep Med. 2010;6:238–43.
18. Van Maanen JP, Richard W, van Kesteren ER, Ravesloot MJ, Laman DM, Hilgevoord AA, De Vries N. Evaluation of a new simple treatment for positional sleep apnea patients. J Sleep Res. 2012;21:322–9.
19. Johns MW. A new method for measuring daytime sleepiness: the Epworth sleepiness scale. Sleep. 1991;14:540–5.
20. Weaver TE, Laizner AM, Evans LK, Maislin G, Chugh DK, Lyon K, et al. An instrument to measure functional status outcomes for disorders of excessive sleepiness. Sleep. 1997;20:835–43.

21. Sher AE, Schechtman KB, Piccirillo JF. The efficacy of surgical modifications of the upper airway in adults with obstructive sleep apnea syndrome. Sleep. 1996;19:156–77.
22. Richard W, Venker W, den Herder C, Kox D, van den Berg B, Laman M, van Tinteren H, de Vries N, et al. Acceptance and long-term compliance of nCPAP in obstructive sleep apnea. Eur Arch Otorhinolaryngol. 2007;264:1081–6.
23. Ravesloot MJL, de Vries N. Reliable calculation of the efficacy of non-surgical and surgical treatment of obstructive sleep apnea revisited. Sleep. 2011;34:105–10.
24. Petit F, Pepin J, Bettega G, Sadek H, Raphael B, Levy P. Mandibular advancement devices: rate of contraindications in 100 consecutive obstructive sleep apnea patients. Am J Respir Crit Care Med. 2002;166:274–8.
25. Kribbs NB, Pack AI, Kline LR, Smith PL, Schwartz AR, Schubert NM, et al. Objective measurement of patterns of nasal CPAP use by patients with obstructive sleep apnea. Am Rev Respir Dis. 1993;147:887–95.
26. Cartwright RD, Lloyd S, Lilie J, Kravtiz H. Sleep position training as treatment for sleep apnea syndrome: a preliminary study. Sleep. 1985;8:87–94.
27. Van Kesteren ER, van Maanen JP, Hilgevoord AA, Laman DM, de Vries N. Quantitative effects of trunk and head position on the apnea hypopnoea index in obstructive sleep apnea. Sleep. 2011;34:1075–81.

Long-Term (6 Months) Effectiveness, Compliance, and Subjective Sleep Outcomes of Treatment with the Sleep Position Trainer in a Large Cohort of Position-Dependent OSA Patients

J. Peter van Maanen, Arjan van der Star, and Nico de Vries

Abbreviations

AHI	Apnea–Hypopnea Index
BMI	Body Mass Index
ESS	Epworth Sleepiness Scale
FOSQ	Functional Outcomes of Sleep Questionnaire
OSA	Obstructive sleep apnea syndrome
POSA	Positional obstructive sleep apnea syndrome
PSQI	Pittsburgh Sleep Quality Index
PT	Positional therapy
SPT	Sleep Position Trainer (with permission from the Associated Professional Sleep Societies, LLC, Darien, IL, USA)

J.P. van Maanen, M.D. (✉)
Department of Otolaryngology, Sint Lucas Andreas Ziekenhuis,
Jan Tooropstraat 164, 1061 AE Amsterdam, The Netherlands
e-mail: p.vanmaanen@slaz.nl

A. van der Star, M.Sc.
NightBalance B.V., Delft, The Netherlands

N. de Vries, M.D., Ph.D.
Department of Otolaryngology, Sint Lucas Andreas Ziekenhuis,
Amsterdam, The Netherlands

Department of Otolaryngology, University Hospital Antwerp, Antwerp, Belgium

N. de Vries et al. (eds.), *Positional Therapy in Obstructive Sleep Apnea*,
DOI 10.1007/978-3-319-09626-1_24

Introduction

Positional therapy (PT) has shown to significantly influence obstructive sleep apnea syndrome (OSA) severity [1]. PT with a bulky mass placed in the patient's back has been proven to be as effective as continuous positive airway pressure (CPAP) in reducing AHI in mild (5 < AHI < 15) and moderate (15 < AHI < 30) position-dependent OSA (POSA) patients [2].

The Sleep Position Trainer (SPT) was introduced in the previous chapter. It has been shown to reduce the median percentage of supine sleep time from 45.6 to 5.3 % and to cure (AHI < 5.0) 48 % of mild and moderate POSA patients who used the SPT for a month [3].

Most of the currently available prospective studies investigating PT in POSA patients have studied short-term effects on AHI and/or subjective sleep parameters during 1 day, week, or month of use [4–9]. However, it is a clinical reality that most OSA treatment options in which a device is used (CPAP, mandibular advancement device (MAD), PT) suffer from long-term compliance problems and hence hamper therapeutic effectiveness [10–12].

This chapter evaluates effectiveness, long-term compliance, and effects on subjective sleep parameters in a group of POSA patients who used the SPT for a period of 6 months.

Methods

Patients

Consecutive adult patients were recruited from 18 major sleep clinics in the Netherlands. Patients who recently, within 3 months, had been diagnosed with mild or moderate POSA by means of a polysomnography (PSG) and who could be followed up digitally and were computer literate were included. Exclusion criteria included prior (P)OSA treatment, central sleep apnea, uncontrolled or serious illness (i.e., cancer, chronic heart failure, chronic obstructive pulmonary disease), comorbid sleep disorders, seizure disorders, cardiac pacemaker, mental retardation, psychiatric disorders, and physical problems causing inability to sleep on the side. Inclusion consisted of enrolment in an online database. All participants signed informed consent prior to the initiation of any research activities.

Measures and Definitions

The SPT has been described in the previous chapter and is shown in Fig. 1. A Dutch medical device distributor company contacted and visited the included patient to deliver the SPT and instruct the patient on its use. The patient was given an online

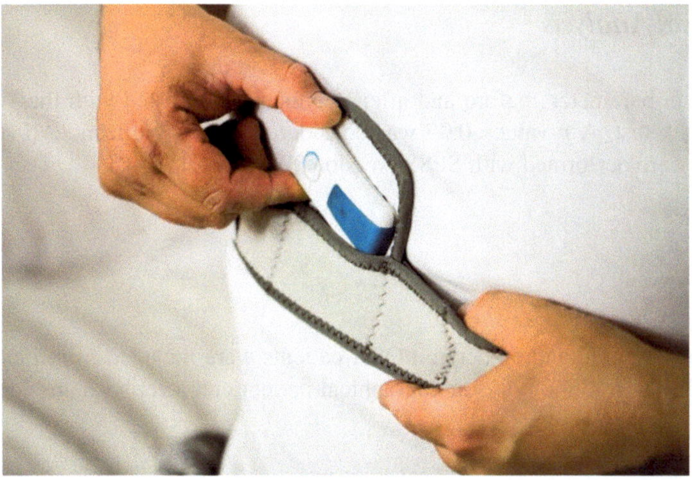

Fig. 1 The Sleep Position Trainer. Used with permission from the Associated Professional Sleep Societies, LLC, Darien, IL, USA [31]

account to be able to upload SPT data after registration of their SPT in the online database. The online inclusion system digitally sent the following questionnaires to all registered subjects at baseline and after the first, third, and sixth month of use: Epworth Sleepiness Scale (ESS, range 0–24) [13], Pittsburgh Sleep Quality Index (PSQI, range 0–21) [14], and the Functional Outcomes of Sleep Questionnaire (FOSQ, range 0–120) [15]. Patients would use the SPT for 6 months and could keep their device after the study period ended. Patients could stop using the SPT at any time. POSA was defined as an AHI $\geq$ 5 and an AHI in supine position at least twice as high when compared to each of the AHI values found in the other positions [16]. Effectiveness was defined in relation to percentage of supine sleep time. The SPT would be considered effective when the use of the device would provide a clinically significant reduction in percentage of supine sleep time. Using SPT's data recording and feedback capability, the number of times in supine position per night, the positional change index, and the response time to the vibrational stimulus were evaluated at baseline, after one, three, and 6 months. The positional change index was defined as the number of positional changes per hour of sleep. Compliance, in line with CPAP's compliance definition, was defined as the nightly use of the SPT for a period of at least 4 h. Additionally, regular SPT use was defined as at least 4 h of SPT usage on 70 % of the days monitored, in line with CPAP's criteria for regular use [17]. Objective data on compliance were obtained through means of the SPT on a day-to-day basis. Subjective compliance was measured using the online questionnaires after 1, 3, and 6 months with the questions "How many hours do you use the SPT per night?" and "How many days per week do you use the SPT?"

Statistical Analysis

Changes in parameters before and after treatment were tested with the Wilcoxon signed-rank test. A *p*-value < 0.05 was considered to be significant. All statistical analyses were performed with SPSS (version 20).

Results

A total of 145 mild and moderate POSA patients were included from February to August 2012. Baseline polysomnographical patient characteristics are depicted in Table 1.

Objective Compliance and Hours of Use

In 39 patients, neither SPT use nor SPT data could be retrieved. For the group ($n = 106$) that did upload SPT data, the distribution of hours of SPT use is shown in Table 2. Median SPT use during 6 months was 5.5 h per night for all nights. As shown in Table 3, 35 patients used the SPT during all 168 nights. Median SPT use for the 106 patients was 163 of the 168 days [interquartile range (IQR)=98]. Figure 2 shows the gradual decrease in the number of patients, from whom SPT data could be retrieved, and shows the eventual number of patients that was using the SPT and uploading the data during the full study period. Objective SPT compliance in this group of 106 patients was 64.4 %. Regular SPT use was 71.2 % over all nights observed.

SPT's Effects on Supine Sleep and on Subjective Sleep Parameters

Figure 3 illustrates that the median percentage (and IQR) of supine sleep time, as measured by the SPT, quickly decreases from baseline to day 9 and that this reduced percentage of supine sleep is maintained over time. SPT's diagnostic and training (day 1 and 2, and 3–9, respectively) and therapeutic phase (from day 10 onwards) can be clearly identified from this figure. Table 4 shows median questionnaire scores and percentage of supine sleep with IQR values for all available SPT users at the different time points. According to a test-by-test exclusion approach on missing data, all parameters showed a significant decrease when compared to baseline. The median percentage of supine sleep time decreased significantly from 21 to 2 % after 1 month ($Z = -8.015$; $p < 0.001$), to 2 % after 3 months ($Z = -7.473$; $p < 0.001$), and to 3 % after 6 months ($Z = -6.251$; $p < 0.001$) (Table 4).

Table 1 Patient characteristics at baseline inclusion polysomnography ($n=145$)

Variable	Median
AHI (/h)	11.5 [9.0]
AHI supine (/h)	28.2 [25.6]
% supine sleep	35.0 [29.0]
Age (years)	53 [14.3]
BMI (kg/m^2)	27.0 [4.0]
Ratio male/female	4.7:1

Values given in brackets represent the interquartile range

Table 2 Distribution of hours of nightly SPT use ($n=106$) as observed over the 6-month study period

Hours of use	*N*	% of patients	Cumulative % of patients
7.5–9.0	10	9.6	9.6
6.0–7.5	32	30.8	40.4
4.5–6.0	23	22.1	62.5
3.0–4.5	8	7.7	70.2
1.5–3.0	15	14.4	84.6
0–1.5	16	15.4	100
Total	104	100	
Missing	2		

Table 3 Distribution of days of SPT use ($n=106$)

Days used	*N*	% of patients	Cumulative % of patients
168	35	33.0	33.0
161–167	19	17.9	50.9
101–160	13	12.3	63.2
51–100	19	17.9	81.1
10–51	10	9.4	90.6
0–9	10	9.4	100
Total	106	100	

ESS values significantly decreased from 11 to 8 after 1 month ($Z=-6.291$; $p<0.001$), to 8 after 3 months ($Z=-6.647$; $p<0.001$), and to 8 after 6 months ($Z=-6.749$; $p<0.001$). FOSQ significantly increased from 87 to 98 after 1 month ($Z=-5.874$; $p<0.001$), to 99 after 3 months ($Z=-5.865$; $p<0.001$), and to 103 after 6 months ($Z=-6.063$; $p<0.001$). PSQI significantly decreased from 8 to 6 after 1 month ($Z=-3.922$; $p<0.001$), to 6 after 3 months ($Z=-4.329$; $p<0.001$), and to 6 after 6 months ($Z=-4.410$; $p<0.001$) (Table 4).

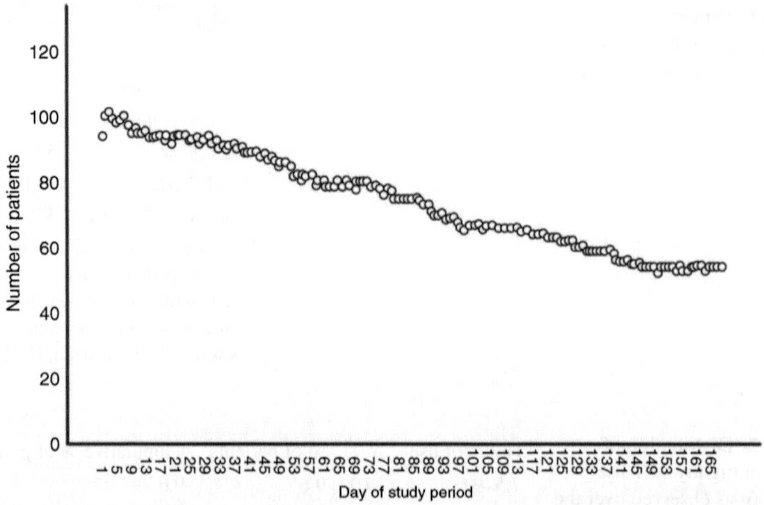

Fig. 2 Patients who used the SPT nightly for 1 h or more during the study period. Used with permission from the Associated Professional Sleep Societies, LLC, Darien, IL, USA [31]

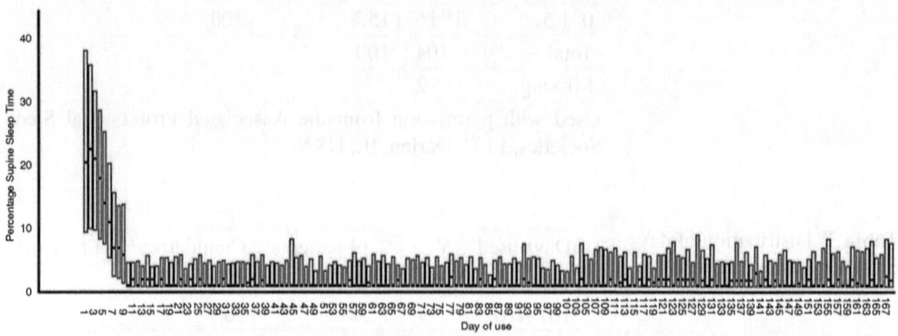

Fig. 3 Median percentage (*dot*) and interquartile range (*bar*) of sleep time in supine position per patient per night. Used with permission from the Associated Professional Sleep Societies, LLC, Darien, IL, USA [31]

Table 4 Questionnaire values and percentage of supine sleep time during 6 months of SPT treatment for all available SPT users

		T=0		T=1 month		T=3 months		T=6 months
Variable	N	Median	N	Median	N	Median	N	Median
ESS	145	11 [8]	114	8 [8]	104	8 [8]	90	8 [6]
FOSQ	145	87 [30]	114	98 [30]	103	99 [32]	90	103 [30]
PSQI	144	8 [6]	113	6 [5]	102	6 [6]	88	6 [6]
% supine	104	21 [30]	94	2 [5]	75	2 [5]	53	3 [5]

Values given in brackets represent the interquartile range
Used with permission from the Associated Professional Sleep Societies, LLC, Darien, IL, USA

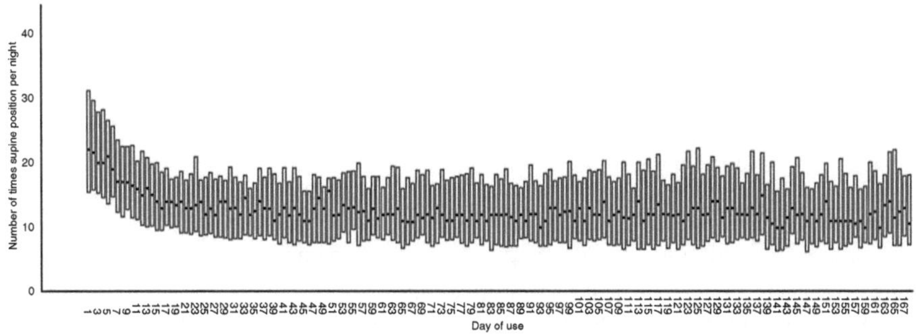

Fig. 4 Median number (*dot*) and interquartile range (*bar*) of times in supine position per patient per night. Used with permission from the Associated Professional Sleep Societies, LLC, Darien, IL, USA [31]

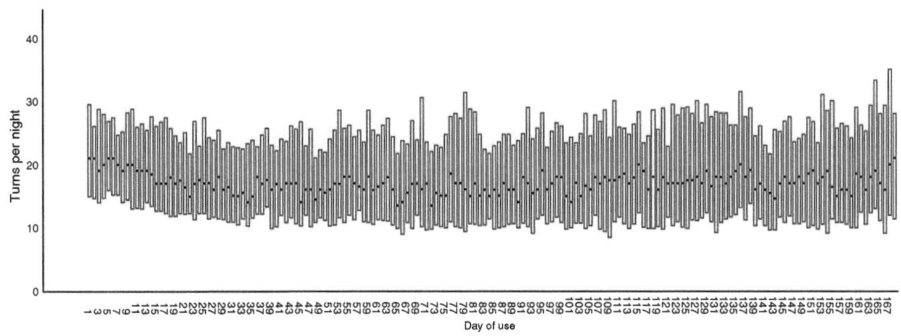

Fig. 5 Median number (*dot*) and interquartile range (*bar*) of positional changes per patient per night. Used with permission from the Associated Professional Sleep Societies, LLC, Darien, IL, USA [31]

Number of Times in Supine Position, Positional Changes and Response to Stimulus

Figure 4 depicts the median number of times in supine position. It seems that the number of times in supine position rapidly decreases during the first 2–3 weeks of treatment (23 times in supine position at baseline vs. 13 times on day 21) and that this value from then onwards is maintained over time.

In Fig. 5, the median number of positional changes per patient per night is shown. Over time, this number of positional changes seems relatively stable (22 at baseline compared to 22 at the end of the study period). The positional change index did not change over time (median positional change index at baseline was 2.9 at baseline compared to 2.8 after 1 month, 2.6 after 3 months, and 3.0 after 6 months).

When studying the time needed to respond to the stimulus, it was found that during the first month of SPT therapy, the median reaction time was 1 s (IQR = 0–3), in the second and third months the reaction time was 0 s (IQR = 0–3), and these values were maintained during the fourth to sixth months.

Table 5 Questionnaire values and percentage of supine sleep time during 6 months of SPT treatment ($n=53$)

	$T=0$	$T=1$ month	$T=3$ months	$T=6$ months
Variable	Median	Median	Median	Median
ESS	11 [6]	9 [8]	8 [8]	7 [6]
FOSQ	91 [29]	98 [19]	99 [27]	103 [21]
PSQI	7 [5]	5 [4]	6 [5]	6 [6]
% supine	21 [30]	2 [4]	2 [5]	3 [5]

Values given in brackets represent the interquartile range

Used with permission from the Associated Professional Sleep Societies, LLC, Darien, IL, USA

Table 6 Distribution of hours of SPT use ($n=53$)

Hours of use	N	% of patients
0–249	0	0
250–499	0	0
500–749	0	0
750–999	13	25
1,000–1,249	30	57
1,250–1,509	10	19
Total	53	100

Used with permission from the Associated Professional Sleep Societies, LLC, Darien, IL, USA

Subjective Compliance

Data on self-reported continued use were obtained using the online questionnaires at three time points. After 1 month of therapy, subjective compliance (>4 h per night, 7 days per week) was 91.8 % ($N=110$). After 3 months of therapy, 74.3 % of the patients were self-reportedly compliant ($N=101$), and after 6 months, the subjective compliance was 59.8 % ($N=87$). Subjective regular SPT use (>4 h per night, 5 days per week) was 96.4 %, after 3 months 89.1 %, and 74.4 % after 6 months.

Follow-Up Cohort

Out of the 106 patients, we chose to further analyze all patients for whom complete records could be collected. Questionnaire scores and percentage of supine sleep time of these 53 patients are shown in Table 5. Distribution of hours of SPT use is shown in Table 6. Median SPT use during 6 months was 1,127 h [IQR=191], or 6.7 h on average per night for all nights. Objective SPT compliance in this group of 53 patients (>4 h per night, 7 days per week) was 100 %.

Discussion

This is the first long-term follow-up study to evaluate a large group of POSA patients sleeping with the SPT during a period of 6 months. The main finding is that selected patients with mild-to-moderate POSA can be effectively treated with the SPT reducing the percentage of supine sleep time persistently over the course of 6 months. In concordance with the results described in the previous chapter, sleeping with the SPT diminishes subjective sleepiness and improves sleep-related quality of life in patients with mild-to-moderate POSA. The long-term decrease in median ESS value from 11 (considered sleepy) to 8 (considered normal) in our group of mild and moderate POSA patients seems comparable to subjective sleep results using the ESS in mild and moderate OSA patients using CPAP (mean ESS decrease from 10 to 8 in 6 months) [18]. Effectiveness of PT and of PT using the SPT in terms of AHI decrease for POSA patients has been demonstrated before [2, 3]. Furthermore, the median percentage of supine sleep quickly decreases from 21 % at baseline to approximately 6 % at day 9 (end of training phase), further decreases during therapy phase (starting day 10) to 2–3 %, and then is maintained over time. This is an interesting finding since the most studied form of PT, the tennis ball technique, has been shown to be little effective in the long term, because more than 80 % of users in the long term neither use it nor avoid the supine position while asleep using tennis ball therapy [10].

Long-term follow-up is important in any study that evaluates treatment with a detachable device, since the device only exerts its effects when in use. CPAP devices nowadays are equipped with built-in counters enabling assessment of the hours of use. Several studies have shown that 29–83 % of CPAP users are noncompliant to therapy (using study periods of 3 months to a year), when compliance is defined as at least 4 h of CPAP use per night. [12] Objective usage data for mandibular advancement device (MAD), until recently [19], have been harder to collect and have been limited to subjective self-report. However, the same group of researchers reported on a high correspondence between objective and subjective long-term MAD compliance data [20]. Long-term subjective MAD compliance rates vary greatly between studies and have shown to be between 4 and 82 % after 1 year of treatment [21–24]. Long-term PT compliance has been hampered by discomfort and low wearing comfort, and reports on compliance so far have been limited to subjective measurements. One study evaluated the tennis ball technique (TBT) and used a follow-up questionnaire in 67 patients who were prescribed TBT with an average follow-up time of 2.5 ± 1.0 years and found long-term compliance to be less than 10 % [10]. Another group studied 14 POSA patients, who were prescribed a supine sleeping position preventive vest, and found subjective compliance at an average time of 24 months to be less than 30 % [25]. To our knowledge, only one study has been conducted evaluating objective long-term use of PT. In this study, 16 patients used a somewhat bulky mass placed in the back for a period of 3 months. Using a built-in actigraphic device, they found that their device, on average, was used during 73.7 % ± 29.3 % of nights for 8.0 ± 2.0 h/night. [26] The SPT is equipped with a built-in sensor enabling assessment of hours of use by both physician and patient. Compliance, using CPAP's compliance criteria [17], was 64.4 % in our current study. Self-reported compliance after 6 months of therapy corresponded well with the objective compliance rate and was 59.8 %. Objective regular SPT use was 71.2 %; subjective regular use was 74.4 %. The high correspondence between subjective and objective compliance data is in line with a recent study focusing on subjective and objective MAD compliance data [20]. Further increased patient guidance and the use of educational and positive reinforcement programs might be used to even further increase SPT compliance since these have been shown to increase CPAP compliance [27–30]. To our knowledge, 64.4 % is the second highest long-term compliance rate of any positional therapy device studied so far. Only the study by Heinzer et al. [26] reported on a higher PT compliance rate. However, the shorter study period (3 vs. 6 months), the smaller sample size ($n = 16$ compared to $n = 106$) and strict inclusion criteria used in that study (prior non-tolerance of either CPAP or oral device therapy and a required <10 % of total sleep time spent in supine sleeping position during a test night with the device) might overestimate their reported compliance rate.

The data presented in Fig. 4 suggest that patients on average only learn to partially avoid the supine position and that continuous positional therapy is needed to prevent them from adopting the supine position throughout the night. However, to truly study a potential learning effect of PT, patients should be treated with PT during a well-defined period and should stop wearing the device during a well-defined period following treatment. During these both well-defined periods, patients and their sleeping positions should be monitored. Any potential learning effect (a trained avoidance of the supine position) [6] of positional therapy in general or in sleeping with the SPT in particular still remains to be investigated.

The median number of positional changes per patient per night seems relatively stable over time (22–22, Fig. 5), as was the case with the positional change index (2.9–3.0). So, contrary to the number of times in supine position per night, the amount of turns per night seems not to be influenced by wearing the SPT. This suggests that patients retain their freedom of movement, which might be beneficial for their sleep architecture.

Reaction time to the stimulus was investigated and found to be stable over time. Patients, therefore, appear not to develop habituation to the vibrational feedback and, when looking at the reaction time, did not ignore the signal structurally. As a result, the vibrational feedback remains effective throughout the therapy.

Methodological Considerations

There are some limitations concerning our study setup and data that need to be addressed. One hundred and forty-five patients were included in our study. Thirty-nine patients did not register their SPT in the online database. No SPT use or SPT data could be retrieved in these patients, despite implementation of protocolled safety nets; registered patients would receive an email reminding them of filling out the questionnaires in case they had not done so in time. When designing this trial, the possibility of patients not registering online was not fully taken into account.

SPT instructions and delivery were taken care of by a Dutch medical device distributor company. The process of registering online was left to the patient, which was not ideal from a research perspective in hindsight. However, the results of this study, in terms of follow-up potential, are likely a good reflection of clinical reality. Of these 106 patients only 53 patients uploaded their SPT data for the full study period and filled in the questionnaires at 2 or more time points. Patients did not receive any other incentives filling out the questionnaires or uploading their data. The data retrieved over the full 6 months might therefore have resulted in a positive selection bias, showing merely the best SPT users. However, the opposite might also be true; some patients reported to have stopped using the SPT because they felt better, did not have any subjective complaints any longer, and learned to avoid sleeping in the supine position. We were not able to collect their subjective experiences in the questionnaires and their objective sleep position and usage data since most of these patients stopped using the SPT already in the first weeks of use and were therefore lost to follow-up.

Another limitation of our study is the lack of a control group. Our results and conclusions could have been stronger had we compared the SPT users to a group of POSA patients with another treatment regimen.

A final limitation of the present study was the lack of an educational program or positive reinforcement program for the patients. Loss to follow-up would probably have been less and compliance would probably have been higher given the positive results in trials with CPAP users [27–30].

Conclusion

Over a period of 6 months, sleeping with the SPT effectively and persistently diminishes percentage of supine sleep time, decreasing supine sleep time from 21 to 3 % within 10 days and maintaining this 3 % supine sleep time over 6 months. The SPT significantly diminishes subjective sleepiness and improves sleep-related quality of life in patients with mild-to-moderate POSA. 64.4 % out of 106 patients using the SPT were considered compliant, defined as SPT use of more than 4 h per night during 7 days per week, and 71.2 % of patients used the SPT on a regular basis, defined as more than 4 h during 5 days per week. Subjective and objective compliance data corresponded well. Future research needs to focus on objective long-term treatment effects, particularly in relation to other already generally accepted POSA treatment modalities.

Clinical Implications

In our opinion, positional therapy (PT) could be the ideal method and maybe should be the initial POSA treatment for patients with mild and moderate POSA. Evidence on effectiveness and long-term compliance of PT in general has been increasing during recent years. SPT's treatment concept, consisting of a small apparatus that is able to register body position as well as provide active feedback effectively to its user during both night and day, seems to be the best, currently available option for treating POSA patients. This cohort of POSA patients using the SPT for a 6-month study period has shown that the SPT is capable of quickly reducing the percentage of supine sleep time within 10 days and maintaining this decreased percentage of supine sleep time over time. Furthermore, SPT usage diminished subjective sleepiness and improved sleep-related quality of life. However, future prospective long-term research is necessary and should focus on objective polysomnographical parameters in direct comparison with other generally accepted treatment modalities as well as objective measurements of continuous usage.

Acknowledgments The authors wish to acknowledge the advice and criticism of Herman Braat, consultant data analytics, and the following persons and the departments they work in for actively being involved in patient enrollment:

R van Uffelen, MD	Albert Schweitzer Ziekenhuis
RJAM van der Hulst, MD, PhD, and JTh Schmidt MD, PhD	Amstelland Ziekenhuis
WJA Wijnands, MD, PhD	Deventer Ziekenhuis
J Dolsma, MD	Diaconessenhuis
F Brijker, MD, PhD	Diakonessenhuis
MAC Klaaver, MD	Havenziekenhuis
AF Kuipers, MD	Isala Klinieken
H Janssen, MD	Kempenhaeghe
LS Hoep, MD	Laurentius Ziekenhuis
JQPJ Claessen, MD, PhD	Martini Ziekenhuis
R Hilgerink, MSc	Medisch Spectrum Twente
PJE Vos, MD, PhD	Rijnstate Ziekenhuis
EFG Kapteijns, MD	Rode Kruis Ziekenhuis
D Kox, MD	Sint Antonius Ziekenhuis
WEJJ Hanselaar, MD	Sint Franciscus Gasthuis
JGM Ribbert, MD	Zuwe Hofpoort Ziekenhuis

References

1. Randerath WJ, Verbraecken J, Andreas S, et al. Non-CPAP therapies in obstructive sleep apnoea. Eur Respir J. 2011;37:1000–28.
2. Permut I, Diaz-Abad M, Chatila W, et al. Comparison of positional therapy to CPAP in patients with positional obstructive sleep apnea. J Clin Sleep Med. 2010;6:238–43.
3. van Maanen JP, Meester KA, Dun LN, et al. The sleep position trainer: a new treatment for positional obstructive sleep apnoea. Sleep Breath. 2013;17:771–9.
4. Berger M, Oksenberg A, Silverberg DS, Arons E, Radwan H, Iaina A. Avoiding the supine position during sleep lowers 24 h blood pressure in obstructive sleep apnea (OSA) patients. J Hum Hypertens. 1997;11:657–64.
5. Bignold JJ, Mercer JD, Antic NA, McEvoy RD, Catcheside PG. Accurate position monitoring and improved supine-dependent obstructive sleep apnea with a new position recording and supine avoidance device. J Clin Sleep Med. 2011;7:376–83.

6. Cartwright RD, Lloyd S, Lilie J, Kravitz H. Sleep position training as treatment for sleep apnea syndrome: a preliminary study. Sleep. 1985;8:87–94.
7. Maurer JT, Stuck BA, Hein G, Verse T, Hormann K. Schlafapnoetherapie mit einer neuartigen rückenlage-verhinderungs-weste. Dtsch Med Wochenschr. 2003;128:71–5.
8. van Maanen JP, Richard W, van Kesteren ER, et al. Evaluation of a new simple treatment for positional sleep apnoea patients. J Sleep Res. 2012;21:322–9.
9. Zuberi NA, Rekab K, Nguyen HV. Sleep apnea avoidance pillow effects on obstructive sleep apnea syndrome and snoring. Sleep Breath. 2004;8:201–7.
10. Bignold JJ, Deans-Costi G, Goldsworthy MR, et al. Poor long-term patient compliance with the tennis ball technique for treating positional obstructive sleep apnea. J Clin Sleep Med. 2009;5:428–30.
11. Clark GT. Mandibular advancement devices and sleep disordered breathing. Sleep Med Rev. 1998;2:163–74.
12. Weaver TE, Grunstein RR. Adherence to continuous positive airway pressure therapy: the challenge to effective treatment. Proc Am Thorac Soc. 2008;5:173–8.
13. Johns MW. A new method for measuring daytime sleepiness: the Epworth sleepiness scale. Sleep. 1991;14:540–5.
14. Buysse DJ, Reynolds 3rd CF, Monk TH, Berman SR, Kupfer DJ. The Pittsburgh Sleep Quality Index: a new instrument for psychiatric practice and research. Psychiatry Res. 1989;28:193–213.
15. Weaver TE, Laizner AM, Evans LK, et al. An instrument to measure functional status outcomes for disorders of excessive sleepiness. Sleep. 1997;20:835–43.
16. Cartwright RD, Diaz F, Lloyd S. The effects of sleep posture and sleep stage on apnea frequency. Sleep. 1991;14:351–3.
17. Kribbs NB, Pack AI, Kline LR, et al. Objective measurement of patterns of nasal CPAP use by patients with obstructive sleep apnea. Am Rev Respir Dis. 1993;147:887–95.
18. Kushida CA, Nichols DA, Holmes TH, et al. Effects of continuous positive airway pressure on neurocognitive function in obstructive sleep apnea patients: the Apnea Positive Pressure Long-term Efficacy Study (APPLES). Sleep. 2012;35:1593–602.
19. Vanderveken OM, Dieltjens M, Wouters K, De Backer WA, Van de Heyning PH, Braem MJ. Objective measurement of compliance during oral appliance therapy for sleep-disordered breathing. Thorax. 2013;68:91–6.
20. Dieltjens M, Braem MJ, Vroegop AV, et al. Objectively measured vs. self-reported compliance during oral appliance therapy for sleep-disordered breathing. Chest. 2013. doi:10.1378/chest.13-0613.
21. Nakazawa Y, Sakamoto T, Yasutake R, et al. Treatment of sleep apnea with prosthetic mandibular advancement (PMA). Sleep. 1992;15:499–504.
22. Walker-Engstrom ML, Wilhelmsson B, Tegelberg A, Dimenas E, Ringqvist I. Quality of life assessment of treatment with dental appliance or UPPP in patients with mild to moderate obstructive sleep apnoea. A prospective randomized 1-year follow-up study. J Sleep Res. 2000;9:303–8.
23. Walker-Engstrom ML, Ringqvist I, Vestling O, Wilhelmsson B, Tegelberg A. A prospective randomized study comparing two different degrees of mandibular advancement with a dental appliance in treatment of severe obstructive sleep apnea. Sleep Breath. 2003;7:119–30.
24. Marklund M, Stenlund H, Franklin KA. Mandibular advancement devices in 630 men and women with obstructive sleep apnea and snoring: tolerability and predictors of treatment success. Chest. 2004;125:1270–8.
25. Wenzel S, Smith E, Leiacker R, Fischer Y. Effektivität und Langzeit-Compliance der Therapie mit Rückenlage-Verhinderungsweste bei obstruktiver Schlafapnoe. Laryngorhinootologie. 2007;86:579–83.
26. Heinzer RC, Pellaton C, Rey V, et al. Positional therapy for obstructive sleep apnea: an objective measurement of patients' usage and efficacy at home. Sleep Med. 2012;13:425–8.
27. Leseux L, Rossin N, Sedkaoui K, et al. Education of patients with sleep apnea syndrome: feasibility of a phone coaching procedure. Phone-coaching and SAS. Rev Mal Respir. 2012;29:40–6.

28. Willemin MC, Fry S, Peres S, Wallaert B, Mallart A. Effects of an educational program in non-adherent apneic patients treated with continuous positive airway pressure. Rev Pneumol Clin. 2013;69:70–5.
29. Fuchs FS, Pittarelli A, Hahn EG, Ficker JH. Adherence to continuous positive airway pressure therapy for obstructive sleep apnea: impact of patient education after a longer treatment period. Respiration. 2010;80:32–7.
30. Ballard RD, Gay PC, Strollo PJ. Interventions to improve compliance in sleep apnea patients previously non-compliant with continuous positive airway pressure. J Clin Sleep Med. 2007;3:706–12.
31. van Maanen JP, de Vries N. Long-term effectiveness and compliance of positional therapy with the sleep position trainer in the treatment of positional obstructive sleep apnea syndrome. Sleep 2014;37:1209–15.

10 Problems and Solutions for Positional Therapy: Technical Aspects of the Sleep Position Trainer

Eline C. Vrijland van Beest

Low Effectiveness Due to Adaptation, Habituation, and Subject Variances

Usually, the tennis ball technique (TBT) is a passive object, a bulky mass attached to the back avoiding people from sleeping supine. For a group of patients, the TBT is not effective however. Research shows that a large group of patients is able to sleep on top of such objects: 25 % of patients sleep on top of TBT up to 30 min [1], 24 % of patients in a self-reported study [2], and 20 % of patients using a ball for TBT [3]; after 8 weeks of use, over 30 % still does sleep supine using a positional device [4]. The reason for the poor effectiveness can be explained by several factors: sensatory adaptation and cognitive habituation to the passive stimulation and variables in subjects. These three main causes will be further explored under problem 1, 2, and 3.

Problem No. 1: Sensory Adaption

TBT Problem: Adaptation to Pressure of a Passive Object (Sensatory Adaptation)

The tennis ball technique (TBT) uses a bulky mass, which is placed into a pocket of a wide cloth band or belt attached around the abdomen such that the ball is positioned in the center of the back. When the patients roll on to their back, they feel the pressure of the "ball" and instinctively roll back on to their side again. The human somatosensory system, however, naturally adapts to pressure stimuli that are applied

E.C.V. van Beest, M.Sc., M.B.I. (✉)
NightBalance B.V., Molengraaffsingel 12-14, 2629 JD Delft, The Netherlands
e-mail: eline@nightbalance.com

N. de Vries et al. (eds.), *Positional Therapy in Obstructive Sleep Apnea*,
DOI 10.1007/978-3-319-09626-1_25

constantly to the skin [5]. The adaptation time is rather short and depends on pressure and size of stimulus; the lower the pressure and the larger the size of the stimulus, the shorter the adaptation [5]. So when turned onto the back using a TBT—generally causing relatively low pressure over a relatively large area—it seems logical that the human body rapidly adapts to the pressure, decreasing its purpose to trigger a position change.

Suggested Solution: Active Stimulation to Avoid Sensatory Adaptation

The only thing needed to restore sensitivity to a tactile stimulus is just a slight change or movement of the stimulus. Try pulling up your socks. The skin is best at detecting a change in pressure. Therefore, a vibrating stimulus with fast pressure changes forms an effective stimulus [5]. As such, a suggested solution should be to provide active feedback through vibrations instead of passive pressure used by the TBT, avoiding adaptation of the skin and enabling a more effective therapy.

Problem No. 2: Cognitive Habituation

TBT Problem: Habituation to Continuous Stimulation (Cognitive Habituation)

Inevitably, a bulky mass strapped to the back, be it a tennis ball, baseball, shark fin, or a special cushion design, is always passive. With it being passive, there is no change in stimulation during use and hence the stimulation given to a subject is always continuous. Research has shown that continuous stimulation causes cognitive habituation during sleep to occur [6, 7]. Specifically for the TBT, this means that when a subject sleeps on top of an object, he/she is able to get used to this stimulation during sleep. The result is that the stimulation can be ignored, resulting in poor effectiveness.

Suggested Solution: Variation of Active Vibration Patterns to Avoid Cognitive Habituation

To avoid cognitive habituation to external stimuli during sleep, researchers have shown that different variations of stimuli help avoid non-reactions. Studies showed that varying interstimulus intervals help avoid habituation [8]. Other studies varied the stimulation by increasing it at nonresponse to avoid habituation [9]. These examples show that in order to evoke reaction, change of stimulus is needed. A suggested solution is to make use of these insights from literature, avoiding cognitive habituation through varying vibration patterns with stimulus intervals and vibration intensity.

Problem No. 3: Individual Adaption

TBT Problem: One Size Doesn't Fit All

Of people that stopped using the TBT, 63 % reported the TBT to be too uncomfortable and 24 % claimed the TBT did not prevent them from sleeping on the back [2]. A similarly report shows that of the study dropouts, 85 % reported discomfort and 20 % reported they were able to sleep on top of the TBT [3]. So where one group of patients feels the TBT is too uncomfortable, the other group reports it is not working for them yet. This all has to do with individual sensitivity and characteristics. Various researchers have shown that the human perceived tactile sensitivity depends on individual subject variances. A study overview based on 20 other papers shows all the personal characteristics that have an influence on the vibrotactile threshold, defined as the smallest displacement that can be detected by the individual undergoing a test [10]. A few of the mentioned variables influencing the vibrotactile sensitivity are BMI (the higher the BMI, the lower the sensitivity), age (the higher the age, the lower the sensitivity), alcohol use (the more alcohol, the lower the sensitivity), skin temperature (the higher the temperature, the lower the sensitivity), and gender (females have higher sensitivity than males). Therefore, one size fits all TBT is not effective for all subjects. And even within one subject, factors like skin temperature and alcohol use can largely vary per night.

Suggested Solution: Continuous Adaptation of Vibration to Individual Strength

Following the logic reasoning of the reported individual sensitivity, the stimuli should be adapted towards this. A suggested solution therefore could be to automatically adjust the intensity of a vibration or other activation depending on the sleep behavior of a user. This should happen automatically; when a subject reacts quickly, the vibration intensity is decreased, whereas it is increased in case of nonresponse. Furthermore, when habituation seems to occur, measurable by long-term nonresponse, the vibration pattern needs to change. That way, personal settings of the device should automatically adapt to the individual. So regardless of age, BMI, gender, skin temperature, or alcohol use, such a solution should change to the effective vibration intensity accordingly.

Compliance Issues Due to Discomfort in Several Areas

Secondly, numerous reports on Positional Therapy state figures for low compliance: 28 % of patients over a period of 24 months [11], 38 % of patients over a period of 6 months [3], 10 % of patients over a period of 30 months [2], 73 % over 3 months [12], and 67 % over 14 days [13]. Reasons mentioned for low compliance are discomfort of the vest/TBT, tightness of the strap attaching the TBT, the object moving around, sleeping on top of the TBT or it not preventing one from sleeping supine, not being able to sleep supine, backache, skin irritation, increased sweating and heat, frequent awakenings, restless sleep, and even interference with bedroom intimacy. These causes will be further explored under problems 4–10.

Problem No. 4: Restricted Movement

TBT Problem: Poor Compliance Due to Restricted Movement

With the TBT, changing position from one side to another is quite a hassle; users have to roll over the bulky mass to be able to switch sides which can cause a significant reduction in quality of sleep or can even cause the patient to wake up. Frequent awakenings and restless sleep have also been reported in research [1–4].

Suggested Solution: 360° Freedom of Movement

The Pittsburgh Sleep Quality Index (PSQI) researches seven areas and has shown to have a diagnostic sensitivity of 89.6 % and specificity of 86.5 % [14]. The researched areas include subjective sleep quality, sleep latency, habitual sleep efficiency, and sleep disturbances. Decreasing these subjective disturbances should improve a subjects' sleep. A suggested solution would therefore be to enable users to change position without disturbance, like one naturally would. This could be for example in form of a light and flat device, so that one can easily change position like one normally would. The device should then only be triggered when patients remain in the supine position and should not provide a stimulus when patients are switching sides during sleep while rolling over their back.

Problem No. 5: Discomfort of Bulky Mass

TBT Problem: Poor Compliance Due to Discomfort Sleeping on Top of a Device

Repeatedly, reports have shown that patients still sleep supine despite sleeping with a bulky mass strapped to their back, on average 20–30 min during sleep, causing significant discomfort and backache [1–4].

Suggested Solution: Flat and Ergonomic Device

Uncomfortable sleeping surfaces can prevent good sleep, for example, the US Department of Health and Human services reports [15]. Encouraging comfortable and natural sleep without any obstacles, the suggested solution should be designed to be as light, thin, small, comfortable, and ergonomic as possible. Even when a subject does not react to a device when in the supine position, sleeping on top of the device should be hardly noticeable.

Problem No. 6: Discomfort While Falling Asleep

TBT Problem: Poor Compliance Due to Discomfort Falling Asleep

In user research we frequently hear people complain about the TBT because it disabled them from sleeping supine. While asking what moments feel most troublesome, users answer that this was mostly the moment of falling asleep and some times during the night when they wake up. While falling asleep, users prefer to lay in their most relaxing position which is often supine. On the other hand, some enjoy reading a book or watching TV while falling asleep; none of them is comfortably possible using a TBT. Also research shows that another reason for stopping therapy with the TBT is due to not being able to sleep supine and restless sleep [1–4].

Suggested Solution: Sleep-In Period

The US National Sleep Foundation states that a sleep-conductive environment is one that is important for sleep onset, including factors like temperature, noise, light, and comfort [16]. To maximize the perceived comfort, a suggested solution would be to enable users to fall asleep in any desired position. The device should only start to work after a sleep-in period of, for example, 30 min, allowing a user to fall asleep on their back if desired. If the user remains in supine position after 30 min, they should be reminded to change position with a vibration. That way, the natural way of falling asleep is maintained, be it reading a book or just relaxing in the supine position.

Problem No. 7: Not Being Able to Get Used to the Bulky Mass

TBT Problem: Poor Compliance Due to Discomfort Getting Used to the Bulky Mass

While testing a TBT in user research, we often saw users drop out after only 1 or 2 days. Reasons that came forward during interviews were numerous like has been seen in research [1–4]. Many patients have difficulty getting used to sleeping with a bulky mass strapped to their backs and may therefore abort the treatment prematurely.

Suggested Solution: Training Program

Change is directly related to the perception of stress in humans. The Holmes and Rahe stress scale is a list of 43 stressful life events that can contribute to illness, also known as the Social Readjustment Rating Scale [17]. This scale includes the event of changing a sleeping habit, which is seen as one of the possible stress factors. To decrease the impact of such a stress factor, the suggested solution should gradually be introduced. It could, for example, slowly train patients to avoid the supine position with a step-by-step buildup and a slow increase of vibration stimuli events. After a certain period it then should be fully active, giving vibrational stimuli every time the user remains in supine position in order to be effective. This slow increase of the amount of time spent in the non-supine positions should allow users to gently get used to their new way of sleeping, avoiding stress.

Problem No. 8: The TBT Is Either ON or OFF

TBT Problem: Poor Compliance Due to Consistent Discomfort During the Night

During in-depth interviews, users also mentioned that sometimes they woke up during the night, just wanting to lay on their back for a little while. Unfortunately with the TBT, there are only two options: you either wear TBT or you don't, and there's no in-between. This often results in users stopping wearing the TBT during the night.

Suggested Solution: Pause Mode

Also decreasing the stress factor of changing a sleeping habit [20], the suggested solution should easily be paused, for example, a 20-min break in which a user can lay in any desired position, providing users with a feeling of comfort and self-control during the night. To enable a sleepy user to activate the pause mode, it should be very easy to do so. After the short break the device should automatically activate again, ensuring Positional Therapy and a decrease in apneas for the rest of the night.

Problem No. 9: Insights in Therapy

TBT Problem: Poor Compliance Due to Poor Monitoring

Compliance has found to be a general problem in TBT as stated earlier [14–16]. Even the most effective medical devices are only effective, when they are used. With an increase in awareness of the importance of compliance, there is an increase in demand for patient therapy monitoring [18, 19]. TBT devices in general have poor monitoring possibilities.

Suggested Solution: Data Readout

Telemonitoring significantly increases patient adherence to their apnea therapy, for example, shown in research and randomized controlled trials [20–22]. Therefore, users should be able to read out their data with special software on their personal computers, which enables them to monitor their sleep behavior and progress of their treatment. The insight in their therapy progress contributes to the effectiveness of the treatment. Furthermore, after informed consent from the patient, the treating physician should be able to view the data and consequently monitor and guide the treatment process.

Problem No. 10: Training and Guidance

TBT Problem: Poor Compliance Due to Poor Guidance

According to research, CPAP adherence can significantly be improved through adequate training and guidance [23]. And this does not necessarily need to be in person. A study, for example, showed that patients were equally satisfied and showed equal adherence when meeting their physician for a follow-up on their CPAP treatment via video or in person [24]. The TBT, generally not being a medical device, does not have any procedures or guidance that will help patients with their therapy management or compliance.

Suggested Solution: Online Support

The effect of interventions (e.g., education or reminders) on direct compliance measures (e.g., losing weight or other measurement results) has shown to be stronger than that for health outcomes overall [25]. Providing this support will help increase adherence. Therefore, the Web application should also provide support in the device's use as well as tips and advice on how to improve their sleep. In addition they should receive reminders, feedback on their training progress, and, for example, monthly reports.

The suggested solutions are all integrated in the NightBalance Sleep Position Trainer (SPT). This active sleep position sensor is a new treatment method for positional sleep apnea, developed following research conducted at the Delft University of Technology and the Sint Lucas Andreas Hospital in Amsterdam, the Netherlands. The SPT is a small, lightweight aid which can be worn around the chest with an ergonomic strap. This effectively and comfortably prevents lying in the supine position and helps reduce sleep apneas.

References

1. Fridel KW. Adherence and effectiveness of positional therapy for obstructive sleep apnea syndrome. Dissertation at the University of Arizona; 2011.
2. Bignold JJ. Poor long-term compliance with the tennis ball technique for treating positional obstructive sleep apnea. J Clin Med. 2009;5:428–30.
3. Oksenberg A, Silverberg DS, Offenbach D. Positional therapy for obstructive sleep apnea patients: a 6-month follow-up study. Laryngoscope. 2006;116:1995–2000.
4. Cartwright R, Ristanovic R, Diaz F, Caldarelli D, Alder G. A comparative study of treatments for positional sleep apnea. Sleep. 1991;14(6):546–52.
5. Krantz JH. Experiencing sensation and perception, 2012. Chapter 12: Skin senses. E-book by Hanover College. http://psych.hanover.edu/classes/sensation/
6. Brackbill Y. Acoustic variation and arousal level in infants. Psychophysiology. 1970;6(5):517–26. doi:10.1111/j.1469-8986.1970.tb02241.
7. Brackbill Y. Cumulative effects of continuous stimulation on arousal level in infants. Child Dev. 1971;42(1):17–26.
8. Lavigne G, Brousseau M, Kato T, Mayer P, Manzini C, Guitard F, Monplaisir J. Experimental pain perception remains equally active over all sleep stages. Pain. 2004;110(3):646–55.
9. Halasz P, Terzano M, Parrino L, Bodizs R. The nature of arousal in sleep. Neurological Department, National Institute of Psychiatry and Neurology, Budapest, Hungary. J Sleep Res. 2004;13(1):1–23.
10. Gandhi MS, Sesek R, Tuckett R, Morris Bamberg SJ. Progress in vibrotactile threshold evaluation. J Hand Ther. 2011. doi:10.1016/j.jht.2011.01.001.
11. Wenzel S, Smith E, Leiacker R, Fischer Y. Efficacy and long-term compliance of the vest preventing the supine position in patients with obstructive sleep apnea. Laryngorhinootologie. 2007;86(8):579–83.
12. Heinzer RC, Pellaton C, Rey V, Rosetti AO, Lecciso G, Haba-Rubio J, Tafti M, Lavigne G. Positional therapy for obstructive sleep apnea; An objective measurement of patients' usage and efficacy at home. Sleep Med. 2012;13:425–8.
13. Svatikova A, Chervin RD, Wing JJ, Sanchez BN, Migda EM, Brown DL. Positional therapy in ischemic stroke patients with obstructive sleep apnea. Sleep Med. 2011;12(3):262–6. doi:10.1016/j.sleep.2010.12.008.
14. Buysse DJ, Reynolds CF, Monk TH, Berman SR, Kupfer DJ. The Pittsburgh Sleep Quality Index: a new instrument for psychiatric practice and research. Psychiatry Res. 1989;28:193–213.
15. US Department of Health and Human Services & National Heart Lung and Blood Institute. Your guide to healthy sleep. NIH publication no. 11-5271; 2011.
16. US National Sleep Foundation, 2013. http://www.sleepfoundation.org/article/how-sleep-works/the-sleep-environment.
17. Holmes TH, Rahe RH. The Social Readjustment Rating Scale. J Psychosom Res. 1967;11(2):213–8. doi:10.1016/0022-3999(67)90010-4. PMID 6059863.
18. Ravesloot MJL, de Vries N. Reliable calculation of the efficacy of non-surgical and surgical treatment of obstructive sleep apnea revisited. Sleep. 2011;34:105–10.
19. Kribbs NB, Pack AI, Kline LR, Smith PL, Schwartz AR, Schubert NM, Redline S, Henry JN, Getsy JE, Dinges DF. Objective measurement of patterns of nasal CPAP use by patients with obstructive sleep apnea. Am J Respir Crit Care Med. 1993;147:887–95.
20. Stepnowsky CJ, Palau JJ, Marler MR, Gifford AL. Pilot randomized trial of the effect of wireless telemonitoring on compliance and treatment efficacy in obstructive sleep apnea. J Med Internet Res. 2007;9(2):e14. doi:10.2196/jmir.9.2.e14.
21. Fox N, Hirsch-Allen AJ, Goodfellow E, Wenner J, Fleetham J, Ryan CF, Kwiatkowska M, Ayas NT. The impact of a telemedicine monitoring system on positive airway pressure adherence in patients with obstructive sleep apnea: a randomized controlled trial. Sleep. 2012;35(4):477–81. doi:10.5665/sleep.1728.

22. Sparrow D, Aloia M, DeMolles DA, Gottlieb DJ. A telemedicine intervention to improve adherence to continuous positive airway pressure: a randomised controlled trial. Thorax. 2012;65(12):1061–6. doi:10.1136/thx.2009.133215. Epub 2010 Sep 29.
23. Pamidi S, Knutson KL, Gohds F, Mokhlesi B. The impact of sleep consultation prior to a diagnostic polysomnogram on continuous positive airway pressure adherence. Chest. 2012;141(1):51–7. doi:10.1378/chest.11-0709. Epub 2011 Jun 23.
24. Parikh R, TouVelle MN, Wang H, Zallek SN. Sleep telemedicine: patient satisfaction and treatment adherence. Telemed J E Health. 2001;17(8):609–14. doi:10.1089/tmj.2011.0025.
25. Roter DL, Hall JA, Merisca R, Nordstrom B, Cretin D, Svarstad B. Effectiveness of interventions to improve patient compliance: a meta-analysis. Med Care. 1998;36(8):1138–61.

Prevalence and Effect of Supine-Dependent Obstructive Sleep Apnea on Oral Appliance Therapy

Marijke Dieltjens, Anneclaire V. Vroegop, Annelies E. Verbruggen, Marc Willemen, Johan A. Verbraecken, Wilfried A. de Backer, Paul H. van de Heyning, Marc J. Braem, Nico de Vries, and Olivier M. Vanderveken

Introduction

Oral appliance (OA) therapy is increasingly prescribed as a noninvasive treatment option for patients with snoring and mild to moderate OSA and as an alternative for patients who do not comply with or refuse CPAP [1]. Oral appliances are designed to prevent upper airway collapse and can be divided into two major classes: (1) a tongue-retaining device (TRD) holding the tongue in a forward position due to a

M. Dieltjens, M.B.S (✉) • M.J. Braem, D.D.S., Ph.D.
Department of Special Care Dentistry, Antwerp University Hospital, University of Antwerp, Wilrijkstraat 10, 2650 Edegem, Antwerp, Belgium
e-mail: Marijke.Dieltjens@uza.be

A.V. Vroegop, M.D., Ph.D.
ENT Department and Head and Neck Surgery, Antwerp University Hospital, University of Antwerp, Edegem, Antwerp, Belgium

Saint Lucas Andreas Hospital, Amsterdam, The Netherlands

A.E. Verbruggen, M.D. • P.H. van de Heyning, M.D., Ph.D. • O.M. Vanderveken, M.D., Ph.D.
ENT Department and Head and Neck Surgery, Antwerp University Hospital, University of Antwerp, Edegem, Antwerp, Belgium

M. Willemen
Multidisciplinary Sleep Disorders Centre, University of Antwerp, Antwerp, Belgium

J.A. Verbraecken, M.D., Ph.D. • W.A. de Backer, M.D., Ph.D.
Department of Pulmonary Medicine, Antwerp University Hospital, Antwerp, Belgium

Multidisciplinary Sleep Disorders Centre, Antwerp University Hospital, Antwerp, Belgium

N. de Vries, M.D., Ph.D.
Department of Otolaryngology, Sint Lucas Andreas Ziekenhuis, Amsterdam, The Netherlands

Department of Otolaryngology, University Hospital Antwerp, Edegem, Antwerp, Belgium

N. de Vries et al. (eds.), *Positional Therapy in Obstructive Sleep Apnea*,
DOI 10.1007/978-3-319-09626-1_26

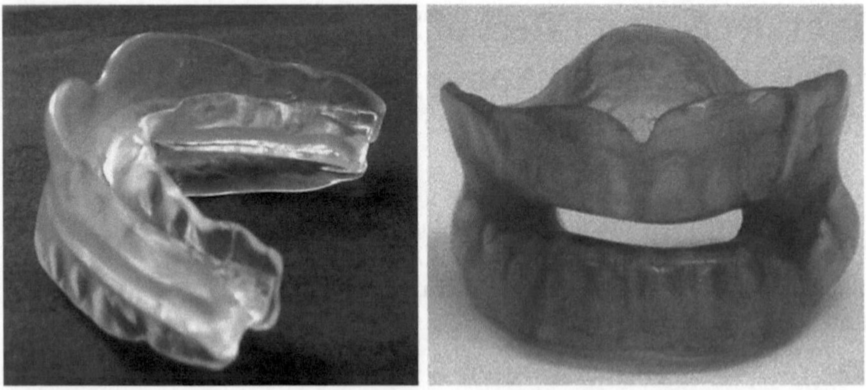

Fig. 1 Two types of oral appliances used for the treatment of obstructive sleep apnea. *Left panel*: prefabricated "boil-and-bite" oral appliance after direct fitting in the patient. *Right panel*: custom-made monobloc oral appliance made on casts of the tooth arcs

negative pressure and resulting suction in a flexible bulb [2] and (2) an oral appliance protruding the mandible during the night (OA_m). It is reported that the TRD appliances have lower tolerance, preference, and compliance when compared to OA_m therapy [3]. Therefore, nowadays, OA_m is the most common type of OA therapy prescribed for the treatment of OSA [4]. Within this group, the custom-made OA_m is reported to give a better overall clinical outcome than prefabricated "boil-and-bite" devices made out of thermoplastic material [5] (Fig. 1). Furthermore, OA_m with an integrated titratable mechanism allowing for gradual mandibular protrusion [6] is superior in their ability to reduce the apnea severity as compared to the monobloc types where upper and lower parts are rigidly interconnected [7]. Different titratable oral appliances with unique design features are currently available (Fig. 2).

When compared to CPAP therapy, OA_m therapy has been proven to reduce the severity of sleep apnea to a lesser or similar extent than CPAP [8–11], although OA_m therapy seems to have a higher acceptance rate and patient preference compared to CPAP [12, 13].

Recently, an objective compliance monitor for OA_m therapy became available, allowing for calculation of the mean disease alleviation as a measure of therapeutic effectiveness [14]. This calculation showed that comparable therapeutic effectiveness between OA_m therapy and the gold standard treatment for patients with OSA, being CPAP, has been reported because the superior efficacy of CPAP in alleviating OSA is offset by inferior acceptance and patient preference relative to OA_m therapy [8, 14, 15].

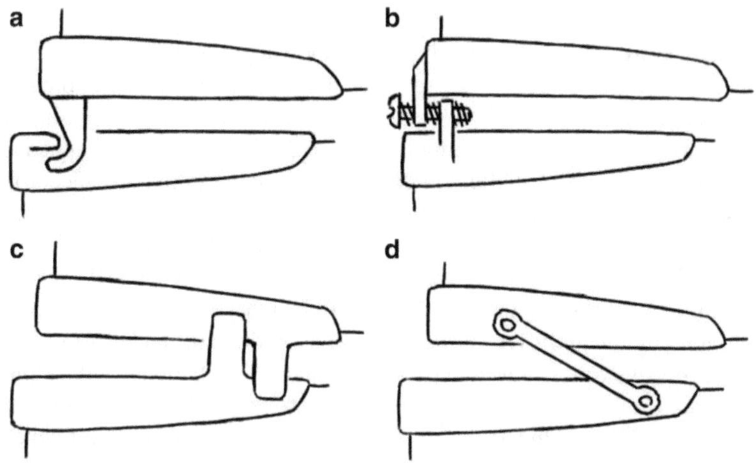

Fig. 2 Schematic overview of titratable, duo-bloc MRA designs used in current clinical practice. (**a**) OAm with an anteriorly articulating component. (**b**) OAm with attachments for adjustment of mandibular protrusion in the frontal teeth area. (**c**) OAm with two lateral positioning attachments for incremental protrusion of the mandible. (**d**) OAm with lateral telescopic rods that force the mandible into an anterior position (taken from [6])

Efficacy of Oral Appliance Therapy

OA_m therapy is effective in reducing the apnea severity in some but not in all patients. In general 65 % of patients respond to the treatment with a ≥50 % reduction in apnea–hypopnea index (AHI) with the OA_m in situ compared to baseline. On average 52 % of patients achieve an AHI < 10 events/h with the OA_m in situ [12]. In the past, retrospective analyses of clinical, physiological, and polysomnographic variables were performed in order to identify predictors of treatment success with OA_m therapy. There is evidence to support the findings that OA_m therapy is more likely to be successful in younger female patients [16], with lower body mass index [17], a smaller neck circumference [11], and less severe sleep apnea [16, 18, 19].

In this chapter, we will focus on studies evaluating the effect of sleep position or the presence of supine-dependent OSA (sdOSA) on OA_m efficacy. Eight [16, 20–26] studies evaluated the effect of sdOSA on the outcome of OA therapy. Six studies [16, 20–24] reported that the efficacy of OA therapy is influenced by sleep position in a way that patients with sdOSA have better treatment outcomes, where two other studies did not find a difference in success rates between non-sdOSA and sdOSA patients [25, 26].

In a study of Cartwright et al. [20], the association between the efficacy of a TRD and the factors obesity, age, supine sleep posture, and severity of sleep apnea was investigated in 16 male patients. The authors concluded that an increase in sleep apnea severity in the supine sleep position was the strongest predictor of success with a TRD.

Marklund et al. [16, 23] evaluated the effect of sdOSA on therapy outcome with success defined as AHI < 10 events/h in both the supine and non-supine sleeping positions with the OA_m in situ. They reported that sdOSA was a strong predictor of successful apnea reduction with OA_m therapy. In addition, it was suggested that a low AHI in the lateral position is important in predicting a successful apnea reduction with OA_m therapy [23]. After subdividing the patient population according to gender, sdOSA remained the strongest predictor of OA_m therapy success in men but did not relate to a successful apnea reduction in female patients [16].

Yoshida [24] assessed a significant decrease in both supine AHI and AHI in prone position under OA_m therapy. The AHI increased in the lateral position, although not significantly. A successful apnea reduction under OA_m therapy (AHI < 10 events/h) was achieved in 61.4, 84.6, and 0 % of patients with respiratory disturbances most frequently observed in supine, prone, and lateral position, respectively. Yoshida [24] concluded that the efficacy of OA_m therapy is influenced by sleep posture.

In a study of Chung et al. [22] using Cartwright's definition [27], the decrease in both total AHI as well as supine AHI under OA_m therapy was significantly higher in sdOSA patients when compared to non-sdOSA patients. The decrease in non-supine AHI did not differ between the two groups. The complete response rate with AHI < 5 events/h under OA_m therapy was higher in sdOSA patients when compared to non-sdOSA patients. Applying a multiple linear regression model, the presence of sdOSA turned out to be the only factor associated with a decrease in overall AHI or with a complete response.

Lee et al. [21] evaluated the efficacy of OA_m therapy in 100 Korean patients in terms of supine dependency. The success rate, defined as a reduction in AHI of 50 % or more and an AHI under OA_m of <10 events/h, was significantly higher in sdOSA compared to the non-sdOSA group.

Fransson et al. [25] subdivided their total patient population in supine-dependent ODI patients if 50 % or more of the estimated sleeping time was in supine position when desaturations were registered. In contrast with the previously described results that suggest that sdOSA is associated with a better treatment response, Fransson et al. [25] did not find a supine-dependent difference in responder rate, defined as patients with a reduction in ODI of at least 50 % or with an ODI value under OA_m therapy of <5 events/h.

Sutherland et al. [26] assessed differences in treatment response among 386 patients with and without sdOSA. In this study, no difference in complete response (AHI < 5 events/h) was noted between sdOSA and non-sdOSA patients.

Several confounders must be taken into account when comparing the studies evaluating the effect of sdOSA on the outcome of OA therapy.

A first confounder is the presence of different criteria for sdOSA in the literature (Table 1). The application of three different criteria for sdOSA makes it hard to compare the prevalence of sdOSA and the effect of sdOSA among the different studies.

A second confounder is the lack of a consensus in literature regarding the definition of successful treatment outcome. Some studies defined success as a reduction

Table 1 Definitions supine-dependent obstructive sleep apnea

Definitions of supine-dependent OSA		Prevalence general population (%)	Prevalence population starting OA_m therapy (%)
Cartwright et al. [27]	Supine AHI at least twice as high as non-supine AHI	50–60	58–80
Mador et al. [32]	Supine AHI at least twice as high as non-supine AHI AHI < 5 events/h 15 min threshold for sleep in both postures	20–35	27
Marklund et al. [16, 23]	Supine AHI ≥ 10 events/h together with non-supine AHI < 10 events/h	N/A	46

in AHI under therapy of ≥50 % compared to baseline, while other studies used a posttreatment AHI of less than 5, 10, or 20 events/h as a successful treatment outcome. In addition, some studies used a combination of a reduction in AHI of ≥50 % compared to baseline combined with a posttreatment AHI of less than 5, 10, or 20 events/h as criteria for success. One study uses the ODI as the main outcome parameter with success defined as a reduction in ODI of at least 50 % or with an ODI value under OA_m therapy of <5 events/h [25].

A third confounder is the use of different types of oral appliances in the discussed studies: one study used a TRD [20] whereas the other studies used an OA_m [16, 21–26]. Furthermore, a monobloc OA_m was used [16, 21, 23–25], whereas only in two studies a titratable OA_m was used [22, 26]. In the studies using a monobloc OA_m, four out of five studies (80 %) did find an association between the efficacy of OA_m therapy and the presence of sdOSA, whereas only one out of two studies (50 %) using a titratable OA_m could confirm these results.

Prevalence of Supine-Dependent Sleep Apnea Under Oral Appliance Therapy

The prevalence of sdOSA in a general population ranges from 20 to 60 %, depending on the definition used (Table 1). This prevalence was also studied in a more restricted population of patients starting OA_m therapy. In order to do so, Marklund et al. [23] defined sdOSA as a supine AHI ≥ 10 events/h with a lateral AHI < 10 events/h. According to this definition, 46 % of patients were diagnosed as having sdOSA. Applying the same definition, Dieltjens et al. [28] found a comparable prevalence of 46 % prior to the start of the OA_m therapy. In three studies, the prevalence of sdOSA as defined by Cartwright's criteria was assessed before starting OA_m therapy and ranged from 58 to 80 % [21, 22, 28]. In a study of Yoshida,

61 % of patients starting OA_m therapy exhibited the respiratory events most frequently in supine sleeping position [24]. Overall, the prevalence of sdOSA found in patients starting OA_m therapy ranged from 27 to 80 % and was comparable to the prevalence of sdOSA in the general population (Table 1). These results however do not reveal the evolution of sdOSA once OA_m has started, and until recently, the prevalence of sdOSA under OA_m therapy was unknown. In a recent study 183 patients with polysomnographic data before and under OA_m therapy were evaluated showing a prevalence under OA_m therapy ranging from 18 to 34 %, depending on the definition used. In addition, it was shown that up to one third of patients shift from non-sdOSA at baseline to sdOSA under OA_m therapy [28].

Positional Therapy in Combination with Oral Appliance Therapy

Patients with sdOSA under OA_m therapy could probably benefit from additional therapy with a supine-avoidance method. Up to this date, there are only two studies comparing the efficacy of positional therapy and OA therapy and assessing whether there is any additional benefit combining positional therapy and OA therapy [29, 30].

In the study of Cartwright et al. [29], the efficacy of a TRD and a posture alarm giving an auditory beep when in supine position were compared, as well as the efficacy of combination therapy of the posture alarm and the TRD. Patients were assigned to either therapy with the posture alarm, the TRD, or combination therapy of the posture alarm and the TRD. Nine out of 15 patients (60 %) and 8 out of 15 patients (53 %) achieved a complete response (AHI < 5 events/h) with the tongue-retaining device and the posture alarm, respectively. The group with combination therapy showed the highest success rate with 11 of 15 patients (73 %) reaching a complete response.

In an ongoing prospective randomized controlled trial [30], the additional effect of a chest-worn Sleep Position Trainer (SPT) (NightBalance™, Delft, the Netherlands) [31] is assessed in patients with sdOSA under OA_m therapy. After a baseline PSG and PSG with OA_m, patients who were unsuccessfully treated (AHI < 5 per hour under OA_m therapy) due to the presence of sdOSA under therapy following both Cartwright's and Marklund's criteria under OA_m therapy were invited for two PSGs in a randomized order: one PSG with SPT alone and one with combination therapy of SPT and OA_m. The SPT used in this study continuously monitors sleep position, vibrating when in supine position. If the patient shifts to non-supine position, vibration of the SPT stops. The results of this randomized controlled trial suggest that combination of a SPT and OA_m therapy in patients with sdOSA under OA_m therapy is effective with a significant and additional reduction in apnea severity as compared to baseline and the individual treatment modalities. The preliminary results of this research seem promising.

Conclusions

Retrospective analyses of clinical, physiological, and polysomnographic variables at baseline were reported in literature, identifying predictors of treatment success with oral appliance therapy.

Six studies observed an association between the efficacy of OA therapy and the presence of supine-dependent OSA (sdOSA), whereas the results of two other studies couldn't confirm this finding. The divergence of defining sdOSA, outcome definitions, and type of oral appliances makes it hard to compare the results with respect to predictive value of sdOSA for a successful OA therapy outcome with a need for larger clinical studies on this topic.

The prevalence of sdOSA in a patient population starting OA_m therapy ranged from 27 to 80 %. In addition, up to 34 % of patients have sdOSA under OA_m therapy and one third of patients shift from non-sdOSA to sdOSA under OA_m therapy.

The combination of an oral appliance with positional therapy shows promising results for this specific combination therapy.

References

1. Kushida CA, et al. Practice parameters for the use of continuous and bilevel positive airway pressure devices to treat adult patients with sleep-related breathing disorders. Sleep. 2006;29(3):375–80.
2. Cartwright RD, Samelson CF. The effects of a nonsurgical treatment for obstructive sleep apnea. The tongue-retaining device. JAMA. 1982;248(6):705–9.
3. Deane SA, et al. Comparison of mandibular advancement splint and tongue stabilizing device in obstructive sleep apnea: a randomized controlled trial. Sleep. 2009;32(5):648–53.
4. Marklund M, Verbraecken J, Randerath W. Non-CPAP therapies in obstructive sleep apnoea: mandibular advancement device therapy. Eur Respir J. 2012;39(5):1241–7.
5. Vanderveken OM, et al. Comparison of a custom-made and a thermoplastic oral appliance for the treatment of mild sleep apnea. Am J Respir Crit Care Med. 2008;178(2):197–202.
6. Dieltjens M, Braem MJ, Van de Heyning PH, Wouters K, Vanderveken OM. Prevalence and clinical significance of supine-dependent obstructive sleep apnea in patients using oral appliance therapy. J Clin Sleep Med. 2014 (in press)
7. Lettieri CJ, et al. Comparison of adjustable and fixed oral appliances for the treatment of obstructive sleep apnea. J Clin Sleep Med. 2011;7(5):439–45.
8. Phillips CL, et al. Health outcomes of continuous positive airway pressure versus oral appliance treatment for obstructive sleep apnea: a randomized controlled trial. Am J Respir Crit Care Med. 2013;187(8):879–87.
9. Gagnadoux F, et al. Titrated mandibular advancement versus positive airway pressure for sleep apnoea. Eur Respir J. 2009;34(4):914–20.
10. Engleman HM, et al. Randomized crossover trial of two treatments for sleep apnea/hypopnea syndrome: continuous positive airway pressure and mandibular repositioning splint. Am J Respir Crit Care Med. 2002;166(6):855–9.
11. Barnes M, et al. Efficacy of positive airway pressure and oral appliance in mild to moderate obstructive sleep apnea. Am J Respir Crit Care Med. 2004;170(6):656–64.
12. Ferguson KA, et al. Oral appliances for snoring and obstructive sleep apnea: a review. Sleep. 2006;29(2):244–62.

13. Ferguson KA, et al. A randomized crossover study of an oral appliance vs nasal-continuous positive airway pressure in the treatment of mild-moderate obstructive sleep apnea. Chest. 1996;109(5):1269–75.
14. Vanderveken OM, et al. Objective measurement of compliance during oral appliance therapy for sleep-disordered breathing. Thorax. 2013;68(1):91–6.
15. Vanderveken OM, et al. Objective measurement of the therapeutic effectiveness of continuous positive airway pressure versus oral appliance therapy for the treatment of obstructive sleep apnea. Am J Respir Crit Care Med. 2013;188(9):1162.
16. Marklund M, Stenlund H, Franklin KA. Mandibular advancement devices in 630 men and women with obstructive sleep apnea and snoring: tolerability and predictors of treatment success. Chest. 2004;125(4):1270–8.
17. Otsuka R, et al. A comparison of responders and nonresponders to oral appliance therapy for the treatment of obstructive sleep apnea. Am J Orthod Dentofacial Orthop. 2006;129(2):222–9.
18. Mehta A, et al. A randomized, controlled study of a mandibular advancement splint for obstructive sleep apnea. Am J Respir Crit Care Med. 2001;163(6):1457–61.
19. Liu Y, et al. Cephalometric and physiologic predictors of the efficacy of an adjustable oral appliance for treating obstructive sleep apnea. Am J Orthod Dentofacial Orthop. 2001; 120(6):639–47.
20. Cartwright RD. Predicting response to the tongue retaining device for sleep apnea syndrome. Arch Otolaryngol. 1985;111(6):385–8.
21. Lee CH, et al. The effect of positional dependency on outcomes of treatment with a mandibular advancement device. Arch Otolaryngol Head Neck Surg. 2012;138(5):479–83.
22. Chung JW, et al. Treatment outcomes of mandibular advancement devices in positional and nonpositional OSA patients. Oral Surg Oral Med Oral Pathol Oral Radiol Endod. 2010; 109(5):724–31.
23. Marklund M, Persson M, Franklin KA. Treatment success with a mandibular advancement device is related to supine-dependent sleep apnea. Chest. 1998;114(6):1630–5.
24. Yoshida K. Influence of sleep posture on response to oral appliance therapy for sleep apnea syndrome. Sleep. 2001;24(5):538–44.
25. Fransson AM, et al. Effects of a mandibular protruding device on the sleep of patients with obstructive sleep apnea and snoring problems: a 2-year follow-up. Sleep Breath. 2003; 7(3):131–41.
26. Sutherland K, Takaya H, Phillips C, Darendeliler A, Qian J, Cistulli P. Polysomnographic phenotypes of OSA and mandibular advancement splint treatment outcome. Abstract presented on the second international conference organised by the European Respiratory Society and the European Sleep Research Society; 2013.
27. Cartwright RD. Effect of sleep position on sleep apnea severity. Sleep. 1984;7(2):110–4.
28. Dieltjens M, Braem MJ, Van de Heyning PH, Wouters K, Vanderveken OM. Prevalence and clinical significance of supine-dependent obstructive sleep apnea in patients using oral appliance therapy. J Clin Sleep Med. 2014 (in press).
29. Cartwright R, et al. A comparative study of treatments for positional sleep apnea. Sleep. 1991;14(6):546–52.
30. Dieltjens M, Vroegop AV, Verbruggen AE, Willemen M, Verbraecken JV, Van de Heyning PH, Braem MJ, de Vries N, Vanderveken OM. Effects of sleep position trainer and mandibular advancement devices on residual positional sleep apnea under MAD therapy: a randomized clinical trial. Sleep Breath. 2013;17:879–94.
31. van Maanen JP, et al. The sleep position trainer: a new treatment for positional obstructive sleep apnoea. Sleep Breath. 2013;17(2):771–9.
32. Mador MJ, et al. Prevalence of positional sleep apnea in patients undergoing polysomnography. Chest. 2005;128(4):2130–7.

Positional Therapy and Palatal Surgery

J. Peter van Maanen, Birgit I. Witte, and Nico de Vries

Introduction

Treatment options for OSA consist of conservative measures (e.g., weight reduction, abstinence from alcohol and sedatives), positional therapy [1], oral device therapy [2], CPAP [3], and surgery. A Cochrane review does not recommend surgery at all for OSA, except in studies [4]. However, it is in concordance with clinical experience that adherence to CPAP, when defined as greater than 4 h of nightly use, is between 17 and 54 % [5], resulting in a significant number of patients abandoning CPAP and seeking alternative treatments, such as oral appliances and surgery. Oral appliances also require sufficient compliance, and roughly one third of patients have contraindications to oral devices [6]. In sum, many patients opt for surgical therapy.

Uvulopalatopharyngoplasty including tonsillectomy (UPPP) was and probably still is the most commonly performed OSA surgery worldwide [7]. Surgical success rates of UPPP range from 30 to 50 % [8, 9]. A variation of the technique, Z-palatoplasty (ZPP), for patients who had undergone tonsillectomy earlier has been described and has similar outcomes [10, 11]. Furthermore, it has been shown that UPPP as single treatment [12, 13] or as part of multilevel surgery [14] may be

J.P. van Maanen, M.D. (✉)
Department of Otolaryngology, Sint Lucas Andreas Ziekenhuis,
Jan Tooropstraat 164, 1061 AE Amsterdam, The Netherlands
e-mail: p.vanmaanen@slaz.nl

B.I. Witte, M.Sc., Ph.D.
Department of Epidemiology and Biostatistics, VU University Medical Centre,
Amsterdam, The Netherlands

N. de Vries, M.D., Ph.D.
Department of Otolaryngology, Sint Lucas Andreas Ziekenhuis,
Amsterdam, The Netherlands

Department of Otolaryngology, University Hospital Antwerp, Antwerp, Belgium

N. de Vries et al. (eds.), *Positional Therapy in Obstructive Sleep Apnea*,
DOI 10.1007/978-3-319-09626-1_27

useful to lower CPAP pressure requirements, thereby improving CPAP compliance in selected patients.

An increasing amount of literature has been published on the role of sleep position in OSA and positional therapy [1, 15–30]. Cartwright was the first to define the current positional OSA (POSA) criteria: an AHI in the worst sleeping position twice or more as high when compared to the AHI in the other positions [17]. It is evident that the overall AHI is affected by the relative proportion of each of the different sleeping positions. However, the effect of UPPP on body position-specific AHI values is not well known. This chapter will describe the effect of UPPP and ZPP on body position-specific AHI values, investigate the efficacy of UPPP/ZPP for both POSA and non-positional OSA (NPOSA) patients, and hypothesize about a possible role for positional therapy to increase treatment efficacy.

Materials and Methods

Patients

Patients with mild to severe OSA and isolated retropalatal collapse or multilevel collapse (retropalatal collapse combined with retrolingual collapse) and refusal or nonacceptance of CPAP treatment were offered surgical treatment. Patients with mild to severe OSA who had undergone UPPP according to Fujita [7] (in patients with tonsils) (or Z-palatoplasty according to Friedman (ZPP [10]) in patients without tonsils) with or without concomitant radiofrequent ablation of the base of the tongue (RFTB [31]) in case of a partial retrolingual collapse were evaluated.

Definitions

Positional OSA (POSA) was defined as an AHI ≥ 5 and an AHI in supine position twice or more as high when compared to each of the AHI values found in the other positions [17]. Full overnight PSG was repeated 3–4 months postoperatively. Surgical success was defined according to Sher's criteria: AHI reduction of at least 50 % and AHI reduction to below 20 [32]. Cure rate was defined as AHI reduction below 5.

Surgical Techniques

UPPP, as first described by Fujita, involves excision of the tonsils and posterior soft palate/uvula and closure of the tonsillar pillars.

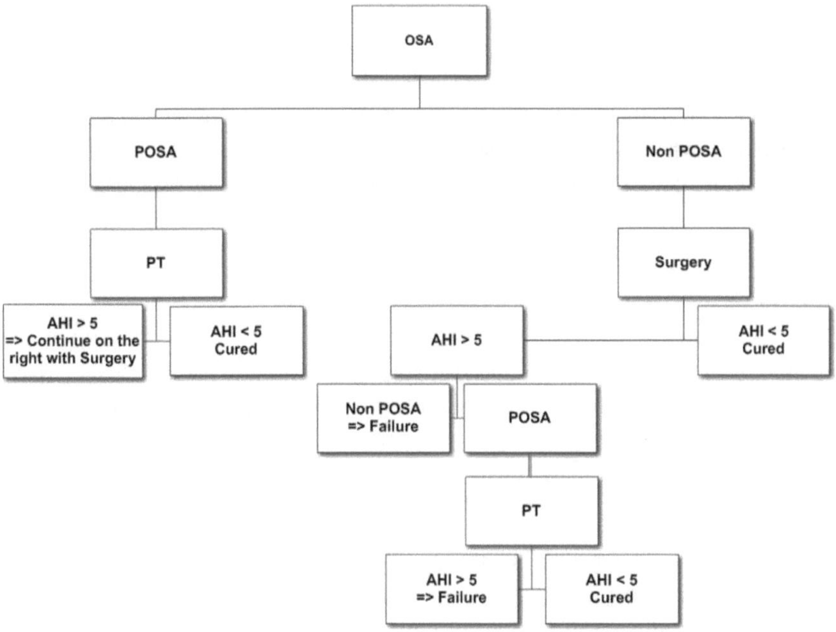

Fig. 1 Flowchart using a theoretical model and an ideal form of positional therapy (PT) in OSA patients. OSA: obstructive sleep apnea, defined as an AHI ≥ 5.0. POSA: positional OSA, defined as an AHI ≥ 5 and an AHI in supine position twice or more as high when compared to each of the AHI values found in the other positions and a supine time between 10 and 90 %. Surgery would be the surgical procedure the patient had undergone. Non POSA: non positional OSA. PT: hypothetical ideal positional therapy, defined as reduction of supine time to 0, thereby reducing the AHI to the non supine AHI

In ZPP a superficial butterfly-shaped mucosal layer is removed. The uvula/soft palate is split and the two flaps are sutured away, thereby closing the previously made wound and creating more space anterior–posterior and sideways.

Depending on the size of the tongue, 6–8 punctures in the region of the circumvallate papillae are performed using Olympus CelonLab ENT and ProSleep Plus using a power setting of 7W. To avoid infections and abscess formation following RFTB, peri- and postoperative administration of broad-spectrum antibiotics (e.g., amoxicillin/clavulanate) is mandatory.

Theoretical Calculations Using an Ideal Form of Positional Therapy (Ideal PT)

Using patients' polysomnographical data, a theoretical model to treat patients was applied (Fig. 1). Patients were considered POSA patients and suitable for ideal PT when suffering from a mild to moderate OSA, sleeping in supine position between 10 and 90 % of total sleep time [30], and showing an AHI in supine position twice or more as high when compared to each of the AHI values found in the other positions. Non-positional (NPOSA) patients would receive surgery (UPPP/ZPP +/− RFTB). POSA patients would start using ideal PT. Ideal PT would reduce the baseline AHI to the baseline non-supine AHI. Additional treatment was considered necessary when the posttreatment AHI exceeded 5. Results in terms of changes in AHI, overall success, and cure rates of this theoretical model were evaluated.

Results

One hundred and thirty-nine patients were included; baseline patient characteristics are shown in Table 1. Fifty-two patients suffered from mild, 62 from moderate, and 25 from severe OSA. Fifty-nine patients were treated with UPPP (mild OSA 21, moderate 25, severe 13), 59 patients with UPPP+RFTB (mild OSA 23, moderate 26, severe 10), and 21 patients with ZPP+RFTB (mild OSA 8, moderate 11, severe 2).

Fifty-five patients (39.6 %) had a successful reduction in AHI, according to Sher's criteria [32]. Twenty-seven out of 139 patients had a postoperative AHI <5 (19.4 %). The median AHI of all 139 patients significantly decreased from 18.0 [range: 5.1–69.6] to 11.2 [1.0–63.0] ($p<0.001$). The median AHI in all separate positions decreased significantly as well. The number of awakenings, total sleep time, and the percentages of total sleep time slept in supine, left, and prone positions did not change significantly after treatment (Table 2).

Treatment

No significant difference between the treatments was found in the number of patients with a successfully reduced AHI; in 27 patients treated with UPPP (CI: 32.7–59.2 %), in 21 patients treated with UPPP+RFTB (CI: 23.6–49.1 %), and in 7 patients treated with ZPP+RFTB (CI: 14.6–57.0 %) ($p=0.432$), treatment was found to be successful. Data of patients treated with either UPPP+RFTB or ZPP+RFTB were pooled in one group ($n=80$) and compared to the patients who underwent UPPP ($n=59$). Between these groups only the percentage in supine position (increase in UPPP group, decrease in the other group) showed a significant difference between groups (Table 3).

Positional OSA (Table 4)

In the 68 patients (48.9 %) with POSA pretreatment, AHI decreased significantly from 15.5 [5.1–46.5] to 11.5 [1.0–40.0] ($p=0.002$), and AHI in supine position decreased significantly from 33.9 [5.1–93.9] to 20.9 [0.0–69.5] ($p<0.001$). No

Table 1 Baseline patient characteristics ($n = 139$) shown as median with full range

Variable	Median [range]
Age (years)	45.0 [25.0–69.0]
BMI (kg/m^2)	27.4 [20.4–38.2]
AHI (/h)	18.0 [5.1–69.6]
AHI supine (/h)	30.2 [0.0–133.1]
% supine	34.1 [0.0–100.0]
Ratio male to female	127:12

Table 2 Median polysomnographical parameters with interquartile range (IQR) before and after surgery ($n = 139$)

	Before		After		
	Median	IQR	Median	IQR	p-value
AHI (/h)	18.0	12.0–27.0	11.2	5.6–20.2	**<0.001**
AHI supine (/h)	30.2	19.1–49.5	20.5	8.3–39.9	**<0.001**
AHI left (/h)	8.1	0.4–17.8	3.1	0.0–11.6	**0.004**
AHI right (/h)	4.4	0.0–17.5	2.6	0.0–7.6	**0.008**
AHI prone (/h)	0.0	0.0–11.1	0.0	0.0–0.9	**0.024**
AHI REM (/h)	21.4	11.3–33.5	12.8	4.9–21.9	**<0.001**
% supine	34.1	17.9–56.4	33.1	20.0–51.1	0.388
% left	24.1	6.2–41.2	29.7	11.0–41.7	0.389
% right	22.5	5.3–37.0	31.8	9.7–42.4	**0.013**
% prone	0.0	0.0–7.6	0.0	0.0–3.9	0.382
Total sleep time (minutes)	418.2	362.5–466.0	424.0	373.5–469.0	0.861
Desaturation index (/h)	5.7	2.1–12.7	3.8	1.4–9.4	**0.001**
Number of awakenings	4.0	2.0–6.0	4.0	2.0–7.0	0.499
Number of position changes	31.0	21.0–55.8	25.0	15.5–46.0	**0.022**
Positional change index (/h)	4.5	3.0–9.0	4.0	2.0–6.0	**0.010**

Bold-faced values represent significant differences

significant decrease was found in the other positions, total sleep time, percentage slept in supine position, or number of awakenings.

In the 71 NPOSA patients' pretreatment, AHI decreased significantly from 23.0 [5.1–69.5] to 11.0 [1.0–63.0] ($p < 0.001$). This difference is significantly higher than the difference in the POSA group ($p = 0.026$). AHI in prone, left, and right positions decreased significantly more in the NPOSA group than in the POSA group ($p = 0.002$, $p = 0.012$, and $p = 0.005$ respectively). No difference was found in the number of patients with a successful reduction of the AHI in both groups: 24 of the 68 patients (35.3 %; CI, 24.1–47.8 %) suffering from POSA versus 31 of the 71 patients (43.7 %; CI, 31.9–56.0 %) suffering from NPOSA ($p = 0.313$). Half of the positional patients remained positional after treatment and more than half of the NPOSA patients remained non-positional after treatment (50.0 and 62.0 %, $p = 0.443$).

Table 3 Median polysomnographical parameters with interquartile range (IQR) before and after palatal surgery with or without concurrent radiofrequent ablation of the base of the tongue

	UPPP ($n = 59$)					UPPP/ZPP + RFTB ($n = 80$)					
	Before		After		*p*-value	Before		After		*p*-value	*p*-value
Treatment	Median	IQR	Median	IQR	(within)	Median	IQR	Median	IQR	(within)	(between)
AHI (/h)	19.0	12.0–27.0	9.0	5.0–15.0	**<0.001**	17.7	12.1–25.1	12.7	6.8–24.4	**0.002**	0.069
AHI supine (/h)	30.6	13.8–50.7	13.7	6.4–34.8	**<0.001**	30.1	21.1–49.3	27.2	9.3–40.5	**0.006**	0.565
AHI left (/h)	8.2	0.0–18.9	2.7	0.0–12.1	**0.005**	6.8	1.1–15.2	3.3	0.2–11.3	0.193	0.199
AHI right (/h)	5.1	0.0–18.0	1.4	0.0–5.6	**0.001**	4.1	0.3–17.3	4.1	0.4–12.7	0.438	0.072
AHI prone (/h)	0.0	0.0–16.0	0.0	0.0–4.2	**0.018**	0.0	0.0–4.7	0.0	0.0–0.0	0.462	0.108
AHI REM (/h)	20.9	11.7–31.3	10.3	4.7–22.5	**<0.001**	21.6	9.7–33.8	13.2	6.2–21.9	**<0.001**	0.505
% supine	24.7	11.8–48.9	33.1	18.4–50.9	0.282	37.3	21.9–62.7	33.0	20.8–51.5	0.066	**0.046**
% left	27.0	0.0–42.9	28.9	12.3–43.6	0.499	23.4	7.0–41.2	30.7	10.8–39.7	0.582	0.823
% right	21.5	0.0–40.1	31.9	1.7–41.4	0.204	22.7	7.9–36.2	31.3	14.4–43.6	**0.030**	0.792
% prone	3.4	0.0–9.3	0.0	0.0–7.3	0.104	0.0	0.0–5.9	0.0	0.0–1.7	0.623	0.087
Total sleep time (minutes)	408.0	354.5–459.0	412.5	352.3–465.0	0.667	431.5	379.3–474.6	436.3	391.1–477.3	0.571	0.535
Number of awakenings	3.0	2.0–6.0	3.0	2.0–7.0	0.742	4.0	2.0–6.0	4.0	2.0–7.0	0.520	0.922
Number of position changes	27.0	18.0–48.5	24.5	15.8–47.5	0.517	33.0	21.0–58.0	30.0	15.0–45.0	**0.015**	0.277
Positional change index (/h)	4.0	2.0–8.5	4.0	2.0–7.0	0.260	5.0	3.0–9.0	4.0	2.0–6.0	**0.014**	0.377

Bold-faced values represent significant differences

Table 4 Median polysomnographical parameters with interquartile range (IQR) before and after surgery for POSA and NPOSA patients

	Yes ($n=68$)					No ($n=71$)					
	Before		After		p-value (within)	Before		After		p-value (within)	p-value (between)
Positional OSA	Median	IQR	Median	IQR		Median	IQR	Median	IQR		
AHI (/h)	15.5	10.9–21.7	11.5	5.0–21.2	**0.002**	23.0	14.3–31.0	11.0	6.1–20.1	**<0.001**	**0.026**
AHI supine (/h)	33.9	22.2–50.6	20.9	8.4–38.3	**<0.001**	27.2	15.0–49.5	20.5	7.8–42.2	**0.014**	0.168
AHI left (/h)	3.1	0.0–9.4	1.9	0.0–8.0	0.567	15.1	4.3–28.1	4.5	1.2–15.6	**0.001**	**0.012**
AHI right (/h)	2.5	0.0–5.8	1.7	0.0–6.2	0.985	14.1	0.0–29.8	4.6	0.0–12.8	**0.001**	**0.005**
AHI prone (/h)	0.0	0.0–0.0	0.0	0.0–0.0	0.438	0.0	0.0–23.0	0.0	0.0–4.2	**0.003**	**0.002**
AHI REM (/h)	18.6	7.7–29.5	12.8	4.4–21.9	**0.011**	24.2	12.7–38.3	12.6	6.5–22.5	**<0.001**	**0.039**
% supine	34.9	18.5–56.3	34.5	22.0–51.1	0.562	31.6	15.1–58.3	29.1	18.6–51.6	0.541	0.948
% left	23.0	4.2–39.0	27.4	4.3–41.6	0.636	27.0	6.9–45.6	30.3	16.5–42.8	0.497	0.861
% right	22.8	5.5–39.8	33.1	11.0–43.4	0.107	22.2	5.3–35.2	30.4	6.3–42.3	**0.049**	0.899
% prone	0.0	0.0–5.8	0.0	0.0–1.8	1.000	1.8	0.0–8.9	0.0	0.0–7.3	0.195	0.266
Total sleep time (minutes)	423.0	379.3–464.8	421.5	373.1–461.3	0.721	416.0	355.0–470.1	425.0	374.0–478.0	0.538	0.559
Number of awakenings	4.0	1.3–7.0	4.0	2.0–7.0	0.758	4.0	2.0–6.0	3.5	2.0–7.0	0.490	0.930
Number of position changes	31.0	20.0–53.3	30.5	16.0–47.8	0.127	31.0	21.0–57.3	25.0	15.0–45.0	0.070	0.685
Positional change index (/h)	4.5	3.0–7.3	4.0	2.0–7.0	0.149	4.5	2.8–10.0	4.0	2.0–6.0	**0.029**	0.420

POSA positional OSA, *NPOSA* non-positional OSA
Bold-faced values represent significant differences

Results of the Theoretical Treatment Flowchart

Fifteen of 68 pretreatment POSA patients were not eligible for ideal PT (four patients had an AHI > 30, six patients in a supine sleep < 10 %, five patients > 90 %). Thirty-two of these 53 patients would have an ideal PT posttreatment AHI < 5. Two patients in the pretreatment POSA group were not eligible for ideal PT but showed a posttreatment AHI < 5 following surgery as initial treatment. Three patients would be cured when, following a non-curative (AHI > 5 posttreatment) trial of ideal PT, surgery would be performed. Five patients (who were not eligible for initial ideal PT treatment) would be cured from their OSA following surgery and additional ideal PT postoperative. Seven patients would ultimately be cured following a non-curative trial of ideal PT, non-curative surgery, and ideal PT. In total 49 patients (72.1 %) were cured from their OSA. Their median AHI decreased significantly from 13.7 [5.1–34] to 2.5 [0.0–4.9] ($p < 0.0001$). For the pretreatment POSA patients who were not cured ($n = 19$) by this protocol median AHI decreased from 21.5 [11.5–46.5] to 10.6 [5.2–47.7] ($p = 0.117$). Twelve of 71 NPOSA patients were cured by surgery alone. Eighteen of 25 pretreatment NPOSA but posttreatment POSA patients were eligible for additional ideal PT. Thirteen patients could be cured by combined therapy. By using this treatment protocol, 25 out of 71 patients (35.2 %) could be cured from their OSA. Their median AHI decreased significantly from 16.0 [5.1–57.2] to 2.1 [0.0–4.9] ($p < 0.0001$). The other 46 non-curatively treated NPOSA patients showed a significant decrease in median AHI from 24.5 [8.0–69.6] to 13.1 [5.1–63.4] ($p = 0.001$).

Overall this treatment regimen would result in a significant decrease in median AHI from 18.0 [5.1–69.6] to 4.5 [0.0–63.4] ($p < 0.0001$). Ninety-nine patients (71.2 %) would have had a successful reduction in AHI according to Sher's criteria and 74 patients (53.2 %) would have been "cured" from their OSA based on AHI < 5.

Discussion

This chapter describes better results of UPPP/ZPP +/− RFTB in NPOSA patients compared to POSA patients (Table 4). Surgery did not enhance the position effect. In contrast, 50 % of POSA patients did not show positional dependency any longer after surgery, whereas only 38 % of NPOSA patients became POSA patients following surgery. Although it has been shown previously that PSG might overestimate the severity of OSA in some patients with POSA because of an increase in time spent supine compared to nights not wearing the PSG apparatus [33], it has also been shown that the correlations between PSG night 1 and 2 for the percentage of time spent supine and the supine AHI are similar and highly significant [34].

AHI and all sleeping position-specific AHI values showed a significant decrease in both the isolated palatal surgery group (Table 3) and the total patient group (Table 2). When studying POSA and NPOSA patients, the POSA patient group AHI showed a significant decrease, which mainly might be due to the significant decrease in AHI supine. In NPOSA patients the significant AHI decrease might be caused by the significant effect on all body-specific AHI values. Since POSA patients have lower non-supine AHI values compared to NPOSA patients, a larger number of patients might be needed to detect the significant decrease in their non-supine AHI values. Studying Table 4 it therefore cannot be concluded that in POSA patients palatal surgery exerts its effects solely in supine position.

Only three earlier studies analyzed the effect of sleep position on outcomes of (isolated) UPPP. [35–37] Katsantonis et al. studied the effect of UPPP on the sleeping position-specific AHI values in 17 patients [35]. They found that following UPPP, the AHI significantly improved in the lateral position and that during sleep in supine position, the AHI did not show significant improvement. They concluded that UPPP enhances the position effect on OSA because it eliminates obstructive events in the lateral sleep position. Although some of the patients described in this chapter also underwent RFTB, both the UPPP and UPPP/ZPP+RFTB groups showed a significant decrease in supine AHI (Table 3). A potential reason for this difference could be the small number of patients Katsantonis et al. studied compared to the number of patients described in this chapter. Lee et al. studied the effect of sleep position on surgical outcomes of UPPP in 69 consecutive patients [36]. After categorizing the patients into four groups according to the change in AHI after surgery, they found that the failure group had a higher proportion of supine position dependency. The patients described here were divided into two groups (success [32]/failure (defined as all other patients)) but no significant differences could be found in position dependency between groups. Statistical significant differences were found in AHI, supine AHI, and non-supine AHI for the successful group, whereas no significant differences were found in AHI, supine AHI, and non-supine AHI for the failure group (data not shown here). In a second paper published by Lee et al., results show that UPPP is a successful treatment for obstructive events occurring in the lateral sleep position, especially in patients without positional dependency [37]. The results described in this chapter are in line with their finding that palatal surgery results seem better in NPOSA patients (success rate [32] for POSA patients was 35.3 %, for NPOSA patients 43.7 %).

There are some limitations of the study described in this chapter which need to be addressed. The study population included patients who concomitantly underwent RFTB. Ideally isolated UPPP or ZPP patients would have been studied. However, most patients suffered from multilevel obstruction (58.3 %), and when comparing outcome of isolated palatal surgery to palatal surgery in combination with RFTB, the percentage of supine sleep time was the only significant difference between groups (Table 3). In addition, overall treatment was successful as defined by Sher in 39.6 % of patients and only 19.4 % of patients were "cured" (AHI < 5). However, data inclusion was biased since many patients with mild OSA who did clinically well after surgery had no repeat PSG at all. This was due to Dutch OSA treatment guidelines which state that in a patient with an initial AHI < 15 and clinical improvement, repeat PSG is not mandatory. Furthermore, reviewing all patients in whom UPPP was performed, a substantial number of patients with an AHI > 15 were found to be not motivated for repeat PSG because of their convincing subjective improvement. The here reported overall clinical outcome might be too low because of this bias. However, evaluating effectiveness of palatal surgery was not the purpose of this study. Using a hypothesized ideal PT flowchart in which ideal positional therapy (PT) was applied in POSA patients, the success rate for the 139 patients increased to 71.2 % and cure rate to 53.2 %. There are some limitations of the hypothesized ideal PT flowchart. It was assumed that AHI values did not change after PT. This could be true but night-to-night variability is a known problem in diagnosing OSA. Furthermore, we assumed an ideal PT compliance of 100 %. Long-term compliance with the tennis ball technique was shown to be less than 10 % [38]. For the recently introduced forms of positional therapy [29, 30], long-term compliance remains to be investigated. Short-term—1 month—compliance, as defined by CPAP's compliance criteria of >4 h per night, 7 days per week, was found to be close to 100 % [29]. Furthermore, the theoretical ideal PT was able to fully eliminate the supine sleep time while not affecting other body-specific AHI values. In two recent studies, it was shown that the median percentage of supine sleep time decreased from 37.9 to 6.5 % [30] and from 49.9 to 0.0 % [29] in two groups of 30 POSA patients. Eliminating supine sleep time to 0 % seems within reach.

Sleep-disordered breathing has been proven to be associated with increased mortality and high cardiovascular risk and therefore needs treatment [39]. In patients who cannot use or simply refuse first-line therapy (CPAP), alternative treatment is indicated. Although surgical therapy does not always cure OSA, it has shown to provide significant benefits. OSA surgery improves disease severity and reduces mortality and cardiovascular risk [40, 41]. However, complications following OSA surgery are not uncommon. Furthermore, efficacy of surgical treatment in terms of AHI decrease leaves room for improvement. Our present study shows palatal surgery to yield better results in terms of AHI decrease in NPOSA than in POSA patients. In line with the good results of the theoretical ideal PT model, we therefore would suggest to use PT as a first-line treatment in POSA patients and especially the mild POSA patients without comorbid conditions (e.g., coronary artery disease, cerebrovascular accident). Only after failing this trial with PT, either based upon symptoms or follow-up PSG with therapy in place, should surgery be considered.

The variable compliance, success, and cure rates seen up to now in OSA treatment in general would not be found acceptable in other prevalent diseases such as hypertension, coronary artery disease, or diabetes. The use of both monotherapy and combined therapies has become standard in the treatment of these other diseases [42]. OSA patients might benefit from these complementary and collaborative treatment regimens as well [43].

Fifty-six percent of patients with OSA are positional; POSA more often occurs in mild to moderate than in severe OSA and an additional 30 % suffers from evident aggravation of their AHI in supine position. Based upon the findings presented in this chapter, we would like to suggest using PT as first treatment in POSA patients (without comorbid conditions as coronary artery disease and cerebrovascular accident) and only after failing this considering them for surgery. The effects of PT combined with surgery need more study.

Conclusion

UPPP or ZPP with or without concomitant RFTB significantly reduces overall and body position-specific AHI values and should be considered in patients who do not tolerate or want CPAP or oral device therapy. In NPOSA patients AHI reduction seems more pronounced when compared to POSA patients. This finding further strengthens the need to consider and when possible apply positional therapy in POSA patients. The hypothesized treatment flowchart described in this chapter in which positional therapy is applied in POSA patients, either as monotherapy or in addition to surgery, seems to improve treatment results dramatically. Future research, preferably prospective and controlled, should focus on the possibility of combining sleep surgery and positional therapy.

References

1. Ravesloot MJ, van Maanen JP, Dun L, de Vries N. The undervalued potential of positional therapy in position-dependent snoring and obstructive sleep apnea – a review of the literature. Sleep Breath. 2013;17:39–49.
2. Lim J, Lasserson TJ, Fleetham J, Wright J. Oral appliances for obstructive sleep apnoea. Cochrane Database Syst Rev. 2006. doi:10.1002/14651858.CD004435.pub3:CD004435.
3. Giles TL, Lasserson TJ, Smith BH, White J, Wright J, Cates CJ. Continuous positive airways pressure for obstructive sleep apnoea in adults. Cochrane Database Syst Rev. 2006. doi:10.1002/14651858.CD001106.pub3:CD001106.
4. Sundaram S, Bridgman SA, Lim J, Lasserson TJ. Surgery for obstructive sleep apnoea. Cochrane Database Syst Rev. 2005. doi:10.1002/14651858.CD001004.pub2:CD001004.
5. Weaver TE, Grunstein RR. Adherence to continuous positive airway pressure therapy: the challenge to effective treatment. Proc Am Thorac Soc. 2008;5:173–8.
6. Petit FX, Pepin JL, Bettega G, Sadek H, Raphael B, Levy P. Mandibular advancement devices: rate of contraindications in 100 consecutive obstructive sleep apnea patients. Am J Respir Crit Care Med. 2002;166:274–8.
7. Fujita S, Conway W, Zorick F, Roth T. Surgical correction of anatomic azbnormalities in obstructive sleep apnea syndrome: uvulopalatopharyngoplasty. Otolaryngol Head Neck Surg. 1981;89:923–34.
8. Holty JE, Guilleminault C. Surgical options for the treatment of obstructive sleep apnea. Med Clin North Am. 2010;94:479–515.
9. Friedman M, Ibrahim H, Bass L. Clinical staging for sleep-disordered breathing. Otolaryngol Head Neck Surg. 2002;127:13–21.
10. Friedman M, Ibrahim HZ, Vidyasagar R, Pomeranz J, Joseph NJ. Z-palatoplasty (ZPP): a technique for patients without tonsils. Otolaryngol Head Neck Surg. 2004;131:89–100.
11. Caples SM, Rowley JA, Prinsell JR, et al. Surgical modifications of the upper airway for obstructive sleep apnea in adults: a systematic review and meta-analysis. Sleep. 2010;33:1396–407.
12. Chandrashekariah R, Shaman Z, Auckley D. Impact of upper airway surgery on CPAP compliance in difficult-to-manage obstructive sleep apnea. Arch Otolaryngol Head Neck Surg. 2008;134:926–30.
13. Khan A, Ramar K, Maddirala S, Friedman O, Pallanch JF, Olson EJ. Uvulopalatopharyngoplasty in the management of obstructive sleep apnea: the mayo clinic experience. Mayo Clin Proc. 2009;84:795–800.

14. Friedman M, Soans R, Joseph N, Kakodkar S, Friedman J. The effect of multilevel upper airway surgery on continuous positive airway pressure therapy in obstructive sleep apnea/hypopnea syndrome. Laryngoscope. 2009;119:193–6.
15. Akita Y, Kawakatsu K, Hattori C, Hattori H, Suzuki K, Nishimura T. Posture of patients with sleep apnea during sleep. Acta Otolaryngol Suppl 2003;(550):41–5.
16. Cartwright RD. Effect of sleep position on sleep apnea severity. Sleep. 1984;7:110–4.
17. Cartwright RD, Diaz F, Lloyd S. The effects of sleep posture and sleep stage on apnea frequency. Sleep. 1991;14:351–3.
18. Chaudhary BA, Chaudhary TK, Kolbeck RC, Harmon JD, Speir Jr WA. Therapeutic effect of posture in sleep apnea. South Med J. 1986;79:1061–3.
19. George CF, Millar TW, Kryger MH. Sleep apnea and body position during sleep. Sleep. 1988;11:90–9.
20. Itasaka Y, Miyazaki S, Ishikawa K, Togawa K. The influence of sleep position and obesity on sleep apnea. Psychiatry Clin Neurosci. 2000;54:340–1.
21. Kavey NB, Blitzer A, Gidro-Frank S, Korstanje K. Sleeping position and sleep apnea syndrome. Am J Otolaryngol. 1985;6:373–7.
22. Mador MJ, Kufel TJ, Magalang UJ, Rajesh SK, Watwe V, Grant BJ. Prevalence of positional sleep apnea in patients undergoing polysomnography. Chest. 2005;128:2130–7.
23. Oksenberg A, Khamaysi I, Silverberg DS, Tarasiuk A. Association of body position with severity of apneic events in patients with severe nonpositional obstructive sleep apnea. Chest. 2000;118:1018–24.
24. Oksenberg A, Silverberg DS, Arons E, Radwan H. Positional vs nonpositional obstructive sleep apnea patients: anthropomorphic, nocturnal polysomnographic, and multiple sleep latency test data. Chest. 1997;112:629–39.
25. Permut I, Diaz-Abad M, Chatila W, et al. Comparison of positional therapy to CPAP in patients with positional obstructive sleep apnea. J Clin Sleep Med. 2010;6:238–43.
26. Richard W, Kox D, den Herder C, Laman M, van Tinteren H, de Vries N. The role of sleep position in obstructive sleep apnea syndrome. Eur Arch Otorhinolaryngol. 2006;263:946–50.
27. Schwab RJ. A quantum advance in PSG recordings: the importance of head position in mediating the AHI. Sleep. 2011;34:985–6.
28. van Kesteren ER, van Maanen JP, Hilgevoord AA, Laman DM, de Vries N. Quantitative effects of trunk and head position on the apnea hypopnea index in obstructive sleep apnea. Sleep. 2011;34:1075–81.
29. van Maanen JP, Meester KA, Dun LN, et al. The sleep position trainer: a new treatment for positional obstructive sleep apnoea. Sleep Breath. 2013;17:771–9.
30. van Maanen JP, Richard W, van Kesteren ER, et al. Evaluation of a new simple treatment for positional sleep apnoea patients. J Sleep Res. 2012;21:322–9.
31. Stuck BA, Kopke J, Maurer JT, et al. Lesion formation in radiofrequency surgery of the tongue base. Laryngoscope. 2003;113:1572–6.
32. Sher AE, Schechtman KB, Piccirillo JF. The efficacy of surgical modifications of the upper airway in adults with obstructive sleep apnea syndrome. Sleep. 1996;19:156–77.
33. Metersky ML, Castriotta RJ. The effect of polysomnography on sleep position: possible implications on the diagnosis of positional obstructive sleep apnea. Respiration. 1996;63:283–7.
34. Levendowski DJ, Zack N, Rao S, et al. Assessment of the test-retest reliability of laboratory polysomnography. Sleep Breath. 2009;13:163–7.
35. Katsantonis GP, Miyazaki S, Walsh JK. Effects of uvulopalatopharyngoplasty on sleep architecture and patterns of obstructed breathing. Laryngoscope. 1990;100:1068–72.
36. Lee CH, Shin HW, Han DH, et al. The implication of sleep position in the evaluation of surgical outcomes in obstructive sleep apnea. Otolaryngol Head Neck Surg. 2009;140:531–5.
37. Lee CH, Kim SW, Han K, et al. Effect of uvulopalatopharyngoplasty on positional dependency in obstructive sleep apnea. Arch Otolaryngol Head Neck Surg. 2011;137:675–9.
38. Bignold JJ, Deans-Costi G, Goldsworthy MR, et al. Poor long-term patient compliance with the tennis ball technique for treating positional obstructive sleep apnea. J Clin Sleep Med. 2009;5:428–30.

39. Young T, Finn L, Peppard PE, et al. Sleep disordered breathing and mortality: eighteen-year follow-up of the Wisconsin sleep cohort. Sleep. 2008;31:1071–8.
40. Friedman M, Wilson M. Re-redefining success in airway surgery for obstructive sleep apnea. Sleep. 2009;32:17.
41. Weaver EM, Maynard C, Yueh B. Survival of veterans with sleep apnea: continuous positive airway pressure versus surgery. Otolaryngol Head Neck Surg. 2004;130:659–65.
42. Eveloff SE. Treatment of obstructive sleep apnea: no longer just a lot of hot air. Chest. 2002;121:674–7.
43. Weaver EM. Sleep apnea devices and sleep apnea surgery should be compared on effectiveness, not efficacy. Chest. 2003;123:961–2. Author reply 2.
44. van Maanen JP, Witte BI, de Vries N. Theoretical approach towards increasing effectiveness of palatal surgery in obstructive sleep apnea: role for concomitant positional therapy? Sleep Breath. 2014;18:341–9.

Positional Therapy and Tongue Base Surgery

J. Peter van Maanen, Madeline Ravesloot, and Nico de Vries

Introduction

Since treatment remains indicated in patients with severe OSA with CPAP failure [1], treatment alternatives are being explored. A variety of site-specific surgical techniques have been developed. The traditional uvulopalatopharyngoplasty (UPPP) or Z-palatopharyngoplasty (ZPP) (see chapter "Positional Therapy and Palatal Surgery") can be applied in patients with a palatal obstruction [2]. In patients with a base of tongue obstruction site, hyoidthyroidpexia [3] (HTP) and radiofrequent ablation of the base of the tongue (RFTB, see chapter "Positional Therapy and Palatal Surgery") are some of the surgical options to be considered.

Success rates of isolated tongue base surgery and of multilevel surgery have been extensively reported and vary between 45 and 62 %, depending on variables such as baseline AHI, BMI, and level and configuration of obstruction and on the definition of surgical success used [4–9].

An increasing amount of literature has been published on the role of sleep position in OSA [10–24]. Cartwright was the first to define the current positional OSA (POSA) criteria: an AHI in the worst sleep position twice or more as compared to

J.P. van Maanen, M.D. (✉)
Department of Otolaryngology, Sint Lucas Andreas Ziekenhuis,
Jan Tooropstraat 164, 1061 AE Amsterdam, The Netherlands
e-mail: p.vanmaanen@slaz.nl

M. Ravesloot, M.D., Ph.D.
Department of Otolaryngology/Head and Neck Surgery, Sint Lucas Andreas Hospital,
Jan Tooropstraat 164, 1061 AE Amsterdam, The Netherlands

N. de Vries, M.D., Ph.D.
Department of Otolaryngology, Sint Lucas Andreas Ziekenhuis,
Amsterdam, The Netherlands

Department of Otolaryngology, University Hospital Antwerp, Antwerp, Belgium

N. de Vries et al. (eds.), *Positional Therapy in Obstructive Sleep Apnea*,
DOI 10.1007/978-3-319-09626-1_28

the AHI in the other positions [12]. In two studies from Israel and the Netherlands, a remarkable steady 56 % of patients suffer from POSA [18, 19, 21].

As early as 1978, Harper and Sauerland suggested that when sleep apnea patients sleep in supine position, the tongue tends to fall backward against the pharyngeal wall, due to gravity [25]. Our group recently reported that base of tongue obstruction or epiglottis obstruction, albeit not statistically significant, is associated with POSA [26]. In sleep surgery literature, rarely attention has been paid to the distribution of the sleep position-specific PSG parameters (e.g., AHI) in the 4 sleep positions, namely, the supine, left, right, and prone sleep positions.

This chapter aims to elucidate the role of sleep position as a confounding factor on AHI and surgical success in tongue base surgery.

Materials and Methods

Patients

A retrospective analysis was performed focussing on patients with moderate to severe OSA and who had undergone a HTP surgery (following usual work-up of polysomnography, physical examination, and drug-induced sleep endoscopy) in our hospital between 2004 and 2011.

Patients with moderate to severe OSA who had undergone a hyoidthyroidpexia [3] with or without additional surgical treatment: an uvulopalatopharyngoplasty according to Fujita [27] (in patients with tonsils) or Z-palatoplasty according to Friedman [28] in patients without tonsils and radiofrequent ablation of the base of the tongue (RFTB) were included for analysis [29].

Surgical Techniques

- UPPP, ZPP, and RFTB (see chapter "Positional Therapy and Palatal Surgery")
- Hyoidthyroidpexia

  After exposure via a horizontal skin incision at the level of the thyrohyoid membrane, the strap muscles (sternohyoid, omohyoid, and thyrohyoid muscles) were divided just below the hyoid. Superior to the hyoid, the tendon of the stylohyoid muscle was divided from the hyoid bone. The hyoid bone was then mobilized in anterocaudal direction and permanently sutured to the thyroid cartilage aiming to create more retrolingual space.

Statistics

Changes in parameters before and after treatment were tested with a paired Wilcoxon signed-rank test. Differences between groups were tested with a χ^2-test in case of categorical variables and with a Wilcoxon rank-sum test in case of continuous variables. All statistical analyses were performed with SPSS (version 15.0). A P-value <0.05 was considered to be significant.

Results

One hundred and thirty patients were included for analysis. Patient characteristics are shown in Table 1. Ninety-four patients underwent a combined procedure of base of tongue and palate, from which 72 underwent concurrent radiofrequent thermotherapy of the base of the tongue (RFTB). Thirty-six patients underwent tongue base surgery alone (HTP), from which 22 underwent concurrent RFTB.

No significant differences in AHI, supine AHI, non-supine AHI, percentage of supine sleep position, total sleep time, arousal index, and awakenings were found between the different surgical groups when divided into solely tongue base surgery (HTP either with or without concurrent RFTB) and combined base of tongue and palate surgery (with either UPPP or ZPP) (Table 2).

The mean AHI of all 130 patients decreased significantly from 36.7 (range 9.0–100.9) to 25.1 ($P<0.001$). AHI in supine position decreased significantly from 51.2 to 39.3 ($P<0.001$). AHI in left position decreased significantly from 23.7 to 11.2 ($P<0.001$). AHI in right position decreased significantly from 21.1 to 14.2 ($P<0.001$). AHI in prone position decreased significantly from 11.2 to 6.4 ($P<0.001$).

A successful reduction in AHI, according to Sher's criteria, was seen in 49 patients (CI: 29.3–46.6 %) and in AI in 54 patients (CI: 33.2–50.9 %). Half of the patients (CI: 41.1–58.9 %) either had a successful reduction in AHI or in AI.

In general, patients who had a successful reduction in AHI slept less often in supine position after treatment than before treatment compared to the patients who did not have a successful reduction in AHI ($P=0.024$). The difference between the percentage of total sleep time (TST) in supine position before and after surgery was not significant within each group ($P=0.126$ and $P=0.124$ for both groups respectively). The mean difference in AHI before and after treatment was 26.3 per hour in the group of patients with a successful reduction in AHI, which is significantly higher than the mean difference in the other group ($P<0.001$). The mean AHI in supine position decreased by 30.2 per hour in the first group, again significantly higher than the difference in the other group ($P<0.001$). The differences in AHI, AHI in supine position, and AHI in non-supine position before and after treatment

Table 1 Baseline characteristics are shown as mean ± standard deviation

Variable	Mean ± SD
Age (year)	49.9±9.7
BMI (kg/m^2)	27.3±2.8
AHI (/h)	36.7±14.4
AHI supine (/h)	51.2±24.8
% AHI supine	37.4±24.7
Ratio male to female	9:1

Table 2 Mean values of AHI and AHI in different positions, before and after surgery for different groups of patients

	Mean (before)	Mean (after)	*P*-value (within)	Mean (before)	Mean (after)	*P*-value (within)	*P*-value (between)
AHI successful[a]	Yes (*n*=49)			No (*n*=81)			
AHI	35.8	9.5	**<0.001**	37.2	34.5	0.099	**<0.001**
AHI supine	49.1	18.9	**<0.001**	52.5	51.6	0.749	**<0.001**
AHI non-supine	23.1	5.1	**<0.001**	27.7	23.9	0.052	**<0.001**
AHI prone	4.9	3.5	0.647	15.0	8.1	**0.033**	0.234
AHI left	18.7	4.9	**<0.001**	26.8	20.3	**0.004**	0.077
AHI right	15.9	4.8	**<0.001**	24.2	19.9	0.137	0.061
% supine sleep position	42.8	36.9	0.126	34.2	37.9	0.124	**0.024**
AI successful[b]	Yes (*n*=54)			No (*n*=76)			
AI	20.0	2.7	**<0.001**	21.0	21.9	0.376	**<0.001**
AHI	34.4	13.1	**<0.001**	38.3	33.9	**0.026**	**<0.001**
AHI supine	51.8	24.1	**<0.001**	51.5	50.5	0.792	**<0.001**
AHI non-supine	22.7	8.7	**<0.001**	28.2	22.8	**0.011**	**0.003**
AHI prone	10.4	3.4	0.154	11.9	8.5	0.161	0.922
AHI left	21.9	8.3	**<0.001**	25.4	19.1	**0.006**	**0.029**
AHI right	18.5	7.5	**0.001**	23.3	19.2	0.098	0.141
% supine sleep position	36.8	37.7	0.679	38.4	37.7	0.886	0.720
AHI or AI successful	Yes (*n*=65)			No (*n*=65)			
AHI	34.8	13.1	**<0.001**	38.5	37.1	0.501	**<0.001**
AHI supine	49.8	23.8	**<0.001**	52.7	54.8	0.498	**<0.001**
AHI non-supine	23.6	8.4	**<0.001**	28.3	25.2	0.152	**<0.001**
AHI prone	9.4	3.5	0.115	12.9	9.2	0.197	0.808
AHI left	20.8	8.2	**<0.001**	26.7	20.9	**0.023**	**0.027**
AHI right	18.0	6.9	**<0.001**	24.2	21.4	0.258	0.071
% supine sleep position	38.2	37.2	0.838	36.7	37.9	0.575	0.565
Positional OSA[c]	Yes (*n*=70)			No (*n*=60)			
AHI	32.7	23.7	**<0.001**	41.3	26.6	**<0.001**	**0.044**
AHI supine	57.9	42.2	**<0.001**	43.5	35.6	0.132	0.107
AHI non-supine	14.9	13.3	0.106	38.8	20.8	**<0.001**	**<0.001**
AHI prone	4.4	6.3	0.793	19.1	6.4	**0.002**	**0.039**
AHI left	16.0	11.6	0.159	32.8	17.9	**<0.001**	**<0.001**
AHI right	12.8	13.0	0.501	30.8	15.6	**<0.001**	**0.001**
% supine sleep position	43.9	43.9	0.654	29.9	30.1	0.853	0.642
Treatment	HTP±RFTB (*n*=36)			HTP+UPPP/ZPP±RFTB (*n*=94)			
AHI	26.7	16.4	**<0.001**	38.4	26.5	**<0.001**	0.744

(continued)

Table 2 (continued)

	Mean (before)	Mean (after)	*P*-value (within)	Mean (before)	Mean (after)	*P*-value (within)	*P*-value (between)
AHI supine	41.4	30.4	0.059	52.9	40.7	**<0.001**	0.837
AHI non-supine	19.8	8.5	**0.001**	27.0	18.2	**<0.001**	0.676
AHI prone	9.6	0.5	**0.043**	11.4	7.4	0.133	0.275
AHI left	15.5	10.8	0.055	25.2	15.2	**<0.001**	0.474
AHI right	19.0	8.5	**0.010**	21.5	15.1	**0.008**	0.365
% supine sleep position	34.2	42.1	0.260	38.0	36.8	0.750	0.162

Bold-faced values are the significant differences before and after treatment within the groups or between the groups
[a]Reduction in AHI of at least 50 % and to below 20
[b]Reduction in AI of at least 50 % and to below 10
[c]AHI supine/AHI non-supine > 2

Table 3 Success rates split for different outcomes of positional OSA

	Percentage	95 % CI	Percentage	95 % CI	
Positional OSA[a]	Yes ($n=70$)		No ($n=60$)		*P*-value
AHI successful	35.7 %	24.6–48.1 %	40.0 %	27.6–53.5 %	0.615
AI successful	42.9 %	31.1–55.3 %	40.7 %	28.1–54.3 %	0.803
AHI or AI successful	48.6 %	36.4–60.1 %	51.7 %	38.4–64.7 %	0.725

The *P*-values denote the difference in these rates between the two groups
[a]AHI supine/AHI non-supine > 2

were all significant for the patients with successful AHI reduction (all $P<0.001$), and not for the patients in the non-successful group ($P=0.099$ total AHI, $P=0.749$ AHI supine, $P=0.052$ AHI non-supine). The AHI in left or right position decreased significantly for the successful group; AHI in prone position did not. In the unsuccessfully treated group, the AHI in prone and left position did decrease significantly after surgery (Table 2). Total sleep time, arousal index and number of awakenings did not change significantly after surgery (data not shown here).

Seventy patients suffered from POSA preoperatively. Within this group the total AHI decreased significantly from 32.7 to 23.7 ($P<0.001$), and the AHI in supine position decreased significantly from 57.9 to 42.2 ($P<0.001$). The percentage of supine sleep position did not change significantly after treatment ($P=0.654$). In 34 of the 70 position-dependent patients, the treatment was successful (CI: 36.4–60.1 %) (Table 3). The other 60 preoperative non-POSA patients had a significantly lower AHI following surgery ($P<0.001$). A significant decrease of the AHI was seen in all positions except the AHI in supine position. The difference in supine AHI before and after treatment between the POSA and non-POSA groups was not significant ($P=0.107$), while the AHI decreased more for the non-POSA patients ($P=0.044$) (Table 2). Furthermore, in the non-POSA patients, the postoperative decrease in non-supine, prone, left, and right AHI was significant when compared to these parameters in the POSA patients ($P<0.001$, $P=0.039$, $P<0.001$, $P=0.001$).

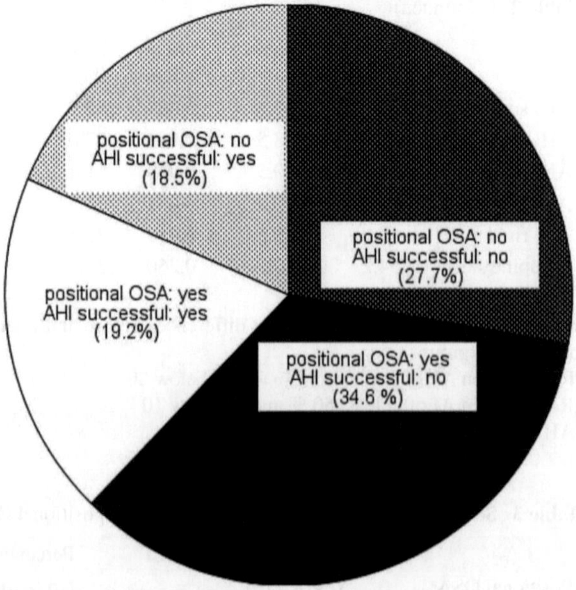

Fig. 1 Distribution of surgical success among POSA and non-POSA patients

Table 4 Effect of surgery on position dependency

		Posttreatment				
		No		Yes		
	Positional OSA[a]	*N*	%	*N*	%	*P*-value
Pretreatment	No	34	57.6	25	42.4	0.451
	Yes	19	27.1	51	72.9	

[a]AHI supine/AHI non-supine > 2

Surgery was not more successful in the group with position-dependent patients than in the other group ($P = 0.615$) (Fig. 1). Most positional patients remained positional after surgery and most non-POSA patients remained non-positional (72.9 % and 57.6 %, $P = 0.451$) (Table 4).

Discussion

The present study is the first which looks into the relation between tongue base surgery either with or without concurrent palatal surgery and sleep position.

The studied patient group did not solely consist of isolated tongue base surgery patients but also included patients who concurrently underwent surgery of the soft palate. This is a limitation of this analysis. Ideally, isolated tongue base surgery patients would have been studied. Most patients who underwent a HTP suffered from multilevel obstruction. When comparing the isolated tongue base surgery group to the combined base of tongue and palate surgery group, no significant differences could be found.

The overall success rate and overall response rate of this series of HTP/tongue base surgery with or without concomitant palatal surgery in patients with moderate to severe OSA and CPAP failure are 38 % and 60 % respectively, which is in the low-normal range compared to previously reported series [4–9]. Improvement of treatment outcome is mandatory if treatment intent is "salvage" in CPAP failures.

It is a clinical reality in sleep surgery that remarkable differences in outcome can occur among patients with comparable preoperative AHI, BMI, and clinical findings such as tongue size, tonsil size, and drug-induced sleep endoscopy (DISE) findings [26, 30]. Patients were divided into a POSA and non-POSA group to study whether discrepancies between expected and actual outcome could be explained by changes in body position before and after treatment.

In general, in both POSA and non-POSA patients, the percentage of supine sleep time remained remarkably constant after surgery and successes or failures could not be explained by considerable changes in percentage of supine sleep time. In conclusion, surgery did not influence patient's position dependency (Table 4).

Hyoidthyroidpexia is traditionally thought to exert its effect by increasing the retrolingual airway space. We hypothesized therefore that in a successful surgery, more outspoken decreases in AHI would be found in the supine position than in other sleep positions.

The results of this retrospective analysis show that HTP did not have better effect on the supine AHI compared to the AHI in the other sleep positions. When surgery was either successful or non-successful, the reduction in AHI was uniform in all sleep positions.

Earlier Stuck et al. reported that MRI studies do not show enlargement of the retrolingual airway space following HTP. These authors concluded that the effect of HTP had to be found in an increased general stabilization of the upper airway, not an enlargement of the retrolingual airway [31]. The present findings further support this concept. However, our follow-up was relatively short (3–4 months). Further research to evaluate long-term results is ongoing.

POSA occurs in 56 % [21] of OSA patients. PT as treatment for POSA is gaining momentum [24]. After surgical failure in positional patients, a further decrease of the AHI can theoretically be accomplished by prevention of the supine sleep position. This leads to the concept of multimodality treatment. Theoretically, in POSA, multilevel surgery with PT would achieve better results than surgery or PT alone. This is in concordance with earlier research papers in palate surgery. Katsantonis et al. studied the effect of UPPP on sleep posture and differences in uvulopalatopharyngoplasty (UPPP) results in various sleep positions in a small series of 17 patients [32]. They found that following UPPP, the AHI significantly improved in the lateral position. They also found that during sleep in a supine position, the AHI did not show significant improvement. They conclude that UPPP enhances the position effect on OSA because it readily eliminates obstructive events in the lateral sleep position. In other words the difference in AHI in supine and non-supine positions is more pronounced postoperatively. They are of opinion that additional positional therapy could significantly improve response to treatment with UPPP. Lee et al. studied the effect of sleep position on surgical outcomes as well [33]. They studied 69 consecutive patients who underwent a UPPP. After categorizing the patients into four groups according to the change in AHI after surgery, they found that the failure group had a higher proportion of supine position dependency than any other group. In a second paper published by the same group, results show that UPPP is a successful treatment for obstructive events occurring in the lateral sleep position, especially in patients without positional dependency [34]. The suggestion is made that patients who have become position dependent may benefit from positional therapy after UPPP.

Until recently, PT consisted of the "tennis ball technique." A variety of tennis balls, squash balls, shark fins, special pajamas, and vests all had the same concept of a bulky mass worn on the back. All these devices have in common that they are not comfortable, they disrupt sleep architecture, and the long-term compliance is a disappointing 10 % [35]. A recent paper by our group for the first time showed that a small buzzing device worn in the neck can prevent supine sleep position without disrupting sleep [24].

Conclusion

The difference between the percentage of total sleep time in supine position before and after surgery was not significant. The differences in AHI, AHI in supine position, and AHI in non-supine position before and after treatment were all significant for the patients with successful AHI reduction (all $P<0.001$), and not significant for the patients in the non-successful group ($P=0.099$ total AHI, $P=0.749$ AHI supine, $P=0.052$ AHI non-supine).

Isolated tongue base or multilevel surgery was as successful on the supine AHI as it was on the AHI in other sleep positions.

Surgery was not more successful in the group with position-dependent patients as compared to the non-POSA patients ($P=0.615$). Successful and non-successful surgical results could not be explained by variations in percentages of supine sleep position.

Surgery was not more successful in the group with POSA patients than in the non-POSA group ($P=0.615$).

From this retrospective analysis, it seems that sleep position is not a confounding factor on surgical outcomes in tongue base surgery.

The results of base of tongue or multilevel surgery in position-dependent OSA patients leave room for improvement, possibly through positional therapy.

References

1. Weaver TE, Grunstein RR. Adherence to continuous positive airway pressure therapy: the challenge to effective treatment. Proc Am Thorac Soc. 2008;5:173–8.
2. Woodson BT. Structural effectiveness of pharyngeal sleep apnea surgery. Sleep Med Rev. 2008;12:463–79.
3. Riley RW, Powell NB, Guilleminault C. Obstructive sleep apnea and the hyoid: a revised surgical procedure. Otolaryngol Head Neck Surg. 1994;111:717–21.
4. Baisch A, Maurer JT, Hormann K. The effect of hyoid suspension in a multilevel surgery concept for obstructive sleep apnea. Otolaryngol Head Neck Surg. 2006;134:856–61.
5. Benazzo M, Pagella F, Matti E, et al. Hyoidthyroidpexia as a treatment in multilevel surgery for obstructive sleep apnea. Acta Otolaryngol. 2008;128:680–4.
6. Kezirian EJ, Goldberg AN. Hypopharyngeal surgery in obstructive sleep apnea: an evidence-based medicine review. Arch Otolaryngol Head Neck Surg. 2006;132:206–13.
7. Richard W, Kox D, den Herder C, van Tinteren H, de Vries N. One stage multilevel surgery (uvulopalatopharyngoplasty, hyoid suspension, radiofrequent ablation of the tongue base with/without genioglossus advancement), in obstructive sleep apnea syndrome. Eur Arch Otorhinolaryngol. 2007;264:439–44.
8. van den Broek E, Richard W, van Tinteren H, de Vries N. UPPP combined with radiofrequency thermotherapy of the tongue base for the treatment of obstructive sleep apnea syndrome. Eur Arch Otorhinolaryngol. 2008;265:1361–5.
9. Yi HL, Sun XQ, Chen B, et al. Z-palatopharyngoplasty plus genioglossus advancement and hyoid suspension for obstructive sleep apnea hypopnea syndrome. Otolaryngol Head Neck Surg. 2011;144:469–73.
10. Akita Y, Kawakatsu K, Hattori C, Hattori H, Suzuki K, Nishimura T. Posture of patients with sleep apnea during sleep. Acta Otolaryngol Suppl. 2003; (550):41–5.
11. Cartwright RD. Effect of sleep position on sleep apnea severity. Sleep. 1984;7:110–4.
12. Cartwright RD, Diaz F, Lloyd S. The effects of sleep posture and sleep stage on apnea frequency. Sleep. 1991;14:351–3.
13. Chaudhary BA, Chaudhary TK, Kolbeck RC, Harmon JD, Speir Jr WA. Therapeutic effect of posture in sleep apnea. South Med J. 1986;79:1061–3.
14. George CF, Millar TW, Kryger MH. Sleep apnea and body position during sleep. Sleep. 1988;11:90–9.
15. Itasaka Y, Miyazaki S, Ishikawa K, Togawa K. The influence of sleep position and obesity on sleep apnea. Psychiatry Clin Neurosci. 2000;54:340–1.
16. Kavey NB, Blitzer A, Gidro-Frank S, Korstanje K. Sleeping position and sleep apnea syndrome. Am J Otolaryngol. 1985;6:373–7.
17. Mador MJ, Kufel TJ, Magalang UJ, Rajesh SK, Watwe V, Grant BJ. Prevalence of positional sleep apnea in patients undergoing polysomnography. Chest. 2005;128:2130–7.
18. Oksenberg A, Khamaysi I, Silverberg DS, Tarasiuk A. Association of body position with severity of apneic events in patients with severe nonpositional obstructive sleep apnea. Chest. 2000;118:1018–24.
19. Oksenberg A, Silverberg DS, Arons E, Radwan H. Positional vs nonpositional obstructive sleep apnea patients: anthropomorphic, nocturnal polysomnographic, and multiple sleep latency test data. Chest. 1997;112:629–39.
20. Permut I, Diaz-Abad M, Chatila W, et al. Comparison of positional therapy to CPAP in patients with positional obstructive sleep apnea. J Clin Sleep Med. 2010;6:238–43.
21. Richard W, Kox D, den Herder C, Laman M, van Tinteren H, de Vries N. The role of sleep position in obstructive sleep apnea syndrome. Eur Arch Otorhinolaryngol. 2006;263:946–50.
22. Schwab RJ. A quantum advance in PSG recordings: the importance of head position in mediating the AHI. Sleep. 2011;34:985–6.

23. van Kesteren ER, van Maanen JP, Hilgevoord AA, Laman DM, de Vries N. Quantitative effects of trunk and head position on the apnea hypopnea index in obstructive sleep apnea. Sleep. 2011;34:1075–81.
24. van Maanen JP, Richard W, van Kesteren ER, et al. Evaluation of a new simple treatment for positional sleep apnoea patients. J Sleep Res. 2012;21:322–9.
25. Harper R, Sauerland E. The role of the tongue in sleep apnea. In: Guilleminault C, Dement WC, editors. Sleep apnea syndromes. New York: A. R. Liss; 1978. p. 219–34.
26. Ravesloot MJ, de Vries N. One hundred consecutive patients undergoing drug-induced sleep endoscopy: results and evaluation. Laryngoscope. 2011;121:2710–6.
27. Fujita S, Conway W, Zorick F, Roth T. Surgical correction of anatomic abnormalities in obstructive sleep apnea syndrome: uvulopalatopharyngoplasty. Otolaryngol Head Neck Surg. 1981;89:923–34.
28. Friedman M, Ibrahim HZ, Vidyasagar R, Pomeranz J, Joseph NJ. Z-palatoplasty (ZPP): a technique for patients without tonsils. Otolaryngol Head Neck Surg. 2004;131:89–100.
29. Stuck BA, Kopke J, Maurer JT, et al. Lesion formation in radiofrequency surgery of the tongue base. Laryngoscope. 2003;113:1572–6.
30. Kezirian EJ, Hohenhorst W, de Vries N. Drug-induced sleep endoscopy: the VOTE classification. Eur Arch Otorhinolaryngol. 2011;268:1233–6.
31. Stuck BA, Neff W, Hormann K, et al. Anatomic changes after hyoid suspension for obstructive sleep apnea: an MRI study. Otolaryngol Head Neck Surg. 2005;133:397–402.
32. Katsantonis GP, Miyazaki S, Walsh JK. Effects of uvulopalatopharyngoplasty on sleep architecture and patterns of obstructed breathing. Laryngoscope. 1990;100:1068–72.
33. Lee CH, Shin HW, Han DH, et al. The implication of sleep position in the evaluation of surgical outcomes in obstructive sleep apnea. Otolaryngol Head Neck Surg. 2009;140:531–5.
34. Lee CH, Kim SW, Han K, et al. Effect of uvulopalatopharyngoplasty on positional dependency in obstructive sleep apnea. Arch Otolaryngol Head Neck Surg. 2011;137:675–9.
35. Oksenberg A, Silverberg D, Offenbach D, Arons E. Positional therapy for obstructive sleep apnea patients: a 6-month follow-up study. Laryngoscope. 2006;116:1995–2000.

Residual POSA After Maxillomandibular Advancement in Patients with Severe OSA

Linda B.L. Benoist, Maurits H.T. de Ruiter, Jan de Lange, and Nico de Vries

Introduction

Various treatment options are available for patients with severe or extreme OSA. There is no clear definition for extreme OSA in the clinical guidelines. We defined extreme OSA when the AHI is >60 per hour. The gold standard therapy entails the use of CPAP, but its compliance is frequently disappointing. 46–83 % of patients are non-compliant and use their CPAP less than 4 h per night [1, 2]. For CPAP to be effective in patients with severe OSA, CPAP must be used more than 80 % per night [2–6]. In patients with severe to extreme OSA and CPAP failure, non-acceptance, or refusal, several surgical therapies are available. These can be considered when CPAP and oral appliance therapy (OAT) are not tolerated and/or if a patient has an anatomical, correctable obstruction in the upper airways. Moreover, younger patients with severe OSA can prefer a permanent (surgical) solution instead of the rather cumbersome appliances for the rest of their lives. Two of these advanced surgical treatments are maxillomandibular advancement (MMA) and multilevel surgery. A variety of interventions, both minimally invasive (radiofrequency-induced thermotherapy (RFTT) of palate and tongue base) and surgical

L.B.L. Benoist, M.D. (✉)
Ear Nose and Throat, Sint Lucas Andreas Ziekenhuis,
Jan Tooropstraat 164, 1061 AE Amsterdam, The Netherlands
e-mail: l.benoist@slaz.nl

M.H.T. de Ruiter, D.D.S. • J. de Lange, D.M.D., M.D., Ph.D.
Department of Oral and Maxillofacial Surgery, Academic Medical Center,
University of Amsterdam, Amsterdam, The Netherlands

N. de Vries, M.D., Ph.D.
Department of Otolaryngology, Sint Lucas Andreas Ziekenhuis,
Amsterdam, The Netherlands

Department of Otolaryngology, University Hospital Antwerp, Antwerp, Belgium

N. de Vries et al. (eds.), *Positional Therapy in Obstructive Sleep Apnea*,
DOI 10.1007/978-3-319-09626-1_29

[uvulopalatopharyngoplasty (UPPP), hyoid suspension (HS), genioglossus advancement (GA)], have been reported as part of multilevel surgery. Success rates of multilevel surgery have been extensively reported and vary between 45 and 62 %, depending not only on the surgical technique applied but also on variables such as baseline AHI, BMI, and level and configuration of obstruction and on the definition of success used [7–10]. Van Maanen et al. showed a success rate of 45 % and an overall response rate of 72 % in one-stage multilevel procedure [11].

In selected patients with severe to extreme OSA, MMA can be indicated, both as primary surgical modality and in case of failure of multilevel surgery. MMA is a highly effective technique, with success rates between 80 and 90 % [12–16].

Surgical Technique

Since the mid-1980s orthognathic surgery was introduced as a treatment modality for patients suffering from severe OSA. MMA surgery resulted in better surgical outcomes compared to other existing pharyngeal enlargement surgeries [12–14].

This surgical technique is a combined Le Fort I osteotomy with advancement and a bilateral sagittal split osteotomy (BSSO). The maxilla is advanced to the desired position (approximately 8–10 mm ventrally) and an intermediate splint is applied to immobilize the advanced maxilla. After fixation of the maxilla with osteosynthesis, dissection and corticotomies for the sagittal split osteotomies are executed. With rigid maxillomandibular fixation, the mandible is repositioned and fixated with osteosynthesis. The maxillomandibular fixation is removed and postoperative functional therapy with elastics is often applied for stabilization of the occlusion [17–20].

MMA has proved its efficacy and should be considered in patients with severe OSA, patients with obvious retrognathia (skeletal class II profile), or patients wishing for a definitive solution for OSA. An adverse effect that has to be considered is paresthesia of the alveolar nerve, which runs through the mandible. This complication occurs in 10–30 % of the patients. Patients often experience a postoperative malocclusion, which can be corrected with orthodontic treatment. Preferably, all orthognathic surgery is performed with orthodontic treatment [15]. The advancement may compromise facial aesthetics. Most patients find these changes to be moderate and only a few patients (around 10–15 %) consider these changes as unfavorable [21].

Residual POSA

We observed that in a number of patients in whom MMA was performed, the total AHI decreased, but not sufficiently to fulfil the criteria for success according to Sher's definition for surgical success [22]. Since MMA is often the *ultimum refugium*, and taking into account its considerable morbidity, this is a very disappointing outcome. However, on closer inspection, in many of these patients, only the AHI in supine sleep position remained high, whereas the AHI in other sleep positions had improved significantly. These patients had reversed from severe non-positional OSA to less severe POSA. In a group of 42 patients who underwent MMA surgery, 9 patients were diagnosed with POSA after MMA surgery.

In this chapter we discuss in detail a small cohort of patients who have residual POSA after MMA surgery for severe OSA. These results will also be published elsewhere; however, in this chapter we describe this new phenomenon for the first time and discuss theoretical considerations.

Methods

Patients

In this study we reviewed the polysomnographic results of nine patients who underwent MMA for severe OSA. All patients had severe OSA and CPAP failure and received overnight polysomnography (PSG) before and after surgery.

Polysomnography

A position sensor (Sleepsense, St Charles, IL, USA) attached to the midline of the abdominal wall was used to differentiate between supine, prone, right lateral, left lateral, and upright positions.

Definition

POSA is diagnosed when having a supine AHI that is at least twice as high as the non-supine AHI [23].

Results

From 2011 to 2014, a total of 42 patients underwent MMA surgery for OSA. All patients had CPAP failure and some had previous surgery (i.e., uvulopalatopharyngoplasty, radiofrequent ablation of the tongue base, or hyoid suspension).

Table 1 Polysomnographic and clinical variables of the study group

Patient no.	AHI		AHI supine		AHI non-supine		% supine position		Desaturation index	
	Baseline	After MMA	Baseline	After MMA	Baseline	After MMA	Baseline	After MMA	Baseline	After MMA
1	46,6	4,9	77,8	13,3	39,3	1,2	18,8	30,7	48,0	3,9
2	35,6	12,5	81,7	24,0	29,2	3,2	12,3	44,8	28,2	7,2
3	68,2	28,2	82,0	31,0	48,4	4,6	59,1	89,3	53,0	25,0
4	82,2	40,9	88,8	69,1	71,8	22,6	62,2	39,3	75,6	13,6
5	38,2	24,0	53,2	49,3	33,1	9,4	28,2	36,5	27,1	19,1
6	50,7	14,9	86,5	28,0	30,8	3,8	35,8	45,9	52,9	14,4
7	64,1	20,6	76,0	36,9	54,4	0,6	45,7	53,4	62,9	17,7
8	66,9	14,8	64,1	18,1	82,1	3,8	84,7	78,0	69,4	9,2
9	57,0	27,0	60,2	62,4	49,1	2,5	70,7	40,9	48,6	22,3

AHI Apnea–Hypopnea Index, *MMA* maxillomandibular advancement

Table 2 Comparison of pre- and post-MMA results

Characteristics	Pre Mean ± SD	Post Mean ± SD	Wilcoxon signed-ranks *p*-value
BMI	28.3 ± 3.3	27.3 ± 3.3	0.123
Total AHI	56.6 ± 15.3	20.9 ± 10.6	<0.01
Total AHI supine	74.5 ± 12.4	36.9 ± 19.5	0.01
Total AHI *non*-supine	48.7 ± 18.4	5.7 ± 6.8	<0.01
Desaturation index	51.7 ± 16.6	14.7 ± 7.0	<0.01

SD standard deviation, *AHI* Apnea–Hypopnea Index

Nine of these 42 patients (8 male and 1 female, age 55.1 ± 6.8 and BMI 28.3 ± 3.3) were diagnosed with residual OSA postoperatively, which was mainly due to an AHI that was still high (in four cases an AHI still above 30) in supine sleep position, i.e., residual POSA. One of these patients had a total AHI of 4.9, but the AHI in supine sleep position was 13.3. In hindsight, two of the nine patients already had POSA before MMA surgery. Table 1 demonstrates the individual values of the polysomnographic and clinical variables of the study group at baseline and after MMA surgery.

Average follow-up interval for the second PSG recording was 5.9 ± 3.9 months after surgery. Table 2 shows the averages of the polysomnographic results pre and post MMA. A significant decrease in all polysomnographic parameters was seen following MMA surgery. However, the mean supine AHI was still >30. The mean supine AHI decreased from 74.5 to 36.9; this is a reduction of 50.5 %. The mean AHI in lateral sleep positions both decreased even more: right sleep position 42.4–7.0 (83.5 %) and left sleep position 52.7–4.8 (90.9 %). These results are shown in Fig. 1. The BMI did not change significantly postoperatively.

The patients' dental characteristics are shown in Table 3. Different parameters of the MMA are demonstrated per patient. The pharyngeal airway space (PAS) is defined as the smallest airway space measured on a lateral cephalogram in millimeters

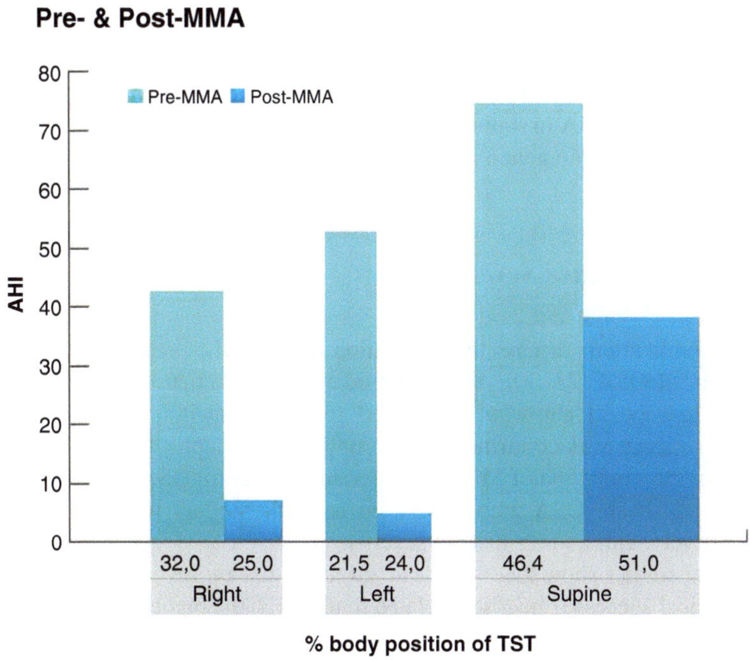

Fig. 1 Pre- and postoperative results of MMA

Table 3 Polysomnographic and clinical variables of the study group

	PAS in mm		Advancement SNA angle		Advancement mandible
Patient no.	Baseline	After MMA	Baseline	After MMA	Baseline
1	4	14	88	102	11
2	6	10	79	89	8
3	7	12	82	87	8
4	4	10	84	85	7
5	8	24	90	94	10
6	5	15	79	85	7
7	4	12	78	85	5
8	10	13	83	84	10
9	7	12	80	82	8

PAS pharyngeal airway space; *SNA* angle between point sella, nasion, and frontal bone of the maxilla

pre- and postoperatively. All patients have an increased PAS after MMA with a mean increase from 6.1 to 13.6 mm. The advancement of the maxilla is shown in the cephalometric angle between point sella, nasion, and frontal bone of the maxilla, defined as SNA in amount of degrees. All patients have an increased angle after MMA with a mean of 82.6–88.1°. The advancement of the mandible is measured on a panoramic radiograph and has a mean increase of 8.2 mm after advancement.

Discussion

The results of this study indicate that persistent OSA after MMA surgery can be caused by residual OSA in supine position. To the best of our knowledge, this is the first time that this phenomenon is described after MMA surgery.

Influence of Disease Severity

Different publications discuss the correlation between the presence of POSA and the severity of OSA [23–30]. All these studies conclude that patients with severe OSA are less positional when compared to patients with mild and moderate OSA. This theory was confirmed by Morong et al. (chapter "Influence of Sleep Position on the Transition of Mild to Moderate and Severe OSA"), who found that patients with severe OSA who underwent bariatric surgery reversed into POSA postoperatively with a lower disease severity.

Different studies show that there is an effect of disease severity on surgical outcome; surgical success is inversely related to the AHI: the higher the AHI preoperatively, the lower the success rate [7, 8, 10, 31–33].

Effect of Gravity

In general the AHI in supine sleep position is usually higher when compared to other sleep positions. Moreover, Oksenberg et al. [34] showed that in patients with severe OSA the apneic events appear to be more severe in supine sleep position than those occurring in other sleep positions. The current results demonstrate the presence of residual OSA after MMA surgery. Thus, in some cases surgery will only have a partial treatment effect (mostly in lateral sleep positions), and it appears that those patients can have residual apneic events only in the supine sleep position. The influence of gravity (i.e., sleep position) has therefore a larger impact on surgical outcome than previously thought.

Sleep Position and Surgical Outcome

Only a few studies have addressed the issue of the influence of sleep position after surgery for OSA.

Katsantonis et al. [35] were among the first to evaluate the effect of UPPP as related to sleep posture. The authors found a significant improvement of the AHI in lateral sleep position following UPPP and suggest that additional PT could significantly improve response to treatment with UPPP.

Lee et al. [36] retrospectively evaluated the effect of sleep position on surgical outcome. Patients who underwent UPPP were categorized into four groups. They showed that the failure group had a higher proportion of OSA supine position dependency compared to the other groups. Furthermore, it was shown that the fluctuation of sleep position in each polysomnography might confound the surgical outcome. A second paper from the same group [37] indicated that UPPP is a successful treatment for obstructive events occurring in the lateral sleep position, especially in patients without positional dependency.

Van Maanen et al. [11] analyzed the results of 130 patients who underwent either isolated tongue base or multilevel surgery for OSA. They concluded that successful and non-successful surgical outcomes could not be explained by variations in percentages of supine sleep position and that sleep position is not a confounding factor on surgical outcomes in tongue base surgery. However, a more recent study by van Maanen et al. [38] (chapter "Positional Therapy and Palatal Surgery") showed that in patients who previously underwent uvulopalatopharyngoplasty/Z-palatoplasty (UPPP/ZPP) +/– radiofrequent ablation of the tongue base (RFTB), the reduction in AHI was significantly higher in non-positional OSA patients compared to POSA patients. They suggest to apply positional therapy (PT) after surgery or even to start with PT as a monotherapy prior to surgery.

They conclude that the effect of UPPP is most successful in decreasing the AHI in the lateral sleep position. Additional PT postoperatively could potentially improve treatment outcome. This conclusion also supports the theory discussed in chapter "Influence of Sleep Position on the Transition of Mild to Moderate and Severe OSA".

It is believed that non-apneic snorers predominantly start snoring in supine position; this progresses into mild OSA which is also positional in nature. When left untreated, a transition from mild to moderate sleep apnea will occur in the supine position (POSA) to a more severe sleep apnea noted in all sleep positions. In patients who have had surgery for OSA, a reversible effect is observed; AHI decreases in most patients but some still have POSA postoperatively.

Conclusion

The same pattern as after UPPP can occur after MMA: the AHI decreases in lateral sleep position, but not sufficiently in supine sleep position. Postoperative residual POSA in theory can be a good indication for additional positional therapy.

Despite the high success rate of MMA reported in medical literature, MMA is more invasive and associated with more risks and adverse events as well as perhaps a greater burden for the patient in comparison to multilevel surgery. For this reason, in many centers in patients with moderate to severe OSA, multilevel surgery is offered first, with MMA in reserve. In patients with extreme OSA, multilevel surgery is frequently not effective and in such patients MMA is often offered as a first-line treatment. With MMA as last resort, and also taking its morbidity in mind, it is extremely disappointing if the effect is not sufficient. In this chapter, we demonstrate that in 20 % of the MMA cases, patients were not cured because of residual POSA. These patients, in theory, may benefit from additional positional therapy or can be offered positional therapy prior to surgery, if POSA is observed at baseline. A study of additional positional therapy after MMA failure is presently ongoing. The results will be published elsewhere. Lastly, more research is required to identify the predictors of residual postoperative OSA.

References

1. Weaver TE, Grunstein RR. Adherence to continuous positive airway pressure therapy: the challenge to effective treatment. Proc Am Thorac Soc. 2008;5(2):173–8.
2. Richard W, Venker J, den Herder C, et al. Acceptance and long-term compliance of nCPAP in obstructive sleep apnea. Eur Arch Otorhinolaryngol. 2007;264(9):1081–6.
3. Weaver TE. Predicting adherence to continuous positive airway pressure – the role of patient perception. J Clin Sleep Med. 2005;1(4):354–6.
4. Weaver TE, Maislin G, Dinges DF, et al. Relationship between hours of CPAP use and achieving normal levels of sleepiness and daily functioning. Sleep. 2007;30(6):711–9.
5. Sin DD, Mayers I, Man GC, Pawluk L. Long-term compliance rates to continuous positive airway pressure in obstructive sleep apnea: a population-based study. Chest. 2002;121(2):430–5.
6. Meurice JC, Dore P, Paquereau J, et al. Predictive factors of long-term compliance with nasal continuous positive airway pressure treatment in sleep apnea syndrome. Chest. 1994; 105(2):429–33.
7. Richard W, Kox D, den Herder C, van Tinteren H, de Vries N. One stage multilevel surgery (uvulopalatopharyngoplasty, hyoid suspension, radiofrequent ablation of the tongue base with/without genioglossus advancement), in obstructive sleep apnea syndrome. Eur Arch Otorhinolaryngol. 2007;264(4):439–44.
8. Riley RW, Powell NB, Guilleminault C. Obstructive sleep apnea syndrome: a surgical protocol for dynamic upper airway reconstruction. J Oral Maxillofac Surg. 1993;51(7):742–7.
9. den Herder C, van Tinteren H, de Vries N. Hyoidthyroidpexia: a surgical treatment for sleep apnea syndrome. Laryngoscope. 2005;115(4):740–5.
10. Verse T, Baisch A, Hormann K. Multi-level surgery for obstructive sleep apnea. Preliminary objective results. Laryngorhinootologie. 2004;83(8):516–22.
11. van Maanen JP, Ravesloot MJ, Witte BI, Grijseels M, de Vries N. Exploration of the relationship between sleep position and isolated tongue base or multilevel surgery in obstructive sleep apnea. Eur Arch Otorhinolaryngol. 2012;269(9):2129–36.
12. Hoekema A, de Lange LJ, Stegenga B, de Bont LG. Oral appliances and maxillomandibular advancement surgery: an alternative treatment protocol for the obstructive sleep apnea-hypopnea syndrome. J Oral Maxillofac Surg. 2006;64(6):886–91.
13. Prinsell JR. Maxillomandibular advancement surgery for obstructive sleep apnea syndrome. J Am Dent Assoc. 2002;133(11):1489–97.
14. Prinsell JR. Maxillomandibular advancement surgery in a site-specific treatment approach for obstructive sleep apnea in 50 consecutive patients. Chest. 1999;116(6):1519–29.
15. Goh YH, Lim KA. Modified maxillomandibular advancement for the treatment of obstructive sleep apnea: a preliminary report. Laryngoscope. 2003;113(9):1577–82.
16. Holty JE, Guilleminault C. Maxillomandibular advancement for the treatment of obstructive sleep apnea: a systematic review and meta-analysis. Sleep Med Rev. 2010;14(5):287–97.
17. Conradt R, Hochban W, Brandenburg U, Heitmann J, Peter JH. Long-term follow-up after surgical treatment of obstructive sleep apnoea by maxillomandibular advancement. Eur Respir J. 1997;10(1):123–8.

18. Hochban W, Conradt R, Brandenburg U, Heitmann J, Peter JH. Surgical maxillofacial treatment of obstructive sleep apnea. Plast Reconstr Surg. 1997;99(3):619–26.
19. Riley RW, Powell NB, Guilleminault C. Maxillary, mandibular, and hyoid advancement for treatment of obstructive sleep apnea: a review of 40 patients. J Oral Maxillofac Surg. 1990;48(1):20–6.
20. Riley RW, Powell NB, Guilleminault C. Maxillofacial surgery and obstructive sleep apnea: a review of 80 patients. Otolaryngol Head Neck Surg. 1989;101(3):353–61.
21. Li KK, Riley RW, Powell NB, Guilleminault C. Patient's perception of the facial appearance after maxillomandibular advancement for obstructive sleep apnea syndrome. J Oral Maxillofac Surg. 2001;59(4):377–80.
22. Sher AE, Schechtman KB, Piccirillo JF. The efficacy of surgical modifications of the upper airway in adults with obstructive sleep apnea syndrome. Sleep. 1996;19(2):156–77.
23. Cartwright RD. Effect of sleep position on sleep apnea severity. Sleep. 1984;7(2):110–4.
24. Mador MJ, Kufel TJ, Magalang UJ, Rajesh SK, Watwe V, Grant BJ. Prevalence of positional sleep apnea in patients undergoing polysomnography. Chest. 2005;128(4):2130–7.
25. Akita Y, Kawakatsu K, Hattori C, Hattori H, Suzuki K, Nishimura T. Posture of patients with sleep apnea during sleep. Acta Otolaryngol Suppl. 2003;550:41–5.
26. Sunnergren O, Brostrom A, Svanborg E. Positional sensitivity as a confounder in diagnosis of severity of obstructive sleep apnea. Sleep Breath. 2013;17(1):173–9.
27. Teerapraipruk B, Chirakalwasan N, Simon R, et al. Clinical and polysomnographic data of positional sleep apnea and its predictors. Sleep Breath. 2012;16(4):1167–72.
28. Oksenberg A, Silverberg DS, Arons E, Radwan H. Positional vs nonpositional obstructive sleep apnea patients: anthropomorphic, nocturnal polysomnographic, and multiple sleep latency test data. Chest. 1997;112(3):629–39.
29. Richard W, Kox D, den Herder C, Laman M, van Tinteren H, de Vries N. The role of sleep position in obstructive sleep apnea syndrome. Eur Arch Otorhinolaryngol. 2006;263(10):946–50.
30. Benoist LB, Morong S, van Maanen JP, Hilgevoord AA, de Vries N. Evaluation of position dependency in non-apneic snorers. Eur Arch Otorhinolaryngol. 2014;271(1):189–94.
31. Hendler BH, Costello BJ, Silverstein K, Yen D, Goldberg A. A protocol for uvulopalatopharyngoplasty, mortised genioplasty, and maxillomandibular advancement in patients with obstructive sleep apnea: an analysis of 40 cases. J Oral Maxillofac Surg. 2001;59(8):892–7.
32. Neruntarat C. Genioglossus advancement and hyoid myotomy: short-term and long-term results. J Laryngol Otol. 2003;117(6):482–6.
33. Miller FR, Watson D, Boseley M. The role of the Genial Bone Advancement Trephine system in conjunction with uvulopalatopharyngoplasty in the multilevel management of obstructive sleep apnea. Otolaryngol Head Neck Surg. 2004;130(1):73–9.
34. Oksenberg A, Khamaysi I, Silverberg DS, Tarasiuk A. Association of body position with severity of apneic events in patients with severe nonpositional obstructive sleep apnea. Chest. 2000;118(4):1018–24.
35. Katsantonis GP, Miyazaki S, Walsh JK. Effects of uvulopalatopharyngoplasty on sleep architecture and patterns of obstructed breathing. Laryngoscope. 1990;100(10 Pt 1):1068–72.
36. Lee CH, Shin HW, Han DH, et al. The implication of sleep position in the evaluation of surgical outcomes in obstructive sleep apnea. Otolaryngol Head Neck Surg. 2009;140(4):531–5.
37. Lee CH, Kim SW, Han K, et al. Effect of uvulopalatopharyngoplasty on positional dependency in obstructive sleep apnea. Arch Otolaryngol Head Neck Surg. 2011;137(7):675–9.
38. van Maanen JP, Witte BI, de Vries N. Theoretical approach towards increasing effectiveness of palatal surgery in obstructive sleep apnea: role for concomitant positional therapy? Sleep Breath. 2014;18(2):341–9.

Impact of Upper Airway Surgery on Positional Change During Sleep

Ji Ho Choi and Seung Hoon Lee

Abbreviations

AASM	American Academy of Sleep Medicine
AHI	Apnea–hypopnea index
OA	Oral appliance
OSAS	Obstructive sleep apnea syndrome
PAP	Positive airway pressure
PCI	Positional change index
RDI	Respiratory disturbance index
RERA	Respiratory event-related arousal
RSI	Restless sleep index
TST	Total sleep time

Introduction (Overview)

Obstructive sleep apnea syndrome (OSAS) is characterized by repetitive partial or complete collapse of the upper airway (e.g., oropharynx, hypopharynx, and larynx) during sleep [1]. The prevalence of pediatric OSAS is estimated to be around 1–3 % and the prevalence of adult OSAS is estimated to be about 2–4 % [2–5].

There are numerous symptoms and signs related with OSAS (e.g., snoring, witnessed apnea, non-refreshing sleep, decreased concentration, restless sleep

J.H. Choi, M.D., Ph.D. • S.H. Lee, M.D., Ph.D. (✉)
Department of Otorhinolaryngology-Head and Neck Surgery, Korea University Ansan Hospital, Korea University College of Medicine, 516 Gojan-dong, Danwon-gu, Ansan-si, Gyeonggi-do 425-707, Republic of Korea
e-mail: shleeent@korea.ac.kr

N. de Vries et al. (eds.), *Positional Therapy in Obstructive Sleep Apnea*,
DOI 10.1007/978-3-319-09626-1_30

[positional change during sleep], daytime fatigue, excessive daytime sleepiness, memory reduction, nasal obstruction, mouth breathing, difficulty with morning arousal, gasping during sleep, nocturia, morning headache, irritability, decreased libido, etc.) [1, 6, 7]. If left untreated, OSAS can lead to various consequences or complications (e.g., hypertension, arrhythmia, ischemic heart disease, myocardial infarction, cor pulmonale, stroke, diabetes, motor vehicle accident, etc.) [8, 9].

Physical examination of the upper airway can be routinely performed in patients with suspected OSAS to reveal the anatomical abnormalities (e.g., nasal septal deviation, inferior turbinate hypertrophy, nasal polyp or mass, adenoid vegetation, high arched/narrow hard palate, tonsillar hypertrophy, enlarged or elongated uvula, redundant soft palate or pharyngeal tissue, high-leveled tongue, laryngeal mass, overjet, overbite, etc.) [10]. In addition, the evaluation of obstructive level may be used for OSAS management such as surgical therapy [11].

Pediatric OSAS is diagnosed if one or more respiratory events (i.e., apnea or hypopnea) are observed per hour of total sleep time (TST) on polysomnography in a patient or caregiver who reports any of the symptoms and signs associated with OSAS [1]. The diagnosis of adult OSAS is established if either of the following criteria is met: (1) 15 or more respiratory events (i.e., apneas, hypopneas, or respiratory event-related arousals [RERAs]) per hour of TST on polysomnography or (2) five or more respiratory events (i.e., apneas, hypopneas, or RERAs) per hour of TST on polysomnography in a patient who complains any of the symptoms and signs related with OSAS [1]. The severity of adult OSAS is determined by apnea–hypopnea index (AHI) or respiratory disturbance index (RDI) on polysomnography and is categorized into three groups including mild ($5 \leq$AHI or RDI<15), moderate ($15 \leq$AHI or RDI<30), and severe (AHI or RDI≥ 30) [12].

Pediatric OSAS is mostly associated with structural problems including adenoid vegetation and/or tonsillar hypertrophy [7]. Therefore, primary treatment for pediatric OSAS is surgical therapy such as adenoidectomy and/or tonsillectomy. According to the recent American Academy of Sleep Medicine (AASM) clinical guideline for adults, OSAS should be considered as a chronic medical condition requiring long-term care and management [10]. There are various OSAS managements (e.g., weight control, positional therapy, oral appliance [OA], positive airway pressure [PAP], surgical modifications of the upper airway, etc.) [13–17]. Of these, OA, PAP, and surgical management are regarded as primary treatments for OSAS in adults [10, 13]. Other management options such as weight loss and positional therapy are included in adjunctive treatments [10, 13].

Restless sleep is one of the common symptoms and signs in pediatric and adult OSAS [7]. It is thought that restless sleep is related with frequent change of sleep position, repetitive movement, or inability to keep consistent position during sleep [7, 18, 19]. Restless sleep is a problem in itself due to its effect on bed partner and may result in numerous symptoms such as daytime sleepiness or impairment [7].

There are little studies about restless sleep in OSAS. The clear definition of restless sleep has not been specified in patients with OSAS. The need of objective assessment of restless sleep has emerged because the measurement of restless sleep has been mostly performed by subjective questionnaire in OSAS. It is not yet well recognized whether OSAS management such as upper airway surgery influences restless sleep. In addition, it is not well known what the effect of OSAS surgery on the distribution of body position during sleep is.

In this chapter, we review a few studies about restless sleep (frequent positional change during sleep) and sleep position in OSAS before and after upper airway surgery and describe the following: (1) the impact of surgical treatment for OSAS on positional change during sleep using an objective measurement (i.e., positional change index [PCI] or restless sleep index [RSI]) and (2) the effect of upper airway surgery on the distribution of sleep position in OSAS patients.

Distribution of Sleep Position

Body positions during sleep are usually categorized into 2–9 types according to various positional sensors. For example, two types consist of supine and non-supine positions. Five types consist of supine, prone, two lateral (left and right), and upright positions (Table 1). Nine types consist of supine, prone, six lateral (left, supine left, prone left, right, supine right, and prone right), and upright positions (Table 2).

Generally, sleep positions in standard (level 1) polysomnography are detected by body position sensor and confirmed by direct monitoring or by a sleep technician using an infrared camera.

In five types of sleep position, four body positions during sleep are classified by 90° ranges and the upright position is defined as a position 30 or 45° above the horizontal plane (Fig. 1). Similarly, in nine types of body position during sleep, eight sleep positions are divided by 45° ranges, and the definition of upright position is the same as stated above (Fig. 2).

Sleep positions are detected by a position sensor on the trunk. The distribution of sleep position is expressed as the proportion of time spent in each sleep position.

Table 1 Five types of sleep position

1.	Supine position
2.	Lateral position (left)
3.	Prone position
4.	Lateral position (right)
5.	Upright position: 30 or 45° above the horizontal plane

Table 2 Nine types of sleep position

1.	Supine position
2.	Supine-lateral position (left)
3.	Lateral position (left)
4.	Prone-lateral position (left)
5.	Prone position
6.	Prone-lateral position (right)
7.	Lateral position (right)
8.	Supine-lateral position (right)
9.	Upright position: 30 or 45° above the horizontal plane

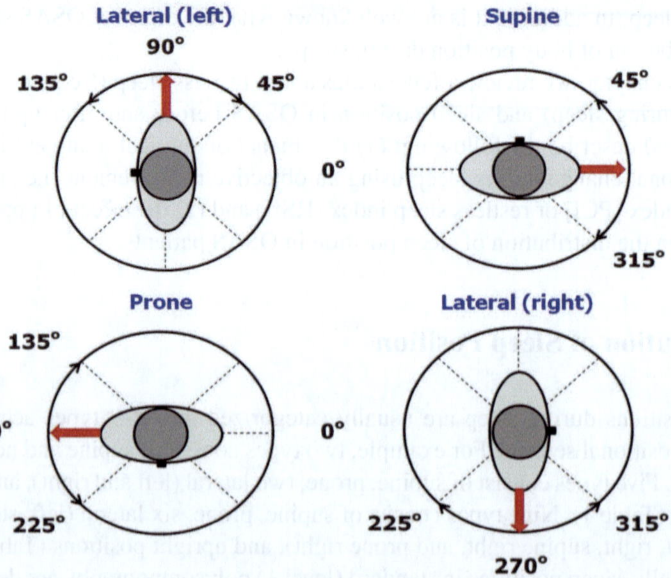

Fig. 1 Four sleep positions divided by 90° ranges

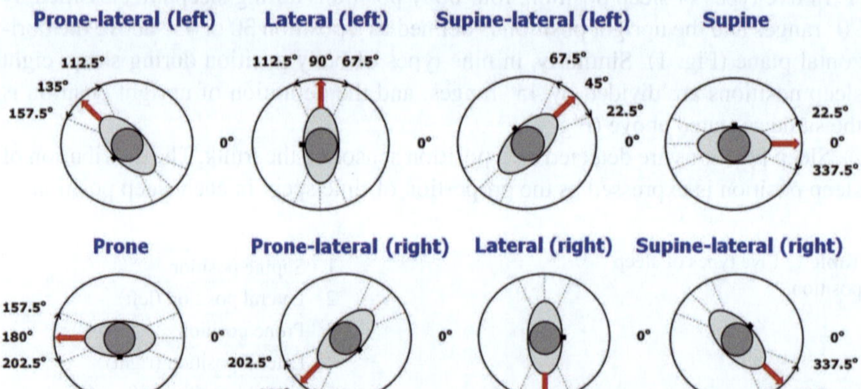

Fig. 2 Eight sleep positions divided by 45° ranges

Positional Change During Sleep (Restless Sleep)

Restless sleep or frequent positional change during sleep is a relatively common clinical manifestation in children and adults with OSAS [7]. In our previous data, snoring was the most severe complaint in both groups (Table 3) [7]. In pediatric OSAS, the second serious complaint was mouth breathing, followed by restless

Table 3 Severe complaints in children and adults with OSAS [7]

	Children with OSAS	Adults with OSAS
1	Snoring	Snoring
2	Mouth breathing	Witnessed apnea
3	Restless sleep	Restless sleep, mouth breathing
4	Nasal obstruction	–
5	Witnessed apnea	Daytime fatigue

OSAS obstructive sleep apnea syndrome

sleep, nasal obstruction, and witnessed apnea [7]. In adult OSAS, the second severe symptom and sign was witnessed apnea, followed by restless sleep, mouth breathing, and daytime fatigue [7].

Although restless sleep is well known as a common symptom and sign related with OSAS, the clear definition or objective assessment of restless sleep has not been established in OSAS. To the best of our knowledge, there has been no research that tried to evaluate the effect of upper airway surgery on restless sleep or positional change during sleep in patients with OSAS except our studies. Therefore, simple definitions of positional change during sleep and index related to positional change or restless sleep were suggested in our researches [18, 19].

Positional change during sleep is defined as change among various sleep positions and the PCI or RSI is defined as the total number of positional change during sleep per hour of TST [18, 19].

Effect of Surgical Treatment for OSAS on Positional Change During Sleep

Effect of Adenotonsillectomy on Positional Change During Sleep in Children with OSAS

In pediatric OSAS, adenotonsillectomy is the first-line treatment because adenotonsillar hypertrophy is the most common etiologic factor [7]. Accumulating studies suggest that adenotonsillectomy is associated with improvements of various symptoms and signs (e.g., snoring, obstructive apnea, behavior, neurocognition, etc.) and OSAS-related quality of life [20, 21]. However, there were few studies in which adenotonsillectomy is objectively related to the alleviation of restless sleep or frequent positional change during sleep in children with OSAS. Therefore, we investigated the effect of adenotonsillectomy on positional change during sleep as determined by an objective sleep test in pediatric patients with OSAS [18].

A total of 22 children (a mean age of 6.6 ± 2.7 years, 16 male and 6 female) with OSAS were included in our study. The frequency of positional change during sleep was estimated using body position sensor (1566-kit, Sleepmate® Technologies) in polysomnography.

Table 4 Study related with PCI during sleep in pediatric OSAS before and after adenotonsillectomy

Study	Group	Before	After	*p*-value
Choi et al. [18]	Total ($N=22$)	9.3±5.4	5.1±2.4	0.001

Data are presented as means ± SD
PCI positional change index, *OSAS* obstructive sleep apnea syndrome

There were significant changes in AHI (from 10.7±11.0 to 1.1±1.0; $p<0.001$) and arousal index (from 19.9±8.6 to 10.0±4.6; $p<0.001$) after adenotonsillectomy. The frequency of position change during sleep reduced in most children (81.8 %) with OSAS, and PCI significantly decreased from 9.3±5.4 to 5.1±2.4 ($p<0.001$) postoperatively (Table 4).

The exact mechanisms or causes of the positional change during sleep in pediatric OSAS are not yet known. Considering the results of this study that frequent positional change during sleep declined with the improvement of AHI and arousal index after adenotonsillectomy, it is thought that respiratory disturbances and/or arousals may be related to positional change during sleep in children with OSAS. It is also postulated that respiratory disturbance and/or arousal may partially contribute to the patient's discomfort, which, in turn, causes positional change to decrease the discomfort.

Effect of Upper Airway Surgery on Positional Change During Sleep in Adults with OSAS

There are several therapeutic options for OSAS (e.g., PAP, OA, upper airway surgery, behavioral therapy, etc.) [13–17]. Each treatment has its indications, advantages, and disadvantages [10]. Surgical treatment for OSAS can be considered in three conditions including primary (e.g., tonsillar hypertrophy, other severe obstructing upper airway structure), secondary (e.g., inadequate or intolerant of PAP or OA therapy), and adjuvant (e.g., to improve tolerance of other therapy) indications [10]. There are various surgical procedures for OSAS according to the site (e.g., nasal, nasopharyngeal, oropharyngeal, hypopharyngeal, laryngeal, and multilevel procedures) [10]. Numerous studies have shown that successful surgical management is related with alleviation of subjective symptoms and objective polysomnographic parameters [22–24]. However, it is not yet recognized what the effect of upper airway surgery on positional change is during sleep in adult OSAS. Therefore, we assessed whether upper airway surgery for OSAS influences positional change during sleep in adults with or without response [19].

A total of 53 adult patients with OSAS were enrolled in this study and were divided into response ($n=28$) and nonresponse ($n=25$) groups. The definition of surgical response was achieving a greater than 50 % reduction in AHI before and

Table 5 Study related with PCI during sleep in adult OSAS before and after upper airway surgery

Study	Group	Before	After	p-value
Choi et al. [19]	Response ($n=28$)	4.2±3.8	2.6±1.6	0.038
	Nonresponse ($n=25$)	3.4±2.0	3.4±2.1	NS

Data are presented as means ± SD
PCI positional change index, *OSAS* obstructive sleep apnea syndrome, *NS* not significant

after surgery. No significant differences were found in baseline data (e.g., age, sex, BMI, AHI, arousal index, PCI, and proportion of time spent in supine position) between the response and nonresponse groups.

In the response group, there were significant changes in AHI (from 45.7±23.9 to 8.6±9.7; $p<0.001$) and arousal index (from 45.6±21.5 to 23.1±10.9; $p<0.001$) after upper airway surgery. In addition, the PCI significantly reduced from 4.2±3.8 to 2.6±1.6 ($p=0.038$) (Table 5). However, in the nonresponse group, no significant postoperative changes were found in AHI, arousal index, and PCI.

In adult OSAS, little is also known about the exact mechanisms or etiologies of positional change during sleep. As mentioned above (section "Effect of Adenotonsillectomy on Positional Change During Sleep in Children with OSAS"), these results suggest that the respiratory disturbances and/or arousals are partially related with restless sleep or frequent positional change during sleep in adult OSAS. Also, it is presumed that respiratory disturbances and/or arousals may influence discomfort of the patient, which, in turn, causes positional change during sleep to alleviate the discomfort.

Effect of Surgical Treatment for OSAS on the Distribution of Sleep Position

Effect of Adenotonsillectomy on the Distribution of Sleep Position in Children with OSAS

In our 2009 study, we also evaluated the effect of adenotonsillectomy on the distribution of sleep positions as determined by positional sensor in pediatric OSAS [18]. After adenotonsillectomy, there were significant changes in the proportion of each sleep position (supine, lateral, and upright position) except prone position (Table 6). The proportion of sleep time spent in the supine position elevated significantly (from 42.0±12.2 to 56.6±21.7; $p=0.001$) and the proportion of sleep time spent in the lateral position reduced significantly after surgery (from 53.1±14.2 to 39.8±21.6; $p=0.003$). Postoperative elongation of the proportion of supine position and reduction of the proportion of lateral position indicated that supine position becomes a more comfortable for breathing after surgery in children with OSAS.

Table 6 Study related with the distribution of sleep position in pediatric OSAS before and after adenotonsillectomy

Study	Group	Position	Before (%)	After (%)	*p*-value
Choi et al. [18]	Total (N = 22)	Supine	42.0 ± 12.2	56.6 ± 21.7	0.001
		Lateral	53.1 ± 14.2	39.8 ± 21.6	0.003
		Prone	4.6 ± 10.4	3.5 ± 8.1	NS
		Upright	0.3 ± 1.0	0.0 ± 0.2	0.018

Data are presented as means ± SD
OSAS obstructive sleep apnea syndrome, *NS* not significant

Table 7 Studies related with the distribution of sleep position in adult OSAS before and after upper airway surgery

Study	Group	Position	Before (%)	After (%)	*p*-value
Katsantonis et al. [25]	Good/moderate responders (*n* = 8)	Supine	43.1 ± 41.0	41.0 ± 22.6	NS
		Lateral	56.9 ± 23.8	59.0 ± 22.7	NS
	Poor responders (*n* = 9)	Supine	31.3 ± 28.9	45.6 ± 38.8	NS
		Lateral	65.4 ± 28.0	51.6 ± 36.5	NS
	Total (*N* = 17)	Supine	36.8 ± 26.5	43.5 ± 31.3	NS
		Lateral	61.4 ± 25.7	55.1 ± 30.1	NS
Lee et al. [26]	Success (*n* = 20)	Supine	66.2 ± 22.6	68.1 ± 24.3	NS
	Response (*n* = 14)	Supine	72.7 ± 23.0	60.5 ± 20.0	NS
	Nonresponse (*n* = 9)	Supine	73.0 ± 24.8	68.1 ± 21.2	NS
	Failure (*n* = 26)	Supine	48.6 ± 25.6	60.8 ± 28.0	.028
Choi et al. [19]	Response (*n* = 28)	Supine	55.5 ± 23.9	60.1 ± 23.1	NS
		Non-supine	44.5 ± 23.9	39.9 ± 23.1	NS
	Nonresponse (*n* = 25)	Supine	62.4 ± 18.1	60.5 ± 21.3	NS
		Non-supine	37.6 ± 18.1	39.5 ± 21.3	NS

Data are presented as means ± SD
OSAS obstructive sleep apnea syndrome, *NS* not significant

Effect of Upper Airway Surgery on the Distribution of Sleep Position in Adults with OSAS

To our best knowledge, there are three studies about the effect of palatal upper airway surgery on the distribution of sleep position in adult OSAS (Table 7) [19, 25, 26].

Katsantonis et al. [25] investigated the effect of uvulopalatopharyngoplasty (UPPP) on sleep position and found that there were no significant changes in the proportion of time spent in the supine (from 36.8 ± 26.5 to 43.5 ± 31.3) and lateral (from 61.4 ± 25.7 to 55.1 ± 30.1) positions in 17 patients with OSAS before and after surgery. To know more details whether UPPP influences sleep posture in subjects with or without response, the patients were divided into two groups (good/moderate responders [*n* = 8] and poor responders [*n* = 9]) according to the alteration in the AHI and severity index. They also showed that the proportion of time spent in the supine (good/moderate responders [from 43.1 ± 41.0 to 41.0 ± 22.6], poor responders [from 31.3 ± 28.9 to 45.6 ± 38.8]) and lateral (good/moderate responders [from 56.9 ± 23.8 to 59.0 ± 22.7], poor responders [from 65.4 ± 28.0 to 51.6 ± 36.5]) positions did not significantly change in both groups after surgery.

Lee et al. [26] evaluated the change of supine sleep time in patients with OSAS before and after UPPP. At first, they categorized the patients into four groups (success [$n = 20$], response [$n = 14$], nonresponse [$n = 9$], and failure [$n = 26$]) according to the change of AHI after surgery. They assessed the difference in each group between pre- and postoperative supine sleep time and also compared the pre- and postoperative supine sleep time among the four groups. They found that in the failure group, preoperative supine sleep time was significantly low among the four groups ($p = 0.010$) and postoperative supine sleep time significantly elongated (from 48.6 ± 25.6 to 60.8 ± 28.0; $p = 0.028$). These results indicated that the variation of sleep posture, especially supine sleep time, in each polysomnography may be a confounding factor for postoperative outcomes.

In our 2011 study, the proportion of sleep time spent in the supine position was estimated in adults with OSAS before and after upper airway surgery [19]. We divided the patient into two groups (response [$n = 28$] and nonresponse [$n = 25$]) according to the change of AHI after surgery. In both groups, there were no significant changes in the proportion of sleep time spent in the supine position (response group [from 55.5 ± 23.9 to 60.1 ± 23.1], nonresponse group [from 62.4 ± 18.1 to 60.5 ± 21.3]) before and after surgery.

Summary

1. Restless sleep or frequent positional change during sleep is a relatively common clinical symptom in pediatric and adult OSAS.
2. Positional change during sleep is defined as change among various sleep positions and the PCI is defined as the total number of positional change during sleep per hour of TST.
3. In children with OSAS, frequent positional change during sleep significantly reduced with the alleviation of respiratory disturbances and arousals after adenotonsillectomy.
4. In adults with OSAS, frequent positional change during sleep significantly decreased with the improvement of respiratory disturbances and arousals after successful upper airway surgery.
5. In children with OSAS, the proportion of sleep time spent in the supine position significantly elongated after adenotonsillectomy.
6. There were no consistent outcomes related to the distribution of sleep position before and after OSAS surgery. Although it seems that no significant postoperative changes in supine sleep time were found in most adults with OSAS, postoperative changes in the proportion of sleep time spent in the supine position may occur in some patient group, especially in the failure group.
7. Further investigations are needed to identify the impact of surgery on positional change during sleep and distribution of sleep position.

References

1. American Academy of Sleep Medicine. The international classification of sleep disorders: diagnostic and coding manual. 2nd ed. Westchester, IL: American Academy of Sleep Medicine; 2005.
2. Brunetti L, Rana S, Lospalluti ML, Pietrafesa A, Francavilla R, Fanelli M, et al. Prevalence of obstructive sleep apnea syndrome in a cohort of 1,207 children of southern Italy. Chest. 2001;120(6):1930–5.
3. Ali NJ, Pitson DJ, Stradling JR. Snoring, sleep disturbance, and behavior in 4-5 year olds. Arch Dis Child. 1993;68(3):360–6.
4. Young T, Palta M, Dempsey J, Skatrud J, Weber S, Badr S. The occurrence of sleep-disordered breathing among middle-aged adults. N Engl J Med. 1993;328(17):1230–5.
5. Kim J, In K, Kim J, You S, Kang K, Shim J, et al. Prevalence of sleep-disordered breathing in middle-aged Korean men and women. Am J Respir Crit Care Med. 2004;170(10):1108–13.
6. Guilleminault C. Obstructive sleep apnea syndrome. A review. Psychiatr Clin North Am. 1987;10(4):607–21.
7. Choi JH, Kim EJ, Choi J, Kwon SY, Kim TH, Lee SH, et al. Obstructive sleep apnea syndrome: a child is not just a small adult. Ann Otol Rhinol Laryngol. 2010;119(10):656–61.
8. Newman AB, Nieto FJ, Guidry U, Lind BK, Redline S, Pickering TG, et al. Relation of sleep-disordered breathing to cardiovascular disease risk factors: the Sleep Heart Health Study. Am J Epidemiol. 2001;154(1):50–9.
9. Sleep apnea, sleepiness, and driving risk. American Thoracic Society. Am J Respir Crit Care Med. 1994;150(5 Pt 1):1463–73.
10. Epstein LJ, Kristo D, Strollo Jr PJ, Friedman N, Malhotra A, Patil SP, et al. Clinical guideline for the evaluation, management and long-term care of obstructive sleep apnea in adults. J Clin Sleep Med. 2009;5(3):263–76.
11. Kezirian EJ, Hohenhorst W, de Vries N. Drug-induced sleep endoscopy: the VOTE classification. Eur Arch Otorhinolaryngol. 2011;268(8):1233–6.
12. Sleep-related breathing disorders in adults: recommendations for syndrome definition and measurement techniques in clinical research. The Report of an American Academy of Sleep Medicine Task Force. Sleep. 1999;22(5):667–89.
13. Morgenthaler TI, Kapen S, Lee-Chiong T, Alessi C, Boehlecke B, Brown T, et al. Practice parameters for the medical therapy of obstructive sleep apnea. Sleep. 2006;29(8):1031–5.
14. Choi JH, Park YH, Hong JH, Kim SJ, Park DS, Miyazaki S, et al. Efficacy study of a vest-type device for positional therapy in position dependent snorers. Sleep Biol Rhythms. 2009;7: 181–7.
15. Kushida CA, Littner MR, Hirshkowitz M, Morgenthaler TI, Alessi CA, Bailey D, et al. Practice parameters for the use of continuous and bilevel positive airway pressure devices to treat adult patients with sleep-related breathing disorders. Sleep. 2006;29(3):375–80.
16. Kushida CA, Morgenthaler TI, Littner MR, Alessi CA, Bailey D, Coleman Jr J, et al. Practice parameters for the treatment of snoring and obstructive sleep apnea with oral appliances: an update for 2005. Sleep. 2006;29(2):240–3.
17. Powell NB. Contemporary surgery for obstructive sleep apnea syndrome. Clin Exp Otorhinolaryngol. 2009;2(3):107–14.
18. Choi JH, Kim EJ, Choi J, Kim TH, Kwon SY, Lee SH, et al. The effect of adenotonsillectomy on changes of position during sleep in pediatric obstructive sleep apnea syndrome. Am J Rhinol Allergy. 2009;23(6):e56–8.
19. Choi JH, Kim EJ, Choi J, Kwon SY, Lee HM, Kim TH, et al. Effect of successful surgical treatment on changes of position during sleep in adults with obstructive sleep apnea syndrome. Ann Otol Rhinol Laryngol. 2011;120(2):104–9.
20. Brietzke SE, Gallagher D. The effectiveness of tonsillectomy and adenoidectomy in the treatment of pediatric obstructive sleep apnea/hypopnea syndrome: a meta-analysis. Otolaryngol Head Neck Surg. 2006;134(6):979–84.

21. Mitchell RB, Kelly J. Behavior, neurocognition and quality-of-life in children with sleep-disordered breathing. Int J Pediatr Otorhinolaryngol. 2006;70(3):395–406.
22. Riley RW, Powell NB, Li KK, Troell RJ, Guilleminault C. Surgery and obstructive sleep apnea: long-term clinical outcomes. Otolaryngol Head Neck Surg. 2000;122(3):415–21.
23. Choi JH, Kim EJ, Cho WS, Kim YS, Choi J, Kwon SY, et al. Efficacy of single-staged modified uvulopalatopharyngoplasty with nasal surgery in adults with obstructive sleep apnea syndrome. Otolaryngol Head Neck Surg. 2011;144(6):994–9.
24. Choi JH, Yi JS, Lee SH, Kim CS, Kim TH, Lee HM, et al. Effect of upper airway surgery on heart rate variability in patients with obstructive sleep apnoea syndrome. J Sleep Res. 2012;21(3):316–21.
25. Katsantonis GP, Miyazaki S, Walsh JK. Effects of uvulopalatopharyngoplasty on sleep architecture and patterns of obstructed breathing. Laryngoscope. 1990;100(10 Pt 1):1068–72.
26. Lee CH, Shin HW, Han DH, Mo JH, Yoon IY, Chung S, et al. The implication of sleep position in the evaluation of surgical outcomes in obstructive sleep apnea. Otolaryngol Head Neck Surg. 2009;140(4):531–5.

Comparison of Positional Therapy to CPAP in Patients with Positional Obstructive Sleep Apnea

Samuel Krachman, Irene Swift, and Maria Elena Vega

Introduction

Obstructive sleep apnea (OSA) is prevalent in the general population, affecting 9 % of females and 24 % of males ages 30–60 years old [1]. When associated with daytime sleepiness, OSA syndrome is reported to be present in 2 % of females and 4 % of males in the same age range [1]. While treatment has always focused on trying to improve patient's symptoms, including daytime sleepiness and cognitive dysfunction, the recognition that OSA is an independent risk factor for a number of cardiovascular disorders has enhanced efforts to appropriately treat the disorder [2–5]. Treatment of OSA needs to be individualized, as there have been major problems with adherence and compliance with all forms of therapy that are presently used [6–10].

An important factor that affects airway patency is the posture of the patient (supine vs. lateral) [11–13] and may explain the entity known as positional OSA, where all or the majority of sleep-disordered breathing events occur while sleeping in the supine position. Positional OSA has been reported to be present in up to 50–60 % of all patients with diagnosed OSA [14–17]. As a result, positional therapy, directed at keeping the patient from sleeping in the supine position, is recognized as an important treatment option in selected patients with OSA [18]. In this chapter, we will discuss the definitions and pathophysiology behind positional OSA and focus on those studies that have compared positional therapy to continuous positive airway pressure (CPAP) therapy, which is considered by many as the primary treatment for OSA.

S. Krachman, D.O. (✉) • I. Swift, M.D. • M.E. Vega, M.D.
Division of Pulmonary, Critical Care and Sleep Medicine, Temple University School of Medicine, 3401 North Broad St, Philadelphia, PA 19140, USA
e-mail: samuel.krachman@tuhs.temple.edu

N. de Vries et al. (eds.), *Positional Therapy in Obstructive Sleep Apnea*,
DOI 10.1007/978-3-319-09626-1_31

Definition of Positional OSA

While positional OSA is reported as being prevalent, many studies defined positional OSA as simply a 50 % reduction in the AHI when sleeping in the non-supine position [14–17]. As a result, many patients still had an elevated AHI while non-supine, often in the range of mild-to-moderate OSA. More recently, Mador et al. [19] used a definition of normalizing the AHI to <5 in addition to a 50 % reduction and reported an overall prevalence of 27 % of all patients having positional OSA. Based on severity, this included 50 % of patients with mild OSA and 19 % of those with moderate OSA having positional OSA. Only 7 % of patients with severe OSA met their criteria for positional OSA. However, as it is defined, many patients with OSA have a positional component that would allow effective positional therapy to be considered as a primary or secondary therapy.

Pathophysiology for Positional OSA

Upper airway patency is normally maintained through a balance between anatomical and physiological forces that tend to collapse the airway and dilating forces that must be present in order to prevent collapse [11]. Major dilating forces include pharyngeal dilator muscle activation (including the genioglossus) and lung inflation-induced caudal traction on the upper airway that stiffens it and reduces collapsibility [11]. The two primary forces that tend toward upper airway collapse are the negative intraluminal pressure generated by the diaphragm during inspiration and the extraluminal pressure from tissues and bony structures surrounding the airway [11].

An important factor that has an effect on airway anatomy and size is the posture of the individual (supine vs. lateral), primarily due to the effects of gravity on airway tissues. When supine, the tongue and palatal structures move posteriorly due to gravity, and if this increase in tissue pressure is not offset by other dilating forces, upper airway collapse will occur [12, 13].

A more specific measurement of the inherent structural collapsibility of the upper airway can be obtained by measuring the critical collapsing pressure (Pcrit), the nasal pressure at which the hypotonic or "passive" pharynx collapses and inspiratory flow is abolished [20]. In normal subjects, the Pcrit is lower (-6.5 ± 2.7 cm H_2O) as compared to snorers (-1.6 ± 1.4 cm H_2O) and those patients with severe OSA (2.5 ± 1.5 cm H_2O) [21]. Of significance is the effect of body posture on Pcrit in patients with OSA. In the lateral position, Pcrit has been found to be dramatically lower, by 2.0–2.9 cm H_2O, than noted while patients are supine, denoting a stiffer less collapsible airway in the lateral position [22–24]. Values while in the lateral position were at or significantly less than 0 cm H_2O (range from 0.3 to 2.9 cm H_2O) consistent with values seen in normal individuals or snorers [21]. These physiological changes noted in the upper airway based on positioning help explain the entity of positional OSA as well as why some patients can be effectively treated with just positional therapy.

CPAP Compliance Issues

CPAP therapy has been demonstrated to be very effective at correcting sleep-disordered breathing [25] and improving cognitive function and daytime sleepiness [26, 27]. However, compliance with CPAP therapy has been poor [6, 28, 29]. In the seminal paper by Kribbs et al. [6], only 46 % of the patients prescribed with CPAP met the criteria that they defined as regular use, which was >4 h/night for 70 % of the nights monitored. More recently, similar findings of poor compliance have been noted in studies that have compared in-lab vs. at-home sleep testing [30, 31]. Rosen et al. [30] noted no difference in compliance between in-lab (39 %) and at-home testing (50 %) when evaluated at 3 months using a similar definition of compliance of >4 h/night for 70 % of the nights evaluated. Kuna et al. [31] reported that only 49 % and 52 % of in-lab- and at-home-tested VA patients, respectively, used CPAP for >4 h/night at the end of 3 months. The reasons for the poor compliance that is seen with CPAP therapy are numerable and include the mask being uncomfortable and burdensome, intolerance to the pressure, side effects such as nasal congestion, and complaints of claustrophobia [32]. In addition, socioeconomic factors also appear to play a role [33, 34]. However, how important each of these factors are in determining CPAP compliance still remains unclear [7, 8]. What is clear is that when patients are not compliant with CPAP therapy, their OSA will go untreated if other forms of therapy are not sorted out by the patient or physician. As a result, patients are symptomatic and continue to have the cardiovascular risks associated with untreated OSA [2–5]. Therefore, it is important to consider effective alternative treatments in these patients, which may include positional therapy if they have positional OSA.

Types of Positional Devices

There have been a number of positional therapy devices that have been used over the years to try and maintain patients with positional OSA in the non-supine position during sleep. Probably, the oldest and most familiar of these devices is the simple tennis ball technique, where patients have a tennis ball sewn into the back of a T-shirt that they would wear at night [35]. Variants of the tennis ball technique have been used in a number of studies [9, 10] including those that have compared this technique to CPAP therapy in patients with positional OSA [36, 37]. Jokic et al. [36] compared CPAP to positional therapy using a backpack with a soft ball placed inside of it. The size of the ball in the backpack was 10×5.5 in., and it was made of semirigid synthetic foam. In another adaptation of the tennis ball technique, Skinner et al. [37] created the thoracic anti-supine band (TASB) (Fig. 1). The device consists of two cotton stockinette-covered pieces of foam rubber with Velcro attachments on each end. A polystyrene ball (8 or 10 cm in circumference) is inserted inside at the level of the sixth thoracic vertebra. The two short ends are draped over the shoulders and fastened with Velcro over the two long ends. In the only other study that has compared positional therapy to CPAP therapy in patients with positional OSA,

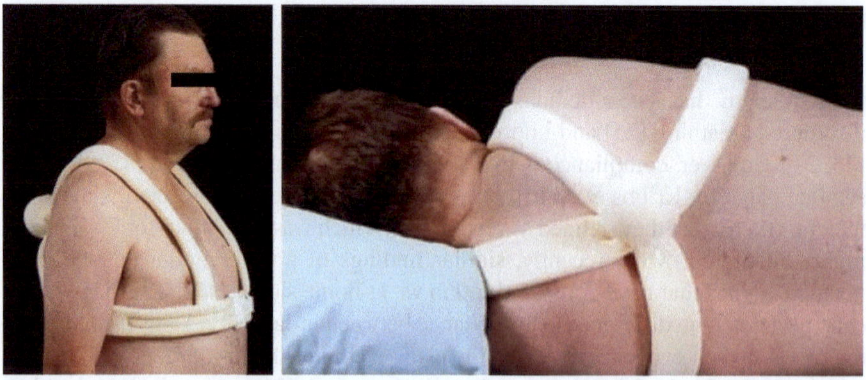

Fig. 1 Thoracic anti-supine band (TASB) (from [37], with permission)

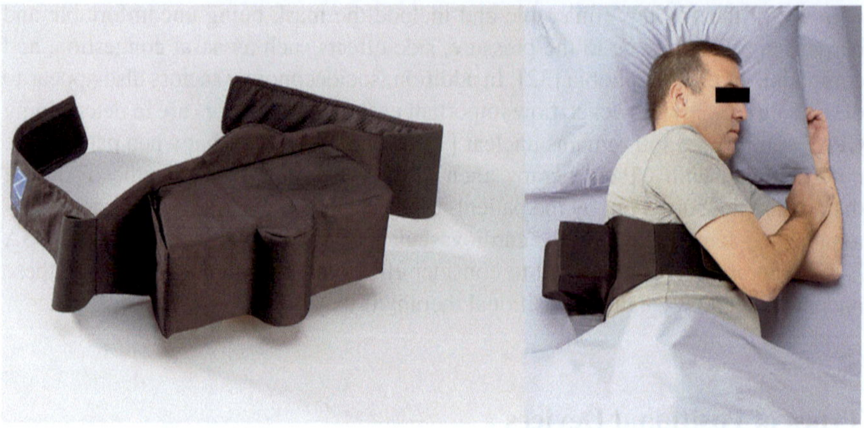

Fig. 2 Zzoma Positional Device (from [38], with permission)

Permut et al. [38] utilized the Zzoma Positional Device, which is 12×5.5×4 in. in size and made of lightweight semirigid synthetic foam (Fig. 2). It is contained in a backpack-type material with an associated Velcro elastic belt. The Zzoma Positional Device is worn on the back, with the elastic belts brought around each side of the patient and secured anteriorly (Fig. 2). The device, with its particular size and wedge-shaped design on both sides, keeps the patient positioned on their side and prevents him/her from assuming the supine position.

Comparison of Positional Therapy to CPAP Therapy

As of this point in time, there have only been three prospective studies that have compared positional therapy to CPAP therapy in patients with positional OSA (Table 1) [36–38]. Jokic et al. [36] in a randomized crossover study of 13 patients

Table 1 Comparison of positional therapy to CPAP therapy

Study	*N*	Length of study	Baseline AHI (events/h)	Effects on AHI	Effects on nocturnal oxygenation	Effects on sleep quality
Jokic et al. [36]	13	2 weeks	18 ± 5	CPAP and PD decreased AHI—but lower with CPAP	Lowest SaO_2 lower with PD	No difference in SE and TST
Skinner et al. [37]	22	1 month	23 ± 12	72 % with PD and 89 % with CPAP had an AHI < 10 events/h	Both PD and CPAP increased the mean SaO_2	No difference in SE and TST
Permut et al. [38]	38	1 night	13 ± 5	92 % with PD and 97 % with CPAP normalized AHI to <5 events/h	No change in mean SaO_2 with PD and increase with CPAP	No difference in SE but TST lower with CPAP

AHI apnea–hypopnea index, *PD* positional device, *SE* sleep efficiency, *TST* total sleep time

with mild-to-moderate OSA (AHI 17 ± 8 events/h) compared positional therapy using their soft ball in a backpack device to CPAP therapy after 2 weeks of using each treatment modality. Positional OSA was defined as an AHI during supine sleep that was two or more times the AHI during sleep in the lateral position. In addition, the AHI in the lateral position had to be <15 event/h, during a minimum duration of 1 h of sleep in the lateral position and the inclusion of at least 1 rapid eye movement (REM) period. In a cross-over designed study, Skinner et al. [37] compared their TASB to CPAP therapy in 22 patients with mild to moderately severe positional OSA (AHI 22.7 ± 12 events/h) after utilizing each treatment modality for 1 month. Positional OSA was defined as an AHI in the supine position that was greater or equal to twice the AHI in other positions. Permut et al. [38] compared the Zzoma Positional Device to CPAP therapy in a crossover designed study after 1 night of use in 38 patients with mild-to-moderate positional OSA (AHI of 13 ± 5 events/h). Positional OSA was defined on the baseline study as an overall apnea–hypopnea index (AHI) of ≥5 events/h with symptoms of excessive daytime sleepiness or an AHI of ≥15 events/h, with a 50 % decrease in the AHI in the non-supine position as compared to the supine position. Additionally, the AHI had to fall to <5 events/h in the non-supine position, and the patient must have slept in the lateral position for a minimum of 1 h during the baseline study.

Sleep-Disordered Breathing

Many would consider the AHI as the most important parameter to be evaluated in regard to assessing the effectiveness of treatment in patient with OSA. That is also the case in regard to studies that have assessed patients with known positional OSA, including those that have compared positional therapy to CPAP therapy. Jokic et al. [36] noted that although 2 weeks of treatment with both their positional device and

CPAP decreased the AHI (from 18 to 10 and 3 events/h, respectively), the decrease with CPAP was statistically more significant and was associated with a normalization of the AHI (<5 events/h). Only 3 of the 13 patients (23 %) slept supine during their study night. Compliance as it relates to use of the positional device and CPAP was not assessed during the study. Skinner et al. [37] noted that both the TASB and CPAP decreased the AHI, from 23 to 12 and 5 events/h, respectively, with a significant difference noted between the two forms of therapy. Using a definition of successful treatment as an AHI of <10 events/h, treatment success was noted in 13/18 subjects using the TASB and 16/18 subjects using CPAP therapy. Supine sleep was significantly decreased but not completely eliminated with the TASB, with 6 % of the total sleep time spent in the supine position. Adherence with the TASB was based on a self-recorded diary, with a significantly higher adherence rate reported for TASB as compared to CPAP therapy. Permut et al. [38] noted that when compared to baseline, both the Zzoma Positional Device and CPAP therapy (mean 10 ± 3 cm H_2O) significantly decreased the AHI, from 11 (9–15, 6–26) events/h to 2 (1–4, 0–8) and 0 (0–2, 0–7) events/h, respectively ($p < 0.001$), with a difference between the two treatments ($p < 0.001$). In addition, the Zzoma Positional Device was equivalent to CPAP (92 % vs. 97 %, respectively [$p = 0.16$]) at normalizing the AHI. The Zzoma Positional Device eliminated supine sleep in 37 of the 38 patients, with only a mean of 1 ± 4 % of total sleep time spent supine. However, the study was only an acute single night intervention, and more long-term results are being examined.

Nocturnal Oxygenation

Jokic et al. [36] noted no difference in mean SaO_2 between their positional device and CPAP therapy. However, the lowest SaO_2 during the night was lower with positional therapy as compared to CPAP. Skinner et al. [37] noted a clinically insignificant difference in mean SaO_2 during the night between CPAP and the TASB. In comparison, Permut et al. [38] noted the mean SaO_2 during the night was unchanged compared to baseline with the use of the Zzoma Positional Device, but was increased with CPAP therapy. In addition, there was an increase in the lowest SaO_2 during the night with both the Zzoma Positional Device and CPAP therapy, with no difference between the two treatment modalities. The percent of total sleep time with a $SaO_2 < 90$ % was significantly decreased compared to baseline with the Zzoma Positional Device and CPAP therapy.

Sleep Quality

Jokic et al. [36] demonstrated no difference in sleep quality between their positional device and CPAP therapy, as measured by total sleep time and sleep efficiency. In addition, the arousal index and sleep architecture were not different between the two treatment modalities. Similar results were noted by Skinner et al. [37] when comparing the TASB to CPAP therapy, with no change in the total sleep time with either form of therapy as compared to baseline. In comparison, Permut el al. [38] noted that when compared to baseline, total sleep time did not change with the Zzoma Positional Device, but decreased with CPAP therapy. There was no change in sleep efficiency noted with either treatment, nor was there any change in the spontaneous arousal index. The sleep architecture, expressed as a percentage of total sleep time, including stage N3 and REM sleep, was not different as compared to baseline for either the Zzoma Positional Device or CPAP therapy.

Other Parameters

In regard to daytime sleepiness, Jokic et al. [36] noted a decrease in the Epworth Sleepiness Scale (ESS) after 2 weeks of therapy with both their positional device and CPAP therapy, but with no difference between the treatment modalities. In addition, similar sleep onset latencies were seen with both treatments as measured on maintenance of wakefulness (MWT) tests. Skinner et al. [37] noted a nonsignificant decrease in ESS with both their TASB and CPAP therapy at the end of 1 month.

Cognitive performance and quality of life changes have also been compared between positional therapy and CPAP therapy. Jokic et al. [36] found no difference in regard to these parameters between the two forms of therapy, and patient preference favored CPAP therapy in this study. Skinner et al. [37] noted no significant difference in any of the quality of life measures that they assessed when the results of their TASB and CPAP therapy were compared. Permut et al. [38] noted that 50 % of their patients preferred the Zzoma Positional Device, 34 % preferred CPAP therapy, and 16 % had no preference.

Future Research

While CPAP compliance has been objectively evaluated in a number of studies [6, 30, 31], there are few studies that have evaluated positional therapy adherence and compliance, with most involving self-reported use or mailed questionnaires [9, 10, 37]. While some of these studies have suggested poor long-term use of positional therapy [9, 10], a more recent prospective study has reported a 3-month compliance rate of 74 % using actigraphy [39]. While this study suggests possible compliance rates that are better than those reported for CPAP therapy, it was uncontrolled. Similar types of studies need to be performed when positional therapy is directly compared to CPAP therapy using methods that allow objective assessment of use.

In addition to compliance, measurement of continued effectiveness should be better evaluated with the use of positional therapy. While some studies have repeated polysomnograms after 1–3 months of using a positional device to demonstrate the device retains its ability to decrease or eliminate supine sleep, studies evaluating continuous nightly effectiveness have not been performed.

Finally, while CPAP therapy has been shown to decrease parameters associated with cardiovascular risk in patients with OSA, the effects of positional therapy on cardiovascular risk are presently unknown [40–44]. CPAP has been demonstrated to decrease endothelial dysfunction as measured by flow-mediated dilation and carotid intima–media thickness measurements [40–42]. In addition, CPAP therapy has been shown to decrease systemic inflammation as measured using biomarkers such as C-reactive protein [43, 44]. At the present time, it is not known whether positional therapy has a similar effect at decreasing cardiovascular risk.

Summary

A large percentage of patients with diagnosed OSA have positional OSA. While CPAP therapy is the most common form of therapy, compliance is poor, and other forms of therapy may be appropriate in these patients, including the use of effective positional therapy. Initial studies that directly compared positional therapy to CPAP therapy suggest that positional therapy can be considered as a primary therapy in patients with positional OSA. However, more long-term studies that use objective measurements of compliance and effectiveness should be performed. Whether positional therapy has the same beneficial effects on cardiovascular risk as seen with CPAP therapy awaits further study.

References

1. Young T, Palta M, Dempsey J, Skatrud J, Weber S, Badr S. The occurrence of sleep-disordered breathing among middle-aged adults. N Engl J Med. 1993;328:1230–5.
2. Nieto FJ, Young TB, Lind BK, et al. Association of sleep-disordered breathing, sleep apnea, and hypertension in a large community-based study: Sleep Heart Health Study. JAMA. 2000;283:1829–36.
3. Peppard PE, Young T, Palta M, Skatrud J. Prospective study of the association between sleep-disordered breathing and hypertension. N Engl J Med. 2000;342:1378–84.
4. Yaggi HK, Concato J, Kernan WN, Lichtman JH, Brass LM, Mohsenin V. Obstructive sleep apnea as a risk factor for stroke and death. N Engl J Med. 2005;353:2034–41.
5. Shahar E, Whitney CW, Redline S, Lee ET, Newman AB, Javier Nieto F, O'Connor GT, Boland LL, Schwartz JE, Samet JM. Sleep-disordered breathing and cardiovascular disease: cross-sectional results of the Sleep Heart Health Study. Am J Respir Crit Care Med. 2001;163:19–25.
6. Kribbs NB, Pack AI, Kline LR, Smith PL, Schwartz AR, Schubert NM, Redline S, Henry JN, Getsy JE, Dinges DF. Objective measurement of patterns of nasal CPAP use by patients with obstructive sleep apnea. Am Rev Respir Dis. 1993;147:887–95.
7. Weaver TE, Grunstein RR. Adherence to continuous positive airway pressure therapy. The challenge to effective treatment. Proc Am Thorac Soc. 2008;5:173–8.

8. Sawyer AM, Gooneratne NS, Marcus CL, Ofer D, Richards KC, Weaver TE. A systematic review of CPAP adherence across age groups: clinical and empiric insights for developing CPAP adherence interventions. Sleep Med Rev. 2011;15:343–56.
9. Oksenberg A, Silverberg D, Offenbach D, Arons E. Positional therapy for obstructive sleep apnea patients: a 6-month follow-up study. Laryngoscope. 2006;116:1995–2000.
10. Bignold JJ, Deans-Costi G, Goldworthy MR, Robertson CA, McEvoy D, Catcheside PG, Mercer JD. Poor long-term compliance with the tennis ball technique for treating positional obstructive sleep apnea. J Clin Sleep Med. 2009;5(5):428–30.
11. White D. Pathogenesis of obstructive and central sleep apnea. Am J Respir Crit Care Med. 2005;172:1363–70.
12. Olson L, Fouke J, Hokje P, Strohl K. A biomechanical view of the upper airway. In: Mathew OP, Saint'Ambroggio G, editors. The respiratory function of the upper airway. New York: Marcel Dekker; 1988. p. 359–90.
13. Fouke J, Strohl K. Effect of position and lung volume on upper airway geometry. J Appl Physiol. 1987;63:375–80.
14. Cartwright RD. Effect of sleep position on sleep apnea severity. Sleep. 1984;7:110–4.
15. Cartwright R, Ristanovic R, Diaz F, Caldarelli D, Alder G. A comparative study of treatments for positional sleep apnea. Sleep. 1991;14:546–52.
16. Oksenberg A, Silverberg DS, Arons E, Radwan H. Positional vs. nonpositional obstructive sleep apnea patients: anthropomorphic, nocturnal polysomnographic, and multiple sleep latency test data. Chest. 1997;112:629–39.
17. Akita Y, Kawakatsu K, Hattori C, Hattori H, Suzuki K, Nishimura T. Posture of patients with sleep apnea during sleep. Acta Otolaryngol. 2003;550(Suppl):41–5.
18. Epstein LJ, Kristo D, Strollo PJ, Friedman NF, Malhotra A, Patil AP, et al. Clinical guideline for the evaluation, management and long-term care of obstructive sleep apnea in adults. J Clin Sleep Med. 2009;5:263–76.
19. Mador MJ, Kufel TJ, Magalang UJ, et al. Prevalence of positional sleep apnea in patients undergoing polysomnography. Chest. 2005;128:2130–7.
20. Schwartz AR, O'Donnell CP, Baron J, et al. The hypotonic upper airway in obstructive sleep apnea: role of structures and neuromuscular activity. Am J Respir Crit Care Med. 1998;157:1051–7.
21. Gleadhill IC, Schwartz AR, Schubert N, Wise RA, Permutt S, Smith PL. Upper airway collapsibility in snorers and in patients with obstructive hypopnea and apnea. Am Rev Respir Dis. 1991;143:1300–3.
22. Boudewyns A, Punjabi N, Van de Heyning PH, De Backer WA, O'Donnell CP, Schneider H, Smith PL, Schwartz AR. Abbreviated method for assessing upper airway function in obstructive sleep apnea. Chest. 2000;118:1031–41.
23. Penzel T, Moller M, Becker HF, Knaack L, Peter JH. Effect of sleep position and sleep stage on the collapsibility of the upper airways in patients with sleep apnea. Sleep. 2001; 24:90–5.
24. Ong JSL, Touyz G, Tanner S, Hillman DR, Eastwood PR, Walsh JH. Variability of human upper airway collapsibility during sleep and the influence of body posture and sleep stage. J Sleep Res. 2011;20:533–7.
25. Gay P, Weaver T, Loube D, Iber C. Evaluation of positive airway pressure treatment for sleep related breathing disorders in adults. Sleep. 2006;29:381–401.
26. Stradling JR, Davies RJ. Is more NCPAP better? Sleep. 2000;23 Suppl 4:S150–3.
27. Antic NA, Catcheside P, Buchan C, Hensley M, Naughton MT, Rowland S, et al. The effect of CPAP in normalizing daytime sleepiness, quality of life and neurocognitive function in moderate-severe OSA. Sleep. 2011;34:111–9.
28. Engleman HM, Martin SE, Douglas NJ. Compliance with CPAP therapy in patients with sleep apnoea/hypopnoea syndrome. Thorax. 1994;49:263–6.
29. Reeves-Hoche MK, Meck R, Zwillich CW. Nasal CPAP. An objective evaluation of patient compliance. Am J Respir Crit Care Med. 1994;149:149–54.

30. Rosen CL, Auckley D, Benca R, Foldvary-Schaefer N, Iber C, Kapur V, Rueschman M, Zee P, Redline S. A multisite randomized trial of portable sleep studies and positive airway pressure autotitration versus laboratory-based polysomnography for the diagnosis and treatment of obstructive sleep apnea: the HomePAP study. Sleep. 2012;35(6):757–67.
31. Kuna ST, Gurubhagavatula I, Malslin G, Hin S, Hartwig K, McCloskey S, Hachadoorian R, Hurley S, Gupta R, Staley B, Atwood CW. Noninferiority of functional outcome in ambulatory management of obstructive sleep apnea. Am J Respir Crit Care Med. 2011;183:1238–44.
32. Pepin JL, Leger P, Veale D, Langevin B, Robert R, Levy P. Side effects of nasal continuous positive airway pressure in sleep apnea syndrome: study of 193 patients in two French sleep centers. Chest. 1995;107:375–81.
33. Platt AB, Field SH, Asch DA, Chen Z, Patel N, Gupta R, et al. Neighborhood of residence is associated with daily adherence to CPAP therapy. Sleep. 2009;32(6):799–806.
34. Simon-Tuval T, Reuveni H, Greenberg-Dolan S, Oksenberg A, Tal A, Tarsiuk A. Low socio-economic status is a risk factor CPAP acceptance among adult OSAS patients requiring treatment. Sleep. 2009;32(4):545–52.
35. Kavey NB, Blitzer A, Gidro-Frank S, Korstanje K. Sleeping position and sleep apnea syndrome. Am J Otolaryngol. 1985;6(5):373–7.
36. Jokic R, Klimaszewski A, Crossley M, Sridhar G, Fitzpatrick MF. Positional treatment vs continuous positive airway pressure in patients with positional obstructive sleep apnea. Chest. 1999;115:771–81.
37. Skinner MA, Kingshott RN, Filsell S, Taylor DR. Efficacy of the 'tennis ball technique' versus NCPAP in the management of position-dependent obstructive sleep apnoea syndrome. Respirology. 2008;13:708–15.
38. Permut I, Diaz-Abad M, Chatila W, Crocetti J, Gaughan J, D'Alonzo GE, Krachman SL. Comparison of positional therapy to CPAP in patients with positional obstructive sleep apnea. J Clin Sleep Med. 2010;6(3):238–43.
39. Heinzer RC, Pellaton C, Rey V, Rossetti AO, Lecciso G, Haba-Rubio J, Tafti M, Lavigne G. Positional therapy for obstructive sleep apnea: an objective measurement of patients' usage and efficacy at home. Sleep Med. 2012;13(4):425–8.
40. Lattimore JL, Wilcox I, Skilton M, Langenfeld M, Celermajer DS. Treatment of obstructive sleep apnoea leads to improved microvascular endothelial function in the systemic circulation. Thorax. 2006;61(6):491–5.
41. Ip MS, Tse HF, Lam B, Tsang KW, Lam WK. Endothelial function in obstructive sleep apnea and response to treatment. Am J Respir Crit Care Med. 2004;169(3):348–53.
42. Imadojemu VA, Gleeson K, Quraishi SA, Kunselman AR, Sinoway LI, Leuenberger UA. Impaired vasodilator responses in obstructive sleep apnea are improved with continuous positive airway pressure therapy. Am J Respir Crit Care Med. 2002;65(7):950–3.
43. Shamsuzzaman ASM, Winnicki M, Lanfranchi P, Wolk R, Kara T, Accurso V, Somers VK. Elevated C-reactive protein in patients with obstructive sleep apnea. Circulation. 2002;105:2462–4.
44. Guo Y, Pan L, Ren D, Xie X. Impact of continuous positive airway pressure on C-reactive protein in patients with obstructive sleep apnea: a meta-analysis. Sleep Breath. 2013;17(2):495–503.

Part VII
Future Developments

Position Training: An Indispensable Therapy

Piet-Heijn J.M. van Mechelen

Introduction

The main problem with OSAS is underdiagnosis. The consequence is that the initially relatively harmless breathing pauses in the night gradually wreak havoc in a person's daily life and sometimes cause physically irreparable damage. This is regrettable because OSAS patients, when diagnosed in a timely manner and treated adequately, can function completely normally in their work, relationships, and family.

International estimates suggest that only around 10–20 % of those suffering from OSAS have been diagnosed so far. Looking at figures and characteristics, one gets the impression that until now mainly those who are being diagnosed are the "usual suspects," the phenotype of the OSAS patient: an overweight man over 50 years of age. With the rising awareness about sleep apnea and an active detection program, we will find a different population, one that is younger, includes more females, is less overweight, and consists largely of those with position-dependent OSAS. Therefore, position training might well become an indispensable therapy.

How Common Is It?

The prevalence study by Young et al. [1] is the most frequently quoted internationally. This study finds that the prevalence of OSAS is 4 % in men aged 30–60 years and 2 % in women of the same age. Applied to the current Dutch population, this

P.-H.J.M. van Mechelen, M.Sc. (✉)
ApneuVereniging (Dutch Apnea Association),
Zandvoorter Allee 5, 2106 BT Heemstede, The Netherlands
e-mail: phvanmechelen@gmail.com

N. de Vries et al. (eds.), *Positional Therapy in Obstructive Sleep Apnea*,
DOI 10.1007/978-3-319-09626-1_32

would mean that there should have been at least 315,000 OSAS patients in 2011. According to the database of the national health insurance system in the Netherlands [2], there are over 74,000 patients being treated with CPAP. Including MAD and ENT surgery, there were a total of 80,000 people treated for OSAS in 2011.This means that approximately 235,000 people are yet untreated. This is a conservative estimate. A lot of research shows that twice that number is defensible. The higher estimates for sleep apnea are based on the growing number of patients in risk groups, such as patients with nocturnal chest pain, hypertension, and diabetes (type 2) and who are overweight. In a recent study in the Netherlands [3] of a normal "healthy" population of working people (Philips employees), a prevalence of 6.4 % was found. This would amount to over 500,000 OSAS patients, of which more than 400,000 are not being diagnosed. This coincides quite well with the finding in the same study that four out of five of those with OSAS did not know that they had it.

It Takes Years Before Diagnosis

In a study of OSAS patients of the Dutch Apnea Association [4], two-thirds of the respondents estimated that in retrospect they had had symptoms of OSAS for more than 5 years before they were diagnosed. For 37 %, it took 8 years or longer before they were diagnosed. A study conducted by Jennum [5] had similar findings. Based on a retrospective cohort study ($N=97{,}180$) of the database of the Danish health insurance system, Jennum concludes that 8 years before the OSAS diagnosis was made, patients can already be identified as having significantly higher medical consumption, higher illness leave, lower average wages, higher unemployment, etc.

The current diagnostic capacity in the Netherlands is 40,000–50,000 sleep studies per year. This results in around 20,000–30,000 OSAS diagnoses [6]. Thus, the underdiagnosis will continue for years to come even if the capacity increases drastically.

The Consequences of Untreated OSAS

The consequences of untreated OSAS can be divided into three categories:

- Personal, which includes the effects on marriage, family, and work
- Medical, as demonstrated by the high rate of comorbidity found in the research reports cited in this book
- Socioeconomic, which includes a wide range of effects from direct costs (e.g., unemployment, health care) to indirect costs and consequences (e.g., travel accidents caused by untreated OSAS)

Relevance: Socioeconomic Implications

The most obvious socioeconomic impacts are increased medical consumption before the correct diagnosis and the costs of illness leave. In the investigation of the aforementioned by Jennum, a calculation was made of the real historic costs that were incurred over those 8 years before diagnosis. The average amounted to €3,860 per undiagnosed OSAS patient per year. For the Netherlands, this would mean a total cost of undiagnosed OSAS of at least €1.5 billion per year. This amount could largely have been saved by timely diagnosis and correct treatment. It is important to note that treatment of this whole group with CPAP would cost only 126 million per year. These are direct and indirect costs and savings. There are no estimates available of the production lost due to a lack of energy and concentration at the workplace, nor for the number of traffic accidents caused by untreated OSAS patients falling asleep at the wheel. We frequently see calculations of this kind in American studies, but reliable figure for the Netherlands and Europe are lacking. We think that we can make our point clearly without them: untreated OSAS is a heavy burden for society. In the remainder of this chapter, we focus on the personal and medical consequences from the patient's perspective.

The Impact of Untreated OSAS on Patients

The consequences of untreated OSAS on a personal level are ultimately quite serious. The known symptoms are everything associated with a lack of sleep. OSAS patients suffer from insufficiently deep restorative sleep, and sometimes they get no restorative sleep at all. Over the years they accumulate a structural and systematic sleep deficit. This means they have less energy, more procrastination, difficulty concentrating, increased daytime sleepiness, irritability, and a short temper. The symptoms are sometimes referred to collectively as a character change. People with these symptoms become, over the years, worse employees, managers, colleagues, partners, and parents. For the partner, there is an extra issue: reduced libido. If this whole process continues long enough, it leads to dysfunctional relationships at work as well as in the marriage and family. The downward spiral is amplified if the patient is sent on sickness leave or becomes unemployed. Sooner or later they will end up with a lack of self-confidence and very low self-esteem. A lot of damage can occur in just 5 years time.

On a physical level, there is fluctuating and declining oxygen saturation during the night, in conjunction with an impaired insulin and hormone metabolism. Repeated arousals from sleep ensure damage to the patient's system. All this means that due to the delayed appropriate diagnosis, the theoretical comorbidity is actually widely manifested among OSAS patients. In our study we asked patients what disease they initially thought they had. As it is a self-reported "disease," we also asked if they had mentioned their suspicion to a doctor, whether the doctor had actually

Table 1 Extent to which OSAS patients have had complaints and disorders prior to treatment for OSAS

	Depression/ burnout (%)	Cardio vascular diseases (%)	Obesity (%)	Diabetes (%)	Overly high blood pressure (%)	Overly high cholesterol (%)
No complaints	56	57	42	72	42	53
Have had complaints	44	43	58	28	58	47
Went to the doctor	31	38	38	25	52	41
I have been treated	22	31	22	22	45	34
Still in treatment	9	23	16	20	39	28

Source: De Apneuketen in Beeld, Van Mechelen, September 2011, $N=2{,}702$

started treatment for the disease mentioned and whether this treatment continued after the diagnosis of OSAS. The answers to all of these questions are shown in Table 1.

This kind of data concerning the comorbidities of OSAS can also be found in the international literature and in the previous chapters of this book. We believe that the above figures significantly underestimate the comorbidity. For example, obesity is both a cause and an effect of OSAS. Ninety percent of the respondents in the same study were overweight (BMI>25). Fifty-two percent had severe to morbid obesity (BMI>30). However, a large number of respondents did not report this as a disease. There can only be one conclusion: many patients suffer from several different diseases at the time of diagnosis. Besides OSAS, they might also be obese and have diabetes and/or hypertension and/or heart problems, etc. In a pilot study conducted at Antonius Hospital (Nieuwegein 2012), we found that OSAS patients had an average of 3.4 comorbidities at the time of their OSAS diagnosis. The majority already had an extensive (often unsuccessful) history of treatment for the other diseases. This should have implications for the treatment of OSAS (see below).

Depression and burnout do not fit completely in this context. Although very high HADS scores are common in OSAS patients at the time of diagnosis, it is possible that this is a consequence of the damage caused by untreated OSAS. One thing is for sure: treatments for depression will not take the OSAS away. Some of the medications prescribed for burnout or depression may even worsen the OSAS (e.g., if they have a muscle relaxant effect). It is very likely, on the other hand, that treatment of OSAS may in many cases eliminate the symptoms of burnout and depression. Therapies for depression and burnout are reduced by more than half after a diagnosis of OSAS.

The consequences of untreated OSAS on a person's work are quite significant. Less than 50 % of the people in the Netherlands that are now treated for OSAS are employed. A large part retired earlier than the normal age of 65 years. The rate of disability is also very high. In the category of 18–39 years of age, 12 % is disabled (compared to 2 % on average in the Netherlands), between 40 and 59 years, 14 % is disabled (6 % is average in the Netherlands), and those over 60 years have doubled the average rate of disability (8 % versus 4 % for the Dutch population). Obviously, a large percentage of those who currently have OSAS are being diagnosed too late. For them, returning to a normal work situation is no longer possible.

To conclude this paragraph on the personal impact of OSAS, we would like to quote Jennum once more. He writes, "Although CPAP treatment reduces mortality, earlier disease detection could have a greater impact on disease complications."

Why Is OSAS Underdiagnosed and Diagnosed So Late?

The disastrous consequences of late diagnosis make it important to determine why OSAS is not being diagnosed in a timely manner. From many conversations at dozens of meetings with those diagnosed with OSAS, a fairly consistent picture emerges.

- *The disease creeps in slowly.* The symptoms are initially not alarming, and they creep in over the years, from a single apnea per night/hour to many apneas per hour after several years. This causes habituation. The clear list of symptoms is misleading because a large number of people did not recognize any of the symptoms at the beginning. Perhaps there was some discomfort, but there was no reason to see a doctor. For example, falling asleep in front of the TV does not prompt many people to visit a GP.
- *Men are often in denial about their health.* The majority of patients are male. In general, men do not know what it means to "listen to your body." Existing symptoms are played down. For example, snoring is not their problem but their partner's problem. Arousals from sleep are often only noticed by the partner. Most men do not want to discuss decreased libido, and they rarely believe that they could be the cause of their poor sex life. Dozing off in traffic is denied or rather looked upon as incidental and not seen as structural. Men do not like their ability (or right) to drive brought under scrutiny. The man's residual energy is used for work because often the activities and adrenaline counteract the effects of untreated OSAS, and therefore the effects are not immediately seen there.
- *Apneas happen during sleep, problems occur during the day.* It is not obvious to relate problems that occur during the day with events at night. In addition, most OSAS patients, in their own words, have no sleeping problem at all. They fall asleep "as soon as their head touches the pillow." While they may have no difficulties falling asleep, they often have difficulties staying asleep early in the morning.
- *There are many other explanations for restless sleep in the morning.* The discovery of OSAS occurs mostly in the second half of someone's life. If any symptoms are observed, there are many aspects of the life of a person over 45 that can explain the symptoms away. For example, the restless sleep in the morning and the short temper might be caused by worries about parents beginning to

struggle with their health or the relationship/marriage that is more than 20 years old and has grown stale and perhaps even troublesome. There are also worries about children's puberty, their results at school, or the fact that they have boyfriends/girlfriends that the parent does not like. Finally, at work there are worries about reorganizations and career moves. Why *would* anyone think about sleep apnea?

- *The accompanying diseases/conditions are more easily recognized (and treated).* When over the years the complaints grow, patients visit a doctor to discuss the problem. By that point OSAS is often in an advanced stage, and comorbidity symptoms overshadow those of OSAS. Therefore, the relationship between the symptoms and OSAS is less likely to be realized by the patient or the doctor. Hypertension, heart disease, diabetes, and obesity are more easily recognized and treated. In more than 20 % of the cases, the symptoms are interpreted as burnout or depression. Patients may be prescribed antidepressants and/or be referred to a psychologist or psychiatrist.
- *The referral is not adequate.* Because of the preoccupation with comorbidity, GPs often refer patients to the wrong specialists in the hospital. Even if OSA is suspected, there is insufficient knowledge about the existence of sleep labs. Referrals are most often (70 %) made to the ENT specialist (snoring), while in the majority of sleep labs in Holland (61 %), the pulmonologist plays the leading role.
- *The organization of most hospitals does not facilitate a multidisciplinary approach.* If the patient is not properly referred, the misunderstanding of the condition and the treatment of comorbidity will persist.

One wonders, after reading numerous cases and the explanations mentioned above, how anybody with OSAS will ever be diagnosed. The answer is simple: in many cases the patient, and more often the partner of the patient, makes the diagnosis. He or she reads something about sleep apnea, or has a relative or a colleague with sleep apnea, and gets the idea that this might be the cause of the other problems and remembers that their partner's breathing stops at night. The patient is often pushed by the partner to see the doctor. After some time and persuasion, he/she visits the doctor and reports the apneas to the GP. Finally, the GP makes the adequate referral for the sleep lab.

Implications for the Treatment

The fact that an OSAS patient is often suffering from several different conditions/diseases at the time of the diagnosis and already has a track record of all kinds of treatments has implications for the OSAS treatment plan.

1. *It is necessary to treat the OSAS patient, not the OSAS.*
   For most of the patients, it is not enough to treat the OSAS by using CPAP or MAD. That will not help the patient enough to take back his or her life. There are different ongoing treatments for other disorders that have to be evaluated in light

of the OSAS. An integrated treatment plan should be made. Some drugs may have to be changed; dosages can possibly be reduced over time. If the patient uses the additional energy he or she gets from the OSAS treatment to make a lifestyle change, some other treatments can be stopped completely. The optimistic message is that while diagnosis of OSAS usually comes after years of downward spiraling, if done in the right way, the treatment for OSAS can be the starting point of years of upward spiraling.

2. *The OSAS patient has to be convinced.*
   The average OSAS patient has heard so many reasons for his complaints and has endured so many ineffective treatments that he or she may be hard to convince. This surely is the case when a doctor cannot provide a cure but can only offer an apparatus to fight the symptoms. It involves a device that is quite obtrusive, even intimidating, and has to be used the whole night, every night, for the rest of your life (20–40 years!). You have to have a good story as a doctor to convince the patient that this device is going to do the trick; otherwise, you will have very low compliance.

The Future Patient

In the Dutch patient population, there is a very significant overrepresentation of the overweight older men. Of the Dutch patients in 2011, 78 % were men,[1] while 84 % were 50 years of age or older. About 90 % had a BMI>25, of which 52 % had a BMI>30, whereas in the Dutch population, 47 % have a BMI>25 and 12 % a BMI>30. Apparently, doctors have been looking for the phenotype of the OSAS patient, and they have found it. These patients can be most easily identified by using the STOP-Bang questionnaire. The Dutch numbers are furthermore influenced by anesthetists, who are very keen to detect OSAS. Knowing whether a patient has OSAS is important for the choice of sedation and the application of intubation. No one wants to see a patient decease in the recovery room after a successful operation because of the removal of the intubation. In the Netherlands, all patients undergoing bariatric surgery are therefore tested for OSAS or treated as OSAS patients.

One of the lessons learned in the foregoing text is that doctors will have to be proactive in hunting down OSAS patients before irreparable damage is done to the patients' social life and/or their health. When doctors start looking for the 80 % of the patients who do not yet know that they have OSAS, they will surely see a different population. According to the prevalence numbers cited in international literature and presented in chapter "OSAS: The Magnitude of the Problem," the true OSAS population is younger, there are more women, and fewer people are obese than the current Dutch OSAS patient population. Most importantly, they will see less severe OSAS (AHI>30). Detecting OSAS early means meeting more patients with moderate OSAS (AHI 15–30). According to the Dutch 2009 guidelines, even those with mild

---

1

OSAS (AHI > 5 with complaints) get insured care. Mild and moderate OSAS cases outnumber severe OSAS cases both absolutely and relatively in the population. Due to the rising awareness about sleep apnea, doctors will encounter more of those patients in the years to come (as they will form a growing part of the patient group).

With mild and moderate apnea cases entering the sleep lab, doctors will get to know a different type of OSAS patient. As presented in chapter "The Contribution of Head Position to the Apnea/Hypopnea Index in Patients with Position-Dependent Obstructive Sleep Apnea," in mild and moderate OSAS, there is a high prevalence of positional OSAS (50–70 %). This will make it necessary to reconsider the treatment palette. Are there appropriate treatments available for the future patients?

The Future Treatment

Let us have a look to the treatment palette for OSAS. See for a summary from patients' perspective Table 2.

CPAP stands for continuous positive airway pressure, and it will remain the first choice for severe OSAS. There is a lot of discussion about compliance, which obscures the fact that today the CPAP treatment saves the lives of more than 74,000 Dutch people, 70 % of whom use the device for every moment of sleep during the night and even for small naps during the day [7]. Is CPAP a successful therapy? The answer depends on how you look at compliance. From the perspective that everyone not being treated for OSAS increasingly suffers from comorbidity, any percentage of noncompliance is too high. Compared to the treatment of those suffering for years from chronic medical problems and using medication, the compliance with the CPAP is not bad at all. Before 2010 every OSAS patient received CPAP therapy, as it was the only insured treatment. We think that compliance numbers will rise if there are different therapies that will enable doctors to prescribe the most appropriate therapy for each patient. On the other hand, real CPAP intolerance is almost unknown

Table 2 Main OSAS therapies and their characteristics (from the patients' perspective)

CPAP: Does not provide a cure but fights the symptoms with intimidating therapy involving a mask on the face blowing air, to be continued every night for the rest of one's life. It is most successful for severe OSAS
MAD: Does not provide a cure but fights the symptoms using a more or less intimidating therapy involving a bit in the mouth pushing the mandible forward, to be continued every night for the rest of one's life. It is most successful for mild and moderate OSAS
ENT surgery: It promises to cure the problem but has variable success stories. It has been successful in limited numbers after careful patient selection in mild and moderate OSAS
Osteotomy: Bimaxillary advancement promises healing after some months of (heavy) discomfort. It can be especially successful for young and female patients with moderate OSAS
Position training: It prevents OSAS after some weeks training and no further treatment is necessary. If it works, it is a very promising option for 50 % of the cases of mild and moderate OSAS

to the Dutch Apnea Association. We only know about patients who are poorly monitored and instructed during the first days and weeks. Many struggle for months with the adjustment and choice of the right mask and how to handle the humidifier. As the research literature confirms, compliance rates improve when good monitoring and information are provided at the start.

MAD therapy is relatively new for the Netherlands. Since January 2010 it has been covered by the national insurance system. In 2011 the number of MADs that are given to patients has risen to record levels of 8,000–10,000 new MADs a year. There have been no reliable compliance studies in the Netherlands so far. According to international research, compliance might be around 55–65 %. This should be no surprise because wearing the bit causes some discomfort. While it is considered less uncomfortable than the CPAP, it still takes some discipline to continue therapy every night.

There is little experience in the Netherlands with osteotomy as a treatment for OSAS. Up to now it has been used as a treatment of last resort, after other treatments were unsuccessful. This might change in the decades to come, as more young female patients do not want to endure 40–50 years of CPAP or MAD usage every night.

For a long time, doctors have known about the existence of position-dependent OSAS in a large percentage of mild and moderate cases. It could be seen in any PSG made in the last decades. However, to be honest, there was really no position therapy. The concept of hindering and preventing the supine position has not worked. Since 1872, patients have tried special mattresses and every variation on the tennis ball technique (TBT), as well as backpacks and vests in many shapes with either steep or shallow slopes. Initially, successful techniques ultimately failed. Discomfort and sleep architecture were the problems, and consequently after some weeks or months, compliance dipped below acceptable levels (less than 10 % [8]).

In contrast to the concept of hindering and preventing a supine position, the concept of training had already proven to be successful in 1991 [9]. With some weeks of training, with or without a device, a great number of patients still avoided sleeping in a supine position even after 6 months. In hindsight, it is easy to explain the success. People need to be able to turn 8–15 times a night from one side to the other. There are some people who want to relax Zen-like for some minutes in a supine position before turning to a lateral position to fall asleep. While this is impossible with the hindering concept, it is possible and does not cause problems with the training concept. In the last years, the training concept has been further elaborated in the Netherlands. A small microchip that is easy to wear is at the heart of the concept. ICT makes it possible to create a personal learning curve, which allows patients to spend short periods in a supine position. The results are presented in previous chapters in this book.

Besides, there is another reason why the Dutch Apnea Association hopes position training will be successful. Its primary goal is to get patients diagnosed at an early stage before too much harm is done and return them to a perfectly normal life as soon as possible. However, there are two reasons why people visit the doctor. First, they come if their symptoms and complaints are quite clear and very disruptive. This is not the case at the onset of OSAS. Second, people come to the doctor if they know that there is a solution and that the therapy is not very frightening. Clearly, CPAP and MAD are not very attractive therapies and the prospect of this intrusive, lifelong treatment scares people away. Therefore, the two conditions that would get people to visit the doctor are not met in the early stage of OSAS. Position training can change this situation. It promises that some groups can get rid of their sleep apnea problem within weeks. We think this will successfully lower the threshold to visit the sleep lab.

Conclusion: Position Training as an Indispensable Treatment

With the rising awareness about sleep apnea and its nasty long-term effects, people will be more inclined to get themselves checked for OSAS. Indeed, to prevent serious damage to their personal life and health, it is necessary to detect and treat OSAS patients at an early stage, when most patients still have mild or moderate OSAS. In a large percentage of cases, at this stage OSAS is position dependent. Unfortunately, so far patients have only been offered very invasive therapies. Position training might be precisely what doctors need to entice patients to come to the sleep lab and then effectively treat many of them.

References

1. Young T, Palta M, Dempsey J, Skatrud J, Weber S, Badr S. The occurrence of sleep-disordered breathing among middle-aged adults. New Engl J Med. 1993;328(17):1230–5.
2. GIP-Database van de zorgverzekeraars in Nederland (basis 16 miljoen verzekerden).
3. Eijsvogel M, November 2012, presentation NSWO congress.
4. van Mechelen PHJM, September 2011, De Apneu-keten in Beeld, ApneuMagazine Extra.
5. Jennum P. BMJ-Thorax. August 2011; 66:560–6 (data from the Danish National Patient Registry (1998–2006)).
6. van Mechelen PHJM, December 2012, Kansrijke klinieken, ApneuMagazine.
7. van Mechelen PHJM , September 2011, De Apneu-keten in Beeld, ApneuMagazine Extra.
8. van Mechelen PHJM, September 2011, De Apneu-keten in Beeld, ApneuMagazine Extra.
9. J Clin Sleep Med. 2009;(5):428–30.
10. Sleep. 14(6):546–52.

Positional Therapy, Consequences for and Implementation in Obstructive Sleep Apnea Guidelines

Nico de Vries and Madeline Ravesloot

There are many national guidelines on diagnosis and treatment of obstructive sleep apnea (OSA) across the world, such as the American Academy of Sleep Medicine (AASM) guideline, the Canadian Thoracic Society (CTS) guideline, the Scottish Intercollegiate Guidelines Network (SIGN) guideline, the Finnish national guideline, the German Society of Ear-Nose-Throat, Head-Neck Surgery (DG HNO KHC) guideline and the Dutch Institute for Health Care (CBO) guideline [1–6].

Interestingly, despite application of a similar systematic approach in answering the same clinical question, the same available medical literature and standardised recommendations concerning quality of evidence, remarkable disagreements exist between evidence-based guidelines. Reasons include citation preference for articles from authors participating in the guideline workgroup or from their own country [7]. Differences in health-care systems, such as organisational structure and financing systems, are another important cause for conflicting recommendations.

In most countries, only costs of CPAP are reimbursed, if at all, or machine rental is subsidised. In some countries such as Austria, Belgium, Cyprus, Greece, Ireland, Latvia, Lithuania, Slovakia and the UK (if undertaken within the National Health Service), no or only partial reimbursement is made available for sleep testing for OSA. Each country has its own internal guideline in mandating at which severity OSA with or without the presence of co-morbidities coverage is provided [8, 9].

N. de Vries, M.D., Ph.D.
Department of Otolaryngology, Sint Lucas Andreas Ziekenhuis, Amsterdam, The Netherlands

Department of Otolaryngology, University Hospital Antwerp, Antwerp, Belgium

M. Ravesloot, M.D., Ph.D. (✉)
Department of Otorhinolaryngology, Sint Lucas Andreas Ziekenhuis, Jan Tooropstraat 164, 1061 AE Amsterdam, The Netherlands
e-mail: m.ravesloot@slaz.nl

N. de Vries et al. (eds.), *Positional Therapy in Obstructive Sleep Apnea*,
DOI 10.1007/978-3-319-09626-1_33

As this book shows, it is to be expected that PT will gain momentum in the scope of OSA treatment. In most guidelines, it is mentioned that patients with POSA may benefit from PT. But there are also guidelines in which the role of sleep position and PT are not mentioned, for example the SIGN guideline.

Future Perspectives

It is to be expected that in future guidelines PT will be included in guideline considerations and will play a more prominent role in treatment recommendations: either as a standalone therapy or in conjunction with other treatment modalities, even though insurance companies often cover only one treatment. Various chapters in this book demonstrate the tremendous potential of combination therapy: PT and oral device therapy PT and palatal surgery, PT and tongue base surgery and, to a lesser extent, PT and CPAP.

In the Netherlands we have the unique situation that both diagnosis and various forms of treatment are subsidised by health insurance companies, dependent on severity of disease. Recommendations of the current Dutch guideline are summarised in Fig. 1 [6]. In brief, behaviour modification is indicated for all patients with a modifiable risk factor such as weight loss, alcohol, tobacco and sedative abstinence and avoidance of the worst sleeping position.

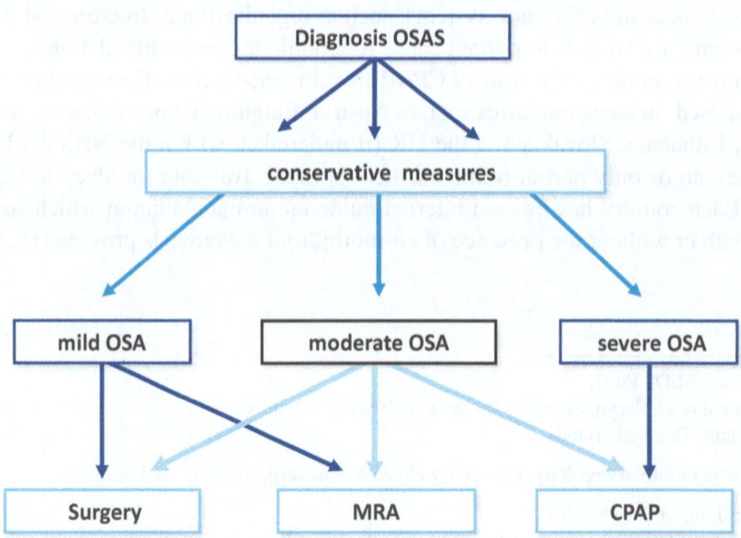

Fig. 1 Recommendations of the current Dutch guideline

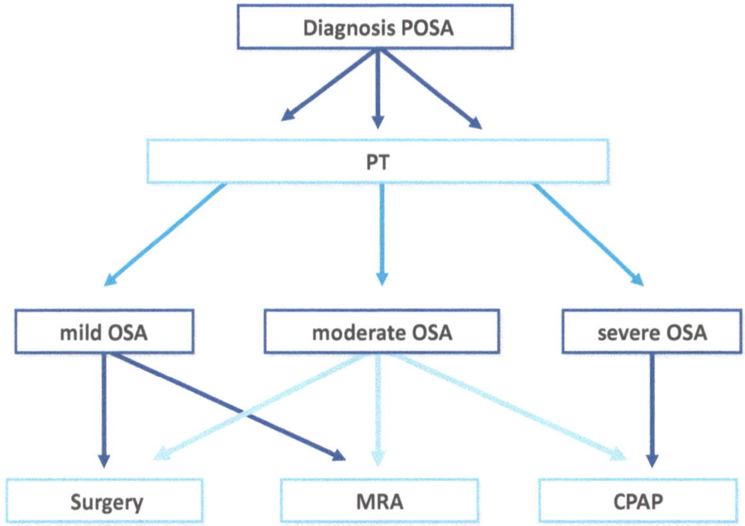

Fig. 2 Alternative is to start with PT, reassess the severity of the disease after PT and subsequently reconsider the treatment options

Patients with severe OSA are recommended to be treated with CPAP, whilst in moderate OSA, MAD or surgery can be considered as well. In patients with mild OSA, CPAP is regarded as overtreatment, especially since evidence suggests that CPAP compliance is reduced considerably in case of mild disease and minor symptoms. MAD or surgery is recommended as an alternative. Choice of treatment depends on patient characteristics, OSA severity, sleep position dependence, co-morbidity, health insurance coverage and patient preference, for instance.

What are the implications for more widespread use of PT for such flow charts? Several possibilities are demonstrated in Figs. 2, 3 and 4.

Figure 2 shows an alternative treatment strategy for patients with POSA, by starting with PT followed by a reassessment of the severity of disease after initiation of treatment and subsequent reconsideration of treatment options. Some cases might be cured by PT alone: a reduction of the AHI to below 5. Whilst PT may result in a reduction in OSA severity in others: from moderate to mild OSA or from severe to moderate OSA, for example. By lowering the OSA severity category, patients could be eligible for less aggressive primary therapy (for example, lower CPAP pressure, less invasive surgery), especially since PT is simple, cheap, well tolerated and reversible. It would be important to accurately identify candidates who will benefit from a clinically significant improvement of their ORA with PT, suing the Amsterdam Positional OSA Classification, for example [10].

A variation on this theme is shown in Fig. 3.

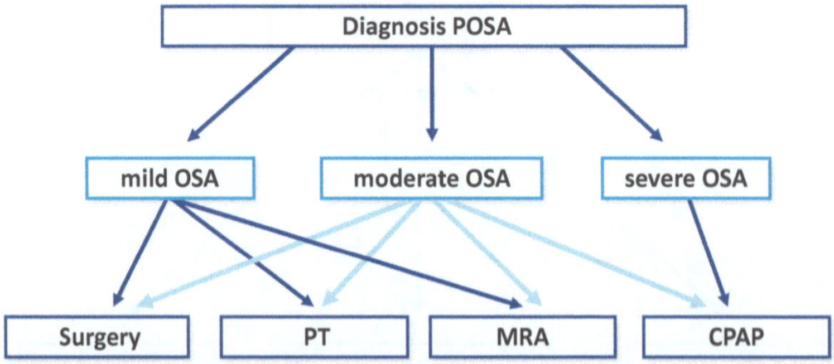

Fig. 3 A variation on the alternative shown in Fig. 2

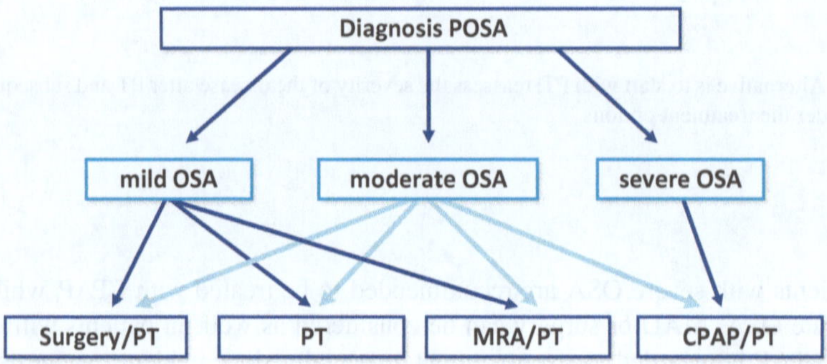

Fig. 4 Shows the situation in an ideal world, in which insurance companies cover multimodality/combined treatment, if indicated

Figure 4 shows the situation in an ideal world, in which insurance companies cover multimodality/combination treatment, if indicated. We are not naive and realise that it might be a long way before such scenarios are implemented. It does no harm, however, to ignore the restraints of the existing guidelines or insurance company dictates, respectively, and to consider future alternative treatment modalities.

References

1. Epstein LJ, Kristo D, Strollo Jr PJ, Friedman N, Malhotra A, Patil SP, Ramar K, Rogers R, Schwab RJ, Weaver EM, Weinstein MD, Adult Obstructive Sleep Apnea Task Force of the American Academy of Sleep Medicine. Clinical guideline for the evaluation, management and long-term care of obstructive sleep apnea in adults. J Clin Sleep Med. 2009;5(3):263–76.

2. Fleetham J, Ayas N, Bradley D, Ferguson K, Fitzpatrick M, George C, et al. Canadian Thoracic Society guidelines: Diagnosis and treatment of sleep disordered breathing in adults. Can Respir J. 2006;13(7):387–92.
3. Scottish Intercollegiate Guidelines Network (SIGN). Management of obstructive sleep apnoea/hypopnea syndrome in adults. A national clinical guideline. SIGN publication No. 73. Edinburgh, UK; 2003. Available at: www.sign.ac.uk. Accessed August 2014.
4. Laitinen LA, Anttalainen U, Pietinalho A, Hamalainen P, Koskela K. Sleep apnoea: Finnish National guidelines for prevention and treatment 2002-2012. Respir Med. 2003;97(4):337–65.
5. Verse T, Bodlaj R, de la Chaux R, Dreher A, Heiser C, Herzog M, et al. Guideline: Treatment of obstructive sleep apnea in adults. HNO. 2009;57(11):1136–56.
6. Dutch Institute for Health Care (CBO). Guideline diagnosis and management of obstructive sleep apnea syndrome in adults. 2009. Available at: www.cbo.nl. Accessed August 2014.
7. Aarts MC, van der Heijden GJ, Rovers MM, Grolman W. Remarkable differences between three evidence-based guidelines on management of obstructive sleep apnea-hypopnea syndrome. Laryngoscope. 2013;123(1):283–91.
8. Ravesloot MJ, de Vries N. Financial coverage of OSAS treatment: an international survey. In: Surgery, sleep & breathing III: an international symposium, Amsterdam, The Netherlands, May 2009. Conference Presentation.
9. Fietze I, Penzel T, Alonderis A, et al. Management of obstructive sleep apnea in Europe. Sleep Med. 2011;12:190–7.
10. Frank MH, Ravesloot MJL, van Maanen JP, Verhagen E, de Lange J, de Vries N. Positional OSA part 1: towards a clinical classification system for position-dependent obstructive sleep apnoea. Sleep Breath. 2014 [Epub ahead of print].

Position-Dependent Sleep Apnea: Implications for Diagnosis and Management

Matt T. Bianchi

Introduction

Obstructive sleep apnea (OSA) is a common problem associated in various clinical and epidemiological studies with cerebrovascular and cardiovascular morbidity and mortality [1–3]. The clinical approach to this treatable disorder begins with accurate assessment of severity, which is important to choose among treatment options as well as to motivate treatment adherence. Current clinical guidelines utilize the summary metric of apneas and hypopneas per hour of sleep (AHI) to make the diagnosis and to categorize severity, typically with overnight polysomnography (PSG) [4]. Although historically it was once felt that the presence of sleepiness was required in addition to an elevated AHI, in more modern evidence-based thinking, the American Academy of Sleep Medicine recommends treatment for patients with AHI > 5 per hour if there are daytime symptoms potentially attributable to sleep or if there are sleep complaints such as snoring (whereas treatment is recommended for AHI > 15 per hour regardless of symptoms) [4, 5]. Having a single metric to guide clinical care can offer important advantages for standardizing clinical practice. However, attention to the complex nature of sleep apnea and the potential impact of various factors on its presence and severity are as critical to individualized clinical care as to research advancement in this field.

Disclosures: Dr Bianchi receives funding from the Department of Neurology, Massachusetts General Hospital, a Young Clinician Award from the Center for Integration of Medicine and Innovative Technology, and the Harvard Catalyst KL2 fellowship. Dr Bianchi has a patent pending on a home sleep monitoring device.

M.T. Bianchi, M.D., Ph.D. (✉)
Neurology Department, Massachusetts General Hospital,
55 Fruit Street, Boston, MA 02114, USA
e-mail: mtbianchi@partners.org

N. de Vries et al. (eds.), *Positional Therapy in Obstructive Sleep Apnea*,
DOI 10.1007/978-3-319-09626-1_34

The Importance of Sleep Apnea Phenotyping

Among the mistakes to avoid in any medical field is to assume that the current standards are sufficient for optimal care. In the field of sleep medicine, there may be a general perception that the hourly rate of apneas and hypopneas in a single-night snapshot of sleep is sufficient for diagnosis and risk stratification of sleep apnea. There may be a sense that what is normal and severe is agreed upon, and the gray areas in between are open for discussion. However, there is substantial and growing evidence that the one-night PSG gold standard is not as shiny as it may seem, with potential to both over- and underestimate OSA severity. Understanding the strengths and limitations of the PSG is crucial for accurate patient phenotyping, whether clinically or for research, especially in light of variable and increasingly restrictive insurance coverage for what is perceived by some as expensive and unnecessary testing that can be accomplished with limited channel home devices. In this chapter, some of the key considerations are reviewed in this regard, with a focus on body position as it pertains to sleep apnea phenotyping. This single factor can allow severe sleep apnea to masquerade as normal and vice versa—a reality of which patients and providers alike should be aware.

Strengths and Limitations of Laboratory Diagnosis of Sleep Apnea

The gold standard for quantifying the presence and severity of OSA remains the attended laboratory PSG. Like any diagnostic test in medicine, there are trade-offs to consider. Clearly the laboratory PSG provides extensive physiological information, including EEG, muscle tone, leg movements, EKG, and typically a combination of seven respiratory channels (two airflow, two effort, oximetry, intercostal EMG, snoring). Video allows manual scoring of body position. Among those patients who exhibit apparent changes in severity despite no change in body position or sleep stage, the video sometimes shows that the head position has changed, which can also influence breathing in some cases [6].

The rich physiological information provided by this array of sensors can offer important insights into a wide range of sleep pathologies. However, for some patients, the presence of these sensors also compromises sleep due to discomfort or restricted positioning. Sensor discomfort and the foreign environment in general may contribute to what is known as the first-night effect, in which laboratory sleep is more fragmented, with increased N1, decreased REM, and decreased sleep efficiency [7–9]. The fact that sleep occurs away from the habitual home environment may, on the other hand, prove to have a positive impact on sleep consolidation if there are factors in the home that contribute to poor sleep consolidation—this is sometimes called the reverse first-night effect.

There are multiple other factors that might not occur in the laboratory setting but could interfere (or help) with sleep consolidation [10, 11]. For example, late or middle of the night consumption of food or alcohol or smoking is typically not permitted in the laboratory. The lack of typical bed partner presence might lead to improved sleep in the lab, if the partner's sleep is disruptive, for example, due to snoring [12]. For other individuals, the absence of a routine of sleeping with a bed partner might itself become a source of stress and thus alter sleep in the laboratory. Finally, the single-night snapshot of sleep presents a limitation of "under-sampling" because some of the aforementioned factors can vary from night to night, in addition to the possibility that sleep may have stochastic variability even when such external factors are held constant. In some publications, night to night variability in OSA severity was partially explained by variability in body position [13–16]. The challenge of night to night variability extends to the possibility that individuals may be differentially vulnerable to the potential impact of body position and other factors impacting severity.

Strengths and Limitations of Home Diagnosis of Sleep Apnea

The main benefit of home sleep apnea testing is that it can be performed in the habitual sleep environment. The widely claimed cost savings of this method are not supported by cost-benefit models except in very specific populations [17–21]. The limitations listed above for laboratory PSG also apply to home testing, many of which are related to the single-night testing paradigm. In addition, there are other key limitations specific to home testing. For example, home-testing devices do not actually measure sleep, with the exception of the Watch-PAT that extracts surrogate sleep stages using an algorithm based on a combination of actigraphy and autonomic signals [22, 23]. This limitation is important from a practical standpoint, as the reported respiratory event index can underestimate the sleep apnea severity simply because the time over which the events are collected may consist of a combination of wake and sleep, and thus the event rate is per hour of recording rather than per hour of sleep (as it is reported in the laboratory PSG). For patients with high sleep efficiency, the approximation has arguably a negligible effect on respiratory event rate calculation. But for patients with insomnia, or who have for any reason excess waking time on the night of testing, this potential for underestimation can impact clinical decision making, depending on the results. For example, a 20 % difference in total sleep time could move a respiratory index from mild to normal or from moderate to mild, which might impact treatment discussions.

Another limitation of failure to measure sleep stages is that REM versus NREM dependence cannot be determined, which may be important for phenotyping (NREM-dominant disease may be a risk for complex apnea), as well as the potential interaction with body position (supine and REM combination may be the most vulnerable combination for many patients). The limited sensor approach of home testing is clearly focused on sleep apnea, but comorbid sleep disorders are not assessed, such as periodic limb movements, REM without atonia, nocturnal seizures, or parasomnia. The potential degree of misperception is also unknown with home devices, which is of key importance in the evaluation and management of the patient with insomnia or comorbid sleep apnea and insomnia. Finally, technical failures and issues of chain of custody represent important considerations when pursuing home sleep apnea testing.

Regarding body position in particular, only some of the currently available devices include this metric. In the 2007 guideline on the use of home sleep apnea testing devices, 10 of 26 devices had position monitoring [24], and in the follow-up technology review of this field, 11 of 20 devices reported position monitoring [25]. Collop et al. listed body position as a main feature in the systematic evaluation scheme (the "C" in the SCOPER framework) [25]. In the published validation studies of these devices, the focus is usually on detecting apneas and hypopneas rather than optimizing the accuracy of body position detection. Thus, among the many reasons why a negative home-testing night should be followed by confirmatory laboratory, PSG is to ensure that supine sleep (and in particular supine-REM sleep) is observed. Yin et al. showed that patients spent somewhat more time supine in the lab than at home, which explained some of the difference between at-home and in-lab assessments of OSA severity [26]. As Collop et al. point out in their manuscript, body position is not formally part of the diagnostic criteria for OSA [25]. This represents a disconnect between the increasingly appreciated importance of body position in phenotyping OSA patients and the tradition of using the full-night AHI as the single-AHI diagnostic answer. Barriers to implementing guidance regarding position include the lack of standard to define position-dependent OSA (what ratio is clinically relevant? does the absolute rate matter as well?) and the lack of readily available techniques to monitor body position longitudinally in the home.

The Importance of Positional OSA Severity: Clinical Scenarios

Consider three patients who undergo laboratory PSG, and each turns out to have the same summary AHI for their night of testing: 20 per hour. Patient A shows marked positional variation in sleep apnea severity and has an AHI of 5 in lateral positions, while the AHI was 35 events per hour in the supine position. He spends half of the night of testing supine, and thus the weighted average of events per hour turns out to be AHI = 20. Patient B also spent half of the night supine, but the AHI was 20 per hour regardless of body position. Patient C spent the entire night supine and has an AHI = 20, with unknown AHI in the lateral positions.

Patient A is reluctant to pursue CPAP despite a supine AHI in the severe range because he maintains that he never sleeps on his back due to back pain. He contends that his lateral AHI, which was borderline, is the more representative value and should guide treatment decisions. This highly positional patient demonstrates two key issues. One is that we do not have reliable and readily available techniques to objectively monitor body position over time in the home, and thus we have little basis for predicting whether any particular patient can successfully and consistently avoid the supine position during sleep. The second issue is that the summary AHI metric is an average of two "extreme" values observed on the single night of testing. This is akin to the satirical comic of a statistician with one hand in ice water and the other in boiling water, saying "the average temperature is perfect," in the sense that the average is not always the relevant metric. In patients with marked positional variability in severity, it makes little sense to formulate decisions based on an AHI that will be weighted toward high or low values based on what happens to occur regarding position on that night. If the sleep position happened to be mainly lateral on testing, and the full-night AHI dictated treatment, then conservative measures might be emphasized. If the position happened to be mainly supine on testing, then the patient would be characterized as severe, and treatment would be strongly emphasized, including the possibility of surgery if PAP were not tolerated. Alternatives such as dental appliance might not be entertained because the AHI was higher than the mild-to-moderate range generally preferred for this strategy. Without repeated measures in the home setting, it remains unknown how the average over months or years impacts associated medical risks. Does an AHI of 20 per night every night carry the same medical risks as alternating nights or weeks at a time with an AHI of 5 and an AHI of 35 based on fluctuations in body position during sleep? Although the "correct" approach depends on many factors and patients' preferences, this hypothetical patient illustrates the uncertainties that can surround the single-night AHI—even when it is obtained from an attended laboratory PSG.

Patient B has OSA that is independent of body position, and the AHI severity is in the moderate range. Although body position does not complicate the discussions and planning as occurred with patient A, there may be other factors that influence the nightly severity in patient B, such as alcohol consumption or nasal congestion. However, given that the night in the lab was "typical" according to his report, he elects to pursue treatment with PAP based on the diagnosis of moderate OSA. This patient, compared to patient A, is a reminder of how clinical counseling and decision making can differ substantially despite the "same AHI value" on testing.

Patient C is reluctant to pursue treatment for sleep apnea. Like patient A, he maintains that he does not sleep on his back at home. He is irritable that the technicians told him he had to sleep supine, and he felt constrained by the wires and sensors. His wife reports he only snores on the rare occasion that he rolls supine, and he strongly suspects on this basis that his breathing is normal so long as he is in the preferred lateral position. Like patient A, he thus thinks that the test is not an accurate representation and treatment should not be guided by it. Sleep labs routinely encourage or enforce supine sleep to avoid the potential for a false-negative interpretation, given that the typically vulnerable combination of supine and REM sleep should be observed before ruling out sleep apnea on a lab PSG. However, this cautionary approach has the potential downside of leaving us unable to counsel patients who happened to sleep supine for the whole PSG, who wish to pursue positional therapy, who believe they can avoid supine sleep as a chronic treatment strategy, or who are reluctant to accept a diagnosis based on a perceived unnatural circumstance. Yet without home monitoring devices to track body position, we cannot objectively confirm that positional therapy is effective. Novel devices are in development to answer this challenge, as described elsewhere in this volume. In the case of patient C, his full night of supine sleep did not allow confirmation of the degree of position dependence, which precludes consideration of positional therapy, even if he and his bed partner note decreased snoring in the lateral position.

How to manage the need to observe different body positions sufficiently in the sleep lab to document position dependence is uncertain. There are competing needs to enforce supine sleep, to decide whether a patient warrants a treatment trial on the same night in the lab (split-night), versus encouraging supine and non-supine time to accurately ascertain the degree of position dependence. It may be that for selected patients, purposeful changing of body position can be pursued either on a single night or having patients such as patient C return for a repeat test for positional evaluation. We recently evaluated the chances of observing all four combinations of sleep stage (REM or NREM) and body position (supine or lateral) and showed that >10 min spent in each possible combination was observed in only a minority of the cohort undergoing clinical PSG [27]. The cohort overall spent about half the time in supine position, while only a minority spent <10 % of the total sleep time in pure non-supine or pure supine position.

The Importance of Body Position During PAP Titration

Clinical practice guidelines suggest that at least 15 min of supine REM be obtained in the successful titration study [28]. Failure to demonstrate that PAP controls apnea due to insufficient supine REM is an indication to repeat the titration study to ensure adequate control. Home auto-titration strategies in lieu of attended laboratory titration have been proposed in several studies [29, 30]. However, auto-titrating machines do not measure sleep stage or body position. Although it may be argued that the pattern obtained over the course of multiple days of auto-titration is a good approximation of pressure requirements because they capture variability and are bound to include supine and supine-REM conditions, there are two points of uncertainty worth mentioning. One is that the possibility of detecting atypical forms of sleep apnea such as complex apnea or RERA-dominant disease is poorly characterized with these machines. Another issue relates to using a machine-determined AHI for the whole night without knowledge of the within-night patterns. For example, what would be concluded for the patient with REM-dominant OSA who spends on average 25 % of the night in REM sleep and has no events in NREM sleep? The full-night AHI value might be "mild" range even if the REM AHI is 30, because REM only occurs for ~25 % of the night; assuming the NREM AHI is negligible, this pattern is predicted to yield a full-night AHI of only ~7.5. Such a value might or might not trigger a pressure change or re-titration, but the challenge is that one does not often know the within-night pattern from data card downloads. Furthermore, similar to the issue of home apnea detection, the event rate is per hour of machine use, not per hour of sleep, and thus the machine-detected residual AHI may be an underestimate.

Practical Implications for Clinical Care and Clinical Research

In our recent study of position and stage dependence of OSA, our sample was similar to prior published work in that just over half showed at least twofold supine dominance of AHI [27]. The range of position dependence was wide, with an interquartile range for a supine to non-supine AHI ratio of 3.5–10.3 among those with at least twofold supine dominance. We estimated that changes in body position resulted in greater risk of apnea severity underestimation (compared to a full-supine night) than adjustment for the commonly observed relative reduction in REM sleep percentage in the laboratory. Thus, one of the most striking findings was that position dependence was predicted to have a greater impact on potential misclassification of OSA severity than REM dependence. In other words, for REM-dominant OSA, if the amount of REM seen in the lab is less than that expected in the home (e.g., due to first-night effect), then the AHI may be underestimated. However, adjusting for this possibility did not substantially alter the predicted AHI values. Although much attention is focused (justifiably) on the observation of REM sleep (and in particular supine REM), the relative importance of body position is not surprising; whereas the amount of REM typically occupies only a minority of the total sleep time, the percentage of the night in lateral versus supine sleep can vary from 0 to 100 %. Of course, this does not suggest that REM dominance can be disregarded. For example, in patients with little or no REM sleep (such as may occur if sleep is greatly fragmented or if certain medications are used), the apnea severity can be underestimated. It is also notable that metrics such as depth of desaturation are commonly considered in assessing the need for treatment, and REM may be more commonly associated with deeper desaturations. However, the findings do indicate that, from a full-night AHI standpoint, body position seems to play a more important role on average (relative to full-supine condition) than lower REM percentages relative to predicted values of 25–30 %.

In our study, the potential for misclassification most commonly involved "adjacent" classes, such as normal-to-mild or mild-to-moderate reassignment based on supine versus whole-night AHI values. However, the data also included an important subset of patients with normal AHI values while lateral but severe AHI values while supine—this setting represents both the greatest risk of false-negative testing and the greatest potential utility of positional therapy. Our data is consistent with prior literature in that the degree of positional OSA suggests the potential utility of positional therapy, as suggested in several other chapters in this book on therapeutics involving body position. It is important to note however that while greater positional dependence ratios might suggest the optimal circumstance to pursue positional therapy, greater ratios suggest that more severe apnea occurs while supine, and thus there is greater risk entailed with incomplete effectiveness of positional therapy.

In addition to utilizing position dependence in clinical care, research-related phenotyping may also benefit from including positional metrics. The perspective may be different however, depending on the research question at hand, as to what the most relevant metric should be for phenotyping. For example, a study of the anatomical determinants of supine-dependent OSA and its potential use for predicting the utility of a dental appliance might not be concerned with the home sleep position tendency of the positional patients enrolling. In other words, the anatomical insights may be apparent during experimental testing even if the positional patients in the study habitually sleep exclusively in the lateral position. An alternative perspective is provided by studies linking sleepiness and OSA, some of which have taken advantage of positional dependence to suggest that the supine AHI was more strongly associated, a reminder of the key role that positional OSA may have and the contexts in which accounting for it may prove important [31]. In contrast, what if a patient enrolling in a randomized clinical trial is labeled "severe OSA" based on an AHI of 40 from the laboratory testing night, in which half was spent lateral with an AHI of 5? If such a patient sleeps exclusively lateral at home, then the home pattern has a far more dominant implication for the trial outcome than, say, the abovementioned study of predictors of dental appliance efficacy. Finally, in epidemiological association studies, one might be more interested in the "average" AHI over several nights in the real world, to capture an individual's actual exposure to OSA and to draw the most firm conclusions about potential morbidity links.

The best metric for quantifying the OSA phenotype thus remains a moving target. Among the important research questions include whether the nightly variability, such as may occur due to fluctuations in body position over time, contains predictive information for symptoms or morbidity. Is the weighted average of the nightly AHI value most relevant on time sales of weeks, months, or years? Could the time of night in which supine versus non-supine body position occurs actually impact the observed OSA severity? For example, it might matter if only the first half versus the second half of the night was spent supine, if there is an apnea-begets-apnea pathophysiological mechanism at work in some individuals. Body position might also interact with factors that differ from night to night, such as alcohol consumption or nasal congestion.

Perhaps the most intriguing aspect of position dependence is whether it can be used, alone or in combination with other factors, to make individualized predictions regarding the potential utility of weight loss, dental appliance, or surgical interventions for OSA [32–34]. Currently, the variability of response to these measures is difficult to predict, and there is a wide range of response in terms of AHI reduction. Predictors for surgical success are of particular importance and hold promise to help balance the potential risks of invasive procedures for patients seeking alternatives to PAP therapy. Ongoing research in this area is showing great progress [35–37] and is described in further detail in chapters "Positional Therapy and Palatal Surgery," "Positional Therapy and Tongue Base Surgery," "Residual POSA After Maxillomandibular Advancement in Patients with Severe OSA," and "Impact of Upper Airway Surgery on Positional Change During Sleep."

Conclusion

The importance of documenting position dependence and incorporating this information into the diagnostic decision making and research phenotyping of patients with sleep apnea cannot be overstated. This information is typically recorded during overnight laboratory PSG, but there is no clinically accepted standard in reporting on this aspect. With the movement toward home-based testing, it is even more important not to lose sight of the utility of this information.

Acknowledgments Dr Bianchi receives support from the department of Neurology, Massachusetts General Hospital, the Young Clinician Award from the Center for Integration of Medicine and Innovative Technology, and the Harvard Catalyst KL2 Medical Research Investigator Fellowship.

References

1. Yaggi HK, Concato J, Kernan WN, Lichtman JH, Brass LM, Mohsenin V. Obstructive sleep apnea as a risk factor for stroke and death. N Engl J Med. 2005;353(19):2034–41.
2. Eastwood PR, Malhotra A, Palmer LJ, et al. Obstructive sleep apnoea: from pathogenesis to treatment: current controversies and future directions. Respirology. 2010;15(4):587–95.
3. Budhiraja R, Budhiraja P, Quan SF. Sleep-disordered breathing and cardiovascular disorders. Respir Care. 2010;55(10):1322–32. Discussion 1330–2.
4. Epstein LJ, Kristo D, Strollo Jr PJ, et al. Clinical guideline for the evaluation, management and long-term care of obstructive sleep apnea in adults. J Clin Sleep Med. 2009;5(3):263–76.
5. International classification of sleep disorders: diagnostic & coding manual. 2nd ed. Westchester: American Academy of Sleep Medicine; 2005.
6. van Kesteren ER, van Maanen JP, Hilgevoord AA, Laman DM, de Vries N. Quantitative effects of trunk and head position on the apnea hypopnea index in obstructive sleep apnea. Sleep. 2011;34(8):1075–81.
7. McCall C, McCall WV. Objective vs. subjective measurements of sleep in depressed insomniacs: first night effect or reverse first night effect? J Clin Sleep Med. 2012;8(1):59–65.
8. Selwa LM, Marzec ML, Chervin RD, et al. Sleep staging and respiratory events in refractory epilepsy patients: is there a first night effect? Epilepsia. 2008;49(12):2063–8.
9. Gouveris H, Selivanova O, Bausmer U, Goepel B, Mann W. First-night-effect on polysomnographic respiratory sleep parameters in patients with sleep-disordered breathing and upper airway pathology. Eur Arch Otorhinolaryngol. 2010;267(9):1449–53.
10. Jaehne A, Unbehaun T, Feige B, Lutz UC, Batra A, Riemann D. How smoking affects sleep: a polysomnographical analysis. Sleep Med. 2012;13(10):1286–92.
11. Peppard PE, Austin D, Brown RL. Association of alcohol consumption and sleep disordered breathing in men and women. J Clin Sleep Med. 2007;3(3):265–70.
12. Blumen M, Quera Salva MA, d'Ortho MP, et al. Effect of sleeping alone on sleep quality in female bed partners of snorers. Eur Respir J. 2009;34(5):1127–31.
13. Bittencourt LR, Suchecki D, Tufik S, et al. The variability of the apnoea-hypopnoea index. J Sleep Res. 2001;10(3):245–51.
14. Aarab G, Lobbezoo F, Hamburger HL, Naeije M. Variability in the apnea-hypopnea index and its consequences for diagnosis and therapy evaluation. Respiration. 2009;77(1):32–7.
15. Levendowski D, Steward D, Woodson BT, Olmstead R, Popovic D, Westbrook P. The impact of obstructive sleep apnea variability measured in-lab versus in-home on sample size calculations. Int Arch Med. 2009;2(1):2.

16. Le Bon O, Hoffmann G, Tecco J, et al. Mild to moderate sleep respiratory events: one negative night may not be enough. Chest. 2000;118(2):353–9.
17. Chervin RD, Murman DL, Malow BA, Totten V. Cost-utility of three approaches to the diagnosis of sleep apnea: polysomnography, home testing, and empirical therapy. Ann Intern Med. 1999;130(6):496–505.
18. Deutsch PA, Simmons MS, Wallace JM. Cost-effectiveness of split-night polysomnography and home studies in the evaluation of obstructive sleep apnea syndrome. J Clin Sleep Med. 2006;2(2):145–53.
19. Benca RM, Peterson MJ. Insomnia and depression. Sleep Med. 2008;9 Suppl 1:S3–9.
20. Pietzsch JB, Garner A, Cipriano LE, Linehan JH. An integrated health-economic analysis of diagnostic and therapeutic strategies in the treatment of moderate-to-severe obstructive sleep apnea. Sleep. 2011;34(6):695–709.
21. Reuven H, Schweitzer E, Tarasiuk A. A cost-effectiveness analysis of alternative at-home or in-laboratory technologies for the diagnosis of obstructive sleep apnea syndrome. Med Decis Making. 2001;21(6):451–8.
22. Bresler M, Sheffy K, Pillar G, Preiszler M, Herscovici S. Differentiating between light and deep sleep stages using an ambulatory device based on peripheral arterial tonometry. Physiol Meas. 2008;29(5):571–84.
23. Herscovici S, Pe'er A, Papyan S, Lavie P. Detecting REM sleep from the finger: an automatic REM sleep algorithm based on peripheral arterial tone (PAT) and actigraphy. Physiol Meas. 2007;28(2):129–40.
24. Collop NA, Anderson WM, Boehlecke B, et al. Clinical guidelines for the use of unattended portable monitors in the diagnosis of obstructive sleep apnea in adult patients. Portable Monitoring Task Force of the American Academy of Sleep Medicine. J Clin Sleep Med. 2007;3(7):737–47.
25. Collop NA, Tracy SL, Kapur V, et al. Obstructive sleep apnea devices for out-of-center (OOC) testing: technology evaluation. J Clin Sleep Med. 2011;7(5):531–48.
26. Yin M, Miyazaki S, Ishikawa K. Evaluation of type 3 portable monitoring in unattended home setting for suspected sleep apnea: factors that may affect its accuracy. Otolaryngol Head Neck Surg. 2006;134(2):204–9.
27. Eiseman NA, Westover MB, Ellenbogen JM, Bianchi MT. The impact of body posture and sleep stages on sleep apnea severity in adults. J Clin Sleep Med. 2012;8(6):655–6A.
28. Kushida CA, Chediak A, Berry RB, et al. Clinical guidelines for the manual titration of positive airway pressure in patients with obstructive sleep apnea. J Clin Sleep Med. 2008;4(2):157–71.
29. Morgenthaler TI, Aurora RN, Brown T, et al. Practice parameters for the use of autotitrating continuous positive airway pressure devices for titrating pressures and treating adult patients with obstructive sleep apnea syndrome: an update for 2007. An American Academy of Sleep Medicine report. Sleep. 2008;31(1):141–7.
30. Ayas NT, Patel SR, Malhotra A, et al. Auto-titrating versus standard continuous positive airway pressure for the treatment of obstructive sleep apnea: results of a meta-analysis. Sleep. 2004;27(2):249–53.
31. Chervin RD, Aldrich MS. Characteristics of apneas and hypopneas during sleep and relation to excessive daytime sleepiness. Sleep. 1998;21(8):799–806.
32. Lee CH, Jung HJ, Lee WH, et al. The effect of positional dependency on outcomes of treatment with a mandibular advancement device. Arch Otolaryngol Head Neck Surg. 2012;138(5):479–83.
33. Randerath WJ, Verbraecken J, Andreas S, et al. Non-CPAP therapies in obstructive sleep apnoea. Eur Respir J. 2011;37(5):1000–28.
34. Li HY, Cheng WN, Chuang LP, et al. Positional dependency and surgical success of relocation pharyngoplasty among patients with severe obstructive sleep apnea. Otolaryngol Head Neck Surg. 2013;149(3):506–12.

35. van Maanen JP, Ravesloot MJ, Witte BI, Grijseels M, de Vries N. Exploration of the relationship between sleep position and isolated tongue base or multilevel surgery in obstructive sleep apnea. Eur Arch Otorhinolaryngol. 2012;269(9):2129–36.
36. Ravesloot MJ, van Maanen JP, Dun L, de Vries N. The undervalued potential of positional therapy in position-dependent snoring and obstructive sleep apnea – a review of the literature. Sleep Breath. 2013;17(1):39–49.
37. Lee CH, Shin HW, Han DH, et al. The implication of sleep position in the evaluation of surgical outcomes in obstructive sleep apnea. Otolaryngol Head Neck Surg. 2009;140(4):531–5.

Positional Therapy in Obstructive Sleep Apnea: For Whom and for Whom Not

Natan Gadoth and Arie Oksenberg

Women (and perhaps also men) have probably noticed many years before positional therapy was formally introduced that their bed partners' snoring is often worse when they sleep on their back. Moreover, they may have also realized that by avoiding the supine posture (positional therapy—PT), they can improve the sleep quality and familial harmony of both their own and their bed partner(s).

In a letter to the editor of Chest entitled "Patient's wife cures his snoring" [1], the writer described what seems to be a layman's innovation of PT for snoring. She wrote:

> I invented a method to prevent my husband from sleeping on his back. I sewed a pocket into the back of a T-shirt and inserted a hollow, lightweight plastic ball (about the size of a tennis ball). I fastened one side of the pocket with safety pins so that the ball can be removed to launder the shirt. It's working beautifully. In about two days, I could see a vast improvement in his energy level, alertness, and interest in life. He no longer falls asleep while sitting straight up in a chair, and the quiet, snoreless nights are great. I thought that this information might be helpful to other patients with similar problems. She also mentioned "the contents of this letter may well prove to be useful for family harmony."

Many snorers date the detection of their problem while serving in the army or even earlier, while at summer camp. Loud snoring may not only impair the sleep quality of soldiers who bunk together but also endanger the whole unit in battle conditions where silence is crucial. It is not surprising that during the American War of Independence and both world wars, soldiers were told to keep their loaded rucksacks on their backs while asleep in an attempt to reduce snoring [2].

The paper by Robin in 1948 [3] was perhaps one of the first to describe the effect of PT for snoring and mentioned that "a cotton reel sewn into the back of the pajamas is efficacious." Gastaut et al. [4] in 1966 reported that in a patient with Pickwick syndrome, sleep apnea events worsened when supine and improved when prone.

N. Gadoth, M.D. • A. Oksenberg, Ph.D. (✉)
Sleep Disorders Unit, Loewenstein Hospital – Rehabilitation Center, POB 3, Raanana, Israel
e-mail: gadoth@post.tau.ac.il; arieo@clalit.org.il

N. de Vries et al. (eds.), *Positional Therapy in Obstructive Sleep Apnea*,
DOI 10.1007/978-3-319-09626-1_35

Only in 1982, two publications in the form of an abstract stated that marked improvement in obstructive sleep apnea (OSA) patient's condition was achieved simply by shifting them from the back to the side position during sleep [5, 6]. Perhaps this was the first time that the tennis ball technique was suggested as a method of avoiding the supine posture during sleep.

In 1984, Cartwright suggested that OSA patients can be divided into positional patients (PP), those who present breathing abnormalities only or mainly in the supine posture (supine apnea–hypopnea index (AHI) at least double the lateral AHI), and non-positional patients (NPP), those who have similar amount of breathing abnormalities in the different postures (supine AHI less than double the lateral AHI) [7].

This distinction between PP and NPP is of major applicability only for PP since the changes in body position have substantial implication for possible candidates for positional therapy.

A next necessary step was to understand the characteristics of PP and how large is the prevalence of PP in patients with OSA.

Characteristics and Prevalence of Positional Patients vs. Non-positional Patients

Traditionally, OSA patients are classified according to their AHI, scored during a nocturnal PSG study. This simple classification does not take into account variables such as the predominant posture for apnea–hypopnea events, the influence of sleep stage on AHI, and additional factors such as age, gender, and BMI.

In the first large study, including 574 consecutive OSA patients diagnosed by polysomnography (PSG) in a sleep disorders unit, it was found that 55.9 % were positional [8]. Thus, it became evident that more than half of the OSA patients seeking treatment are positional patients (PP). The PP were leaner and younger and had fewer and less severe breathing abnormalities as compared to the NPP. Thus, it was not surprising that they enjoyed a better sleep quality (they slept better than NPP in the lateral postures), and according to Multiple Sleep Latency Test, they were less sleepy during daytime than NPP. The respiratory disturbance index (RDI) was the most dominant parameter that predicted the positional dependency followed by BMI and age. The authors also showed that the prevalence of PP was much higher in the milder forms of the disease (mild–moderate). In these OSA patients, the prevalence of PP ranged from 65 to 69 %. The portion of patients with positional dependency decreased with increasing BMI, while age played only a minor role.

In a study on a larger population of 2,077 adult OSA patients by the same group, it was shown that 54 % were PP [9]. In this study, 60.4 % and 56.2 % were PP in mild and moderate OSA, respectively. Other authors have published similar findings [10, 11].

Furthermore, during the last years, several studies of different Asian populations have showed that the prevalence of positional OSA patients is even higher than in Caucasians. In a study of 1,170 OSA patients from Korea who underwent PSG [12], nearly 75 % of the study population were PP. However, in mild and moderated OSA, the prevalence increased to 87 % and 84.2 %, respectively. In another study on 263 OSA patients from Thailand [13], the prevalence of PP reached almost 70 %, and in a study evaluating the effect of positional dependency on outcomes of treatment with mandibular advancement device (MAD), 80 out of a total of 100 Korean OSA patients showed positional dependency [14]. Thus, the majority of Asian as well as non-Asian OSA patients are positional.

Since patients with mild-to-moderate OSA are the prevailing group of OSA patients [15], it can be concluded from the above that positional OSA comprises the vast majority of OSA patients. Thus, if PT will turn out to be a successful mode of therapy for sleep apnea patients, it will eventually be used by a large number of patients.

The high prevalence of positional OSA in the less severe forms of OSA is important, because mild OSA patients are less likely to succeed with the treatment by continuous positive airway pressure (CPAP) [16] and therefore might be good candidates for positional therapy.

The low rate of success of surgical interventions for snoring and in particular for OSA [17] and the fact that untreated patients with mild OSA might eventually progress from moderate to severe OSA [18] are additional reasons why PT should be advocated to the milder form of OSA.

Moreover, several studies performed during the last years have indicated that the worsening effect of the supine posture during sleep is valid also for patients with central sleep apnea. The first report on this issue described a patient with cerebrovascular accident (CVA) in whom a clear-cut detrimental effect on breathing abnormalities in the supine posture during sleep was found [19]. Several studies have shown that the supine posture has an aggravating effect on central sleep apnea in patients with heart failure, with or without Cheyne–Stokes breathing [20–22]. Although PT may be a new and valuable treatment tool for this particular group of patients, there is a need for additional research on this topic.

Pathophysiology Basis for Positional Therapy

The effect of gravity on the upper airway (UA) when adopting the supine posture is most probably the dominant factor responsible for the anatomical and physiological changes in th UA observed in this posture [23]. The effect of gravity on breathing during sleep was nicely shown by Elliot et al. [24] They have analyzed 77 PSG obtained from five healthy astronauts either at normal or microgravity and found that both the severity of AHI and the severity of snoring significantly decreased in zero gravity conditions.

Several studies have suggested that sleep and posture may work synergistically to compromise the UA in OSA patients, and by adopting the supine position, one major physiological change occurs, i.e., an increase in the UA resistance [25, 26]. As a consequence, breathing during sleep becomes more labored, leading to an increased rate of episodes of partial or complete airway obstruction. The critical pressure at which the pharynx collapses (Pcrit) is an objective measurement of upper airway collapsibility. The fact that in comparison to the supine posture, Pcrit decreases in the lateral posture indicates that changing body posture from supine to lateral significantly decreases passive pharyngeal collapsibility. This fact provides a physiological support for positional therapy [27, 28].

The establishment of the concept of PP and NNP was followed by attempts to explain the anatomical basis for this concept. Pevernagie et al. have studied with fast CT scanning the size and shape of the UA in 6 PP and 5 NPP while awake [29]. The main anatomical differences between the two types of patients were present at the velopharyngeal segment of the UA. The minimal cross-sectional area (MCA) of the velopharynx for the PP group was almost twice that of the NPP group in both the supine and right lateral positions. Moreover, the shape of the tract was elliptical (with the long axis oriented laterally) in the PP group while it was circular in the NPP group. The differences in shape were predominantly due to the significantly greater lateral diameter in the PP group while the anteroposterior (AP) dimensions were similar in both groups. These data suggest that during sleep in the supine position, both PP and NPP will have breathing abnormalities mainly due to the gravity effect on the UA soft tissues which reduces the AP diameter significantly. However, when the PP group adopts the lateral position, the AP diameter is increased, and since the lateral walls are far enough apart, sufficient airway space is preserved to avoid the complete collapse of the UA. In the NPP group, changing to the lateral position will still generate pharyngeal collapse since the lateral diameter in these patients is not sufficient enough to allow significant airflow via the collapsed pharynx. Walsh et al. [30] have corroborated and extended the abovementioned concepts by studying 11 males with OSA and 11 age- and BMI-matched control subjects during wakefulness with anatomical optical coherence tomography.

In a more recent study [31], the 3D morphological features of the UA tract in positional and non-positional OSA patients matched for BMI, age, and AHI were studied by pharyngeal CT and MRI. It was found that the dominant determinant for positional dependence was the volume of the lateral pharyngeal wall. The authors noted that positional OSA patients had a smaller volume of the lateral pharyngeal wall soft tissues. Therefore, when OSA patients sleep in the lateral posture, it is the width of the lateral pharyngeal wall that will determine if the gravitational forces acting on the pharyngeal lumen are sufficient to keep it open, as it occurs in positional patients, or insufficient, as it occurs in non-positional patients, to prevent the collapse of the pharyngeal space during sleep.

The above studies provide an anatomical basis for the phenotype distinction between positional (PP) and non-positional (NPP) OSA patients. In addition, it offers an anatomo-physiological explanation for the beneficial effect of assuming the lateral position in patients with sleep apnea.

It should be mentioned that there are at least two additional factors which appear to play an important role in breathing function and are affected by positional changes during sleep:

Lung volume decreases during sleep, and when assuming the supine posture, this decrease produces a narrower upper airway which will further increases UA resistance [32]. Although the influence of assuming the lateral position during sleep was studied only in normal subjects, it should be noted that when they turn from the lateral to the supine position, the expiratory reserve volume decreases [33], and the functional residual capacity [34] and the dynamic lung compliance [35] are increased.

The genioglossus muscle is the main dilator of the UA. As such, its activity is increased in OSA patients, perhaps, in an effort to compensate for the narrower UA, decreased lung volume, and subsequent increased Pcrit [36]. It was also found that the activity of the genioglossus is decreased in the lateral as compared to the supine position in normal subjects as well as in OSA patients [37].

Although the vestibular system could theoretically play a role in increasing the activity of the genioglossus due to its role in maintaining posture, it was suggested that the postural-related changes in the activity of the genioglossus are secondary to the displacement of the hyoid bone when moving from the sitting to supine and from supine to lateral recumbent position [38].

Additional Forms of Positional Therapy

The effect of changes in body posture during sleep on breathing function is not limited to the changes from supine to the lateral posture. For example, some OSA patients claim that the prone posture is a much better position during sleep than the supine posture. Only few studies have provided data on the effect of the prone posture on breathing abnormalities (perhaps mainly due to the fact that to sleep in the prone posture with the equipment used during PSG is almost impossible) during sleep [39, 40].

Nevertheless, a number studies have investigated the effect of elevated posture and knee up posture and the effect of head extension on breathing abnormalities during sleep.

Elevated Posture

Few studies have evaluated the effect of elevating the head and upper body posture on breathing abnormalities during sleep. Skinner et al. [41] used a shoulder–head elevation pillow (SHEP), designed to standardize the elevated posture at 60° above the horizontal plan. It was found that 29 % (4/14) of their mild-to-moderate OSA patients were considered as achieving success judged by AHI ≤ 10 and 21 % (3/14) a partial success (AHI > 10 < 16). In a previous study on 13 patients with OSA, McEvoy et al. [42] found that assuming the elevated posture of about 60° from horizontal was associated with a reduction of AHI from 48.9 ± 5.4 when supine to 19.6 ± 6.9. Neill et al. [43] studied the upper airway stability in eight patients with severe OSA by measuring upper airway closing pressure (UACP) in three postures (supine, elevated to 30°, and lateral). They concluded that in severely affected OSA patients, upper body elevation and, to a lesser extent, lateral positioning significantly improve upper airway stability during sleep. Lee et al. [44] in a group of 16 mild-to-moderate OSA patients found that a reduction of AHI by 80 % can be achieved if the patient assumes a lateral position at an angle greater than 30° and/or a 20 mm. elevation of the upper trunk.

Knee Up Posture

To the best of our knowledge, only a single-case report [45] and a subsequent study by Greer et al. [46] which followed the experience obtained from the reported case mentioned above were published in regard to the "knee up" posture as a form of PT for OSA. The authors of the study asked 24 volunteers with OSA to sleep supine with a foam wedge underneath their knees which provided approximately a 60° elevation. In some patients, this maneuver improved the AHI and the desaturation index. The study was summarized as showing a trend of improvement of the examined position as compared to the knee down position. The mechanism underlying this improvement is unknown, but since this position allows for a greater displacement of the diaphragm during expiration, the net effect in the form of an increase in lung volumes may induce a decrease in pharyngeal resistance.

Head Extension

In two small studies on mild-to-moderate OSA patients (12 and 18 patients, respectively) [47, 48], a cervical pillow which promotes head extension similar to that used in cardiopulmonary resuscitation (CPR) to create an open airway in an unconscious victim was used. A significant trend toward improvement was found, despite spending more time in the supine position and having similar amounts of REM sleep.

The mechanism by which the cervical pillow improves sleep-disordered breathing in patients with mild-to-moderate OSA is most likely related to the increased cross-sectional area of the airway associated with head extension.

Positional Therapy: For Whom and for Whom Not

In order to increase the likelihood of success with any treatment modality, it is essential to identify the group of patients who will benefit mostly from this particular treatment. With this in mind, we need to be able to recognize easily what are the main characteristics that will determine if a particular patient **is or is not** the suitable candidate for this specific treatment. This issue is of importance also for the successful outcome of positional therapy.

The distinction between PP and NPP is crucial for the successful use of PT since only PP are the OSA patients who may significantly benefit from this form of treatment.

Positional therapy is not a good option for NPP who continue to show a relative high amount of breathing abnormalities in the non-supine postures. However, it could somehow improve their condition because breathing abnormalities while sleeping in the supine posture are much more severe that those occurring in the lateral postures [49]. In the supine posture, the apneas are longer, leading to steeper desaturations, producing longer arousals and larger increases in heart rate and loudness of snoring events at the end of the episodes. Moreover, obstructive apneas in the supine posture have been associated with a more significant degree of daytime sleepiness [50]. Nevertheless, in contrary to PP who have almost none or only a small amount of breathing abnormalities while sleeping in the lateral posture, NPP will still show a relative high amount of apneas and hypopneas while sleeping in this position. For those patients, CPAP is undoubtedly the therapy of choice.

A crucial issue for PP is the fact that the *severity of the disease is totally dependent on the time spent or not spent in the supine posture*, and thus, positional therapy is for those patients a valuable therapeutic option.

Self-Avoidance of the Supine Posture During Sleep

Some severe and very severe OSA patients avoid the supine posture without the need for special therapy since they feel and know that this is the worse posture for their breathing function during sleep. In addition, some severe OSA patients, almost immediately after adopting the supine posture, even during wakefulness, may sense difficulties in breathing.

Many patients, but mostly patients with COPD who suffer also from OSA (overlap syndrome), avoid spontaneously the supine posture during sleep and tend to sleep in a sitting posture or in a semi-recumbent position, mainly in a couch or even in a chair. If they sleep in bed, they usually require 2–3 or even more pillows.

These patients should be firmly encouraged to place their legs in an elevated position to avoid legs edema secondary to impaired venous return.

Unfortunately, there are no data on the abovementioned topics to the extent that we do not know how common this phenomenon is. Research regarding those issues is at need and will be very welcomed.

Guidelines for Positional Therapy

Who Are the Sleep Apnea Patients That Could Benefit from PT?

1. One should offer this mode of therapy to supine-related obstructive sleep apnea (OSA) patients (positional patients—PP) whose breathing abnormalities are present mainly (predominant) or only (exclusive) when they are sleeping in the supine posture, while when sleeping in the lateral postures (and sometimes in the prone posture), the breathing abnormalities disappear or are significantly reduced to a non-pathological level.
2. Patients with mixed and central apnea (with or without Cheyne–Stokes breathing) and probably also patients with upper airway resistance syndrome who have most of their breathing abnormalities while sleeping in the supine posture. By sleeping in other positions, the number of these events is reduced to a non-pathological level.
3. PT could be also a therapy for patients without sleep apnea who only snore, but mainly in the supine posture (positional snoring). It should be mentioned that the snoring mainly in the supine posture appears to be the initial stage of the natural history of OSA. It is quite common to hear from bed partners of OSA patients that "*at the beginning he used to snore only when he slept in the supine posture and when he was very tired. Now he snores in all body postures and also I noticed the occurrence of scary breathing pauses when he sleeps on his back.*" [23].
4. Any OSA patient who was not helped or could not tolerate CPAP or oral device and have mainly breathing abnormalities in the supine posture.
5. Patients who had upper airway surgery and still have breathing abnormalities mainly while sleeping in the supine posture.

   It is worth mentioning that any treatment of sleep-disordered breathing that is not capable to eliminate in a radical form the breathing abnormalities during sleep will not eliminate some abnormalities present mainly when the patient sleeps in the supine posture.
6. Pregnant positional OSA women. Although no data on this topic exist in the literature, it is quite possible that a certain number of pregnant women have positional sleep apnea (also see chapter "Sleep Position and Pregnancy" by Morong et al.). Louis et al. [51] found that the prevalence of sleep-disordered breathing in obese pregnant women is 15.4 %. It is known that the incidence of snoring increases during pregnancy, reaching up to 85 % in preeclampsia [52]. Although nasal CPAP treatment had been considered as efficient in pregnant women with OSA [53], it is possible that at least some of them who could not comply with CPAP could benefit from PT.

The fact that the prevalence of the "supine hypertensive syndrome" in pregnant women is about 60 % [54] may suggest that PT could serve an additional simple behavioral solution for women suffering from this syndrome.

Who Are the Sleep Apnea Patients That Should Refrain from PT?

1. All non-positional patients (NPP) with breathing abnormalities not only in the supine posture but also in other body positions. Those patients have the most severe form of sleep apnea, and for most of them, CPAP is certainly the treatment of choice.

   It is important to mention that overweight NPP may convert into PP if they lose weight since weight reduction leads to a major improvement of breathing function during sleep in the lateral posture. As a consequence, these patients could successfully use PT and enjoy a significant improvement in their condition. Indeed, changes in body weight may modulate the reciprocal interaction between PP and NPP, i.e., increased weight may convert a PP into an NPP and vice versa [55]. Thus, close follow-up of such patients is mandatory in order to guarantee that they remain PP and PT still provides them with a good solution.
2. Patients who have most breathing abnormalities in the supine posture but in the lateral or prone postures present with loud and continuous snoring. For them PT could improve their condition, but it is certainly not a radical solution for their breathing abnormalities during sleep.
3. Obviously, all patients who are good candidates for PT, as stated above, but are unable to sleep in the lateral position due to shoulder problems or any other physical disability that interfere with their sleep in the lateral position.
4. PP who enjoy very much sleeping in the supine posture and are not willing to abandon their favorite sleep position.

The Agenda for Future Research

1. Research on the effect of age, gender, and ethnicity on the successful use of positional therapy is needed.
2. Research that will provide information on the characteristics of positional patients that will comply vs. those that will not comply with this therapy is required.
3. Research on adherence to this form of therapy is obviously a requisite.
4. Research that will evaluate the effect of using positional therapy on daytime sleepiness, health-related quality of life, cardiovascular, metabolic, and cognitive parameters is urgently needed.
5. Until now, one of the major problems of positional therapy was that patients refer to it as an uncomfortable technique. Thus, a major effort should be made in order to develop a comfortable, simple, cheap, and effective device that also will have the capabilities of long-term recording, to allow a close follow-up of the compliance as well as efficacy of this technique.

6. Multicenter, high-quality studies are at need, in order to evaluate thoroughly the efficacy of this behavioral simple therapy in the treatment of sleep apnea.
7. It is clear that until large, randomized, controlled, and long-term studies will be available, the exact therapeutic value of this behavioral therapy will be debatable.

References

1. Editor's note. Patient's wife cures his snoring. Chest. 1984; 582.
2. Ravesloot MJL, van Maanen JP, Dun L, de Vries N. The undervalued potential of positional therapy in position-dependent snoring and obstructive sleep apnea- review of the literature. Sleep Breath. 2013;17:39–49.
3. Robin IG. Snoring. Proc R Soc Med. 1948;41:151–3.
4. Gastaut H, Tassinari CA, Duran B. Polygraphic study of the episodic diurnal and nocturnal (hypnic and respiratory B.) manifestations of the pickwick syndrome. Brain Res. 1966;1: 167–86.
5. Jackson EI, Schmidt HS. Modification of sleeping position in the treatment of obstructive sleep apnea. Sleep Res. 1982;11:149.
6. Kavey NB, Gidro-Frank S, Sewitch DE. The importance of sleeping position and a simple treatment technique. Sleep Res. 1982;11:152.
7. Cartwright RD. Effect of sleep position on sleep apnea severity. Sleep. 1984;7:110–4.
8. Oksenberg A, Silverberg DS, Arons E, Radwan H. Positional vs. nonpositional obstructive sleep apnea patients: anthropomorphic, nocturnal polysomnographic, and multiple sleep latency test data. Chest. 1997;112:629–39.
9. Oksenberg A, Arons E, Greenberg-Dotan S, Nasser K, Radwan H. The significance of body posture on breathing abnormalities during sleep: data analysis of 2077 obstructive sleep apnea patients [Article in Hebrew]. Harefuah. 2009;148:157–62.
10. Mador MJ, Kufel TJ, Magalang UJ, Rajesh SK, Watwe V, Grant JB. Prevalence of positional sleep apnea in patients undergoing polysomnography. Chest. 2005;128:2130–7.
11. Richard W, Kox D, den Herder C, Laman M, van Tinteren H, de Vries N. The role of sleep position in obstructive sleep apnea syndrome. Eur Arch Otorhinolaryngol. 2006;263:946–50.
12. Mo JH, Lee CH, Rhee CS, et al. Positional dependency in Asian patients with obstructive sleep apnea and its implication for hypertension. Arch Otolaryngol Head Neck Surg. 2011;137:786–90.
13. Teerapraipruk B, Chirakalwasan N, Simon R, Hirunwiwatkul P, Jaimchariyatam N, Desudchit T, et al. Clinical and polysomnographic data of positional sleep apnea and its predictors. Sleep Breath. 2012;16:1167–72.
14. Lee CH, Jung HJ, Lee WH, Rhee CS, Yoon IY, Yun PY, et al. The effect of positional dependency on outcomes of treatment with a mandibular advancement device. Arch Otolaryngol Head Neck Surg. 2012;138:479–83.
15. Peppard PE, Young T, Barnet JH, Palta M, Hagen EW, Hla KM. Increased Prevalence of Sleep-Disordered Breathing in Adults. Am J Epidemiol. 2013;177:1006–14.
16. Rosenthal L, Gerhardstein R, Lumley A, Guido P, Day R, Syron ML, et al. CPAP therapy in patients with mild OSA: implementation and treatment outcome. Sleep Med. 2000;1:215–20.
17. Elshaug AG, Moss JR, Hiller JE, Maddern GJ. Upper airway surgery should not be first line treatment for obstructive sleep apnoea in adults. BMJ. 2008;336:44–5.
18. Berger G, Berger R, Oksenberg A. Progression of snoring and obstructive sleep apnea: the role of increasing weight and time. Eur Respir J. 2009;33:338–45.
19. Oksenberg A, Arons E, Snir D, Radwan H, Soroker N. Stokes respiration during sleep: a possible effect of body position. Med Sci Monit. 2002;8:CS61–5.

20. Sahlin C, Svanborg E, Stenlund H, Franklin KA. Cheynes-Stokes respiration and supine dependency. Eur Resp J. 2005;25:829–33.
21. Szollosi I, Roebuck T, Thompson B, Naughton MT. Lateral sleeping position reduces severity of Central Sleep Apnea/Cheyne-Stokes respiration. Sleep. 2006;29:1045–51.
22. Joho S, Oda Y, Hirai T, Inoue H. Impact of sleeping position on central sleep apnea/Cheyne-Stokes respiration in patients with heart failure. Sleep Med. 2010;11:143–8.
23. Oksenberg A, Silverberg DS. The effect of body posture on sleep-related breathing disorders: facts and clinical implications. Sleep Med Rev. 1998;2:139–62.
24. Elliot AR, Shea SA, Dijk DJ, Wyatt JK, Riel E, Neri DF, et al. Microgravity Reduces Sleep-disordered Breathing in Humans. Am J Respir Crit Care Med. 2001;164:478–85.
25. Anch AM, Remmers JE, Bunce H 3rd. Supraglottic airway resistance in normal subjects and patients with occlusive sleep apnea. J Appl Physiol. 1982;53:1158–63.
26. Tvinnereim M, Cole P, Mateika S, Haight J, Hoffstein V. Postural changes in respiratory airflow pressure and resistance in nasal, hypopharyngeal, and pharyngeal airway in normal subjects. Ann Otol Rhinol Laryngol. 1996;105:218–21.
27. Isono S, Tanaka A, Nishino T. Lateral position decreases collapsibility of the passive pharynx in patients with obstructive sleep apnea. Anesthesiology. 2002;97:780–5.
28. Ong JS, Touyz G, Tanner S, Hillman DR, Eastwood PR, Walsh JH. Variability of human upper airway collapsibility during sleep and the influence of body posture and sleep stage. J Sleep Res. 2011;20:533–7.
29. Pevernagie DA, Stanson AW, Sheedy PE 2nd, et al. Effects of body position on the upper airway of patients with obstructive sleep apnea. Am J Respir Crit Care Med. 1995;152:179–85.
30. Walsh JH, Leigh MS, Paduch A, Maddison KJ, Armstrong JJ, Sampson DD, et al. Effect of body posture on pharyngeal shape and size in adults with and without obstructive sleep apnea. Sleep. 2008;31:1543–9.
31. Saigusa H, Suzuki M, Higurashi N, Kodera K. Three-dimensional morphological analyses of positional dependence in patients with obstructive sleep apnea syndrome. Anesthesiology. 2009;110:885–90.
32. Sériès F, Cormier Y, la Forge J. Role of lung volumes in nocturnal postapneic desaturations. Eur Respir J. 1989;2:26–30.
33. Behrakis PK, Baydur A, Jaeger MJ, Milic-Emili J. Lung mechanics in sitting and horizontal body positions. Chest. 1983;83:643–6.
34. Barnas GM, Green MD, Mackenzie CF, Fletcher SJ, Campbell DN, Runcie C, et al. Effect of posture on lung and regional chest wall mechanics. Anesthesiology. 1993;78:251–9.
35. Tanskanen P, Kyttä J, Randell T. The effect of patient positioning on dynamic lung compliance. Acta Anaesthesiol Scand. 1997;41:602–6.
36. Mezzanotte WS, Tangel DJ, White DP. Waking genioglossal electromyogram in sleep apnea patients versus normal controls (a neuromuscular compensatory mechanism). J Clin Invest. 1992;89:1571–9.
37. Malhotra A, Trinder J, Fogel R, Stanchina M, Patel SR, Schory K, et al. Postural effects on pharyngeal protective reflex mechanisms. Sleep. 2004;27:1105–12.
38. Otsuka R, Ono T, Ishiwata Y, Kuroda T. Respiratory-related genioglossus electromyographic activity in response to head rotation and changes in body position. Angle Orthod. 2000; 70:63–9.
39. Matsuzawa Y, Hayashi S, Yamaguchi S, et al. Effect of prone position on apnea severity in obstructive sleep apnea. Intern Med. 2005;34:1190–3.
40. Afrashi A, Ucar Z. Is pure prone positioning an effective therapy for the patients with mild to moderate OSAS? Chest. 2011;140(meeting abstract):1072A.
41. Skinner MA, Kingshott RN, Jones DR, Homan SDR, Taylor DR. Elevated Posture for the Management of Obstructive Sleep Apnea. Sleep Breath. 2004;8:193–200.
42. McEvoy RD, Sharp DJ, Thornton AT. The effect of posture on Obstructive Sleep Apnea. Am Rev Respir Dis. 1986;133:662–6.
43. Neill AM, Angus SM, Sajkov D, McEvoy RD. Effects of sleep posture on upper airway stability in patients with obstructive sleep apnea. Am J Respir Crit Care Med. 1997;155:199–204.

44. Lee JB, Park YH, Hong JH, Lee SH, Jung KH, Kim JH, et al. Determining optimal sleep position in patients with positional sleep-disordered breathing using response surface analysis. J Sleep Res. 2009;18:26–35.
45. Bliwise DL, Irbe D, Schulman DA. Improvement in obstructive sleep apnea in the supine "knees-up" position. Sleep Breath. 2004;8:43–7.
46. Greer S, Straight LB, Schulman DA, Bliwise DL. Effect of supine knee position on obstructive sleep apnea. Sleep Breath. 2006;10:98–101.
47. Kushida CA, Rao S, Guilleminault C, Giraudo S, Hsieh J, Hyde P, et al. Cervical positional effects on snoring and apneas. Sleep Res Online. 1999;2:7–10.
48. Kushida CA, Sherrill CM, Hong SC, Palombini L, Hyde P, Dement WC. Cervical positioning for reduction of sleep disordered breathing in mild-to-moderate OSAS. Sleep Breath. 2001;2:71–8.
49. Oksenberg A, Khamaysi Y, Silverberg DS, Tarasiuk A. Association of body position with severity of apneic events in patients with severe nonpositional obstructive sleep apnea. Chest. 2000;118:1018–24.
50. Chervin RD, Aldrich MS. Characteristics of apneas and hypopneas during sleep and relation to excessive daytime sleepiness. Sleep. 1998;21:799–806.
51. Louis J, Auckley D, Bolden N. Management of obstructive sleep apnea in pregnant women. Obstet Gynecol. 2012;119:864–8.
52. Bourjeily G. Sleep disorders in pregnancy. Obstet Med. 2009;2:100–6.
53. Guilleminault C, Kreutzer M, Chang JL. Pregnancy, sleep disordered breathing and treatment with nasal continuous positive airway pressure. Sleep Med. 2004;5:43–51.
54. Kato J, Tanaka T. Shock due to supine hypotensive syndrome. [Article in Japanese]. Sanfujinka No Jissai. 1967;16:118–23.
55. Oksenberg A, Dynia A, Nasser K, Gadoth N. Obstructive sleep apnoea in adults: body postures and weight changes interactions. J Sleep Res. 2012;21:402–9.

Summary and Future Perspectives

Nico de Vries, Madeline Ravesloot, and J. Peter van Maanen

The Wagnerian leitmotif in this book on OSA is sleep position. OSA is a serious, highly prevalent disease with major health implications (chapters "Introduction" and "OSAS: The Magnitude of the Problem"). In the beginning of the book, the finding is highlighted that mild OSA in the majority of cases is positional (chapters "The Contribution of Head Position to the Apnea/Hypopnea Index in Patients with Position-Dependent Obstructive Sleep Apnea", "Influence of Sleep Position on the Transition of Mild to Moderate and Severe OSA" and "Positional Therapy: Left Lateral Decubitus Position Versus Right Lateral Decubitus Position"). With progression of the disease from mild via moderate to eventually severe OSA, positional OSA progresses into non-positional severe OSA. In later chapters the observation is made that patients with insufficient response to therapy, such as can happen in palatal surgery, maxillomandibular advancement or bariatric surgery, severe non-positional OSA can reverse to less severe positional OSA (chapters "Positional OSA in the Morbidly Obese and the Effect of Weight Loss on OSA Severity", "Positional Therapy and Tongue Base Surgery", "Residual POSA After Maxillomandibular Advancement in Patients with Severe OSA", "Impact of Upper Airway Surgery on Positional Change During Sleep" and "Comparison of Positional Therapy to CPAP in Patients with Positional Obstructive Sleep Apnea"). The circle is complete.

N. de Vries, M.D., Ph.D. (✉)
Department of Otolaryngology, Sint Lucas Andreas Ziekenhuis,
Jan Tooropstraat 164, 1061 AE Amsterdam, The Netherlands

Department of Otolaryngology, University Hospital Antwerp,
Antwerp, Belgium
e-mail: n.vries@slaz.nl

M. Ravesloot, M.D., Ph.D.
Department of Otorhinolaryngology, Sint Lucas Andreas Ziekenhuis, Amsterdam,
The Netherlands

J.P. van Maanen, M.D.
Department of Otolaryngology, Sint Lucas Andreas Ziekenhuis, Amsterdam, The Netherlands

N. de Vries et al. (eds.), *Positional Therapy in Obstructive Sleep Apnea*,
DOI 10.1007/978-3-319-09626-1_36

It has become clear that sleep position deserves a larger role in the management of sleep-disordered breathing, especially habitual snoring and OSA. In the first place, polysomnography positional sensing should routinely be included. Separate positional measurements for head and trunk during polysomnography should be seriously considered (chapter "The Contribution of Head Position to the Apnea/Hypopnea Index in Patients with Position-Dependent Obstructive Sleep Apnea"). Polysomnographic observations in various populations, sleep positions and sleep stages are discussed in chapters "Prevalence of Positional Obstructive Sleep Apnea in Patients Undergoing Polysomnography and the Effect of Sleep Stage", "Clinical Characteristics of Positional Obstructive Sleep Apnea Among Asians" and "Positional Therapy: Left Lateral Decubitus Position Versus Right Lateral Decubitus Position". Next in order, improvement of current drug induced sedated endoscopy methods by taking sleep position into account. For example, in cases with positional OSA undergoing DISE, observations in lateral sleeping position are mandatory (chapters "Drug-Induced Sleep Endoscopy and Sleep Position" and "Changes in Site of Obstruction in Obstructive Sleep Apnea Patients According to Sleep Position"). It is a clinical reality that, as yet, this is rarely done. Perhaps, tilting of the head during DISE is sufficient (chapter "Drug-Induced Sleep Endoscopy and Sleep Position").

Generally accepted definitions of POSA are urgently needed, as well as algorithms and formulas to predict if positional therapy might be considered as part of the overall treatment plan (chapters "Towards a Clinical Classification System (APOC) for Position-Dependent Obstructive Sleep Apnea", "Retrospective Cohort Analysis with the APOC System" and "Correlation Between Calculated/Predicted and Actual AHI After Positional Therapy").

It can be concluded that variations on the tennis ball technique have become obsolete since the introduction of smart positional therapy (chapters "History of Positional Therapy: Transition from Tennis Balls to New Devices", "Long-Term Results and Compliance of a Special Vest Preventing the Supine Position", "Results of a First-Generation New Device for Positional Therapy", "Short-Term (4 Weeks) Results of the Sleep Position Trainer for Positional Therapy", "Long-Term (6 Months) Effectiveness, Compliance, and Subjective Sleep Outcomes of Treatment with the Sleep Position Trainer in a Large Cohort of Position-Dependent OSA Patients", "10 Problems and Solutions for Positional Therapy: Technical Aspects of the Sleep Position Trainer" and "Prevalence and Effect of Supine-Dependent Obstructive Sleep Apnea on Oral Appliance Therapy"). Positional therapy can be offered as single treatment or supplementary to oral device treatment or surgery (chapters "Prevalence and Effect of Supine-Dependent Obstructive Sleep Apnea on Oral Appliance Therapy", "Positional Therapy and Palatal Surgery", "Positional Therapy and Tongue Base Surgery", "Residual POSA After Maxillomandibular Advancement in Patients with Severe OSA" and "Impact of Upper Airway Surgery on Positional Change During Sleep"). CPAP and positional therapy have been compared (chapter "Comparison of Positional Therapy to CPAP in Patients with Positional Obstructive Sleep Apnea"), but the value of adding positional therapy to CPAP remains to be studied.

It can be speculated that positional therapy might have a role in other populations and diseases other than obstructive sleep-disordered breathing (chapters "Clinical Characteristics of Positional Obstructive Sleep Apnea Among Asians", "The Effect of Body Position on Sleep Apnea in Children", "Sleep Position and Pregnancy", "Positional OSA in Down Syndrome" and "Positional OSA in the Morbidly Obese and the Effect of Weight Loss on OSA Severity"). Rare cases of central sleep apnea have been shown to be positional as well; the pathophysiology remains unclear (chapter "Positional Central Sleep Apnea").

Concerning future perspectives, much remains to be studied, for example, the promising potential value of positional therapy during pregnancy or patients with Down's syndrome.

There is much debate about the postoperative care of patients with OSA. The epidemic of OSA puts serious strain on IC units. Should all patients be admitted to IC units and treated with CPAP? Relatively new is the insight that most patients sleep on their back after surgery—the worst sleeping position—more than in the normal situation. In such patients, it might be better to look at the AHI in supine position rather than at the overall AHI. Can a role for postoperative positional therapy be envisaged or is postoperative tilting of the head sufficient? There are open questions with potential new fields of research.

In case combined positional and surgical treatment (or oral device therapy) is considered, one has to consider the sequence of the treatments. Some patients will need both forms of therapy simultaneously because the combined treatment is clearly better than one of the two therapies alone. While sleep surgeons are presently often offering positional therapy in case of surgical failure because of residual positional dependency, a future development would be to offer positional therapy before surgery, upfront. In some patients who undergo maxillomandibular advancement however, the different effects of MRA on supine and lateral become apparent only after surgery. Here it would not be logical to begin with positional therapy.

Guidelines might need to be adapted (chapter "Positional Therapy, Consequences for and Implementation in OSA Guidelines").

If one tries to define the features of the ideal treatment for OSA (or for that matter, any other disease), they would include **effectiveness, patient friendliness, good compliance, wide availability, reversibility, cost-effectiveness, absence of (major) side effects and possibility to combine with other treatments**. New forms of positional therapy have the potential to fulfil these criteria to a large degree. For this reason, positional therapy is supported by patient societies (chapter "Position Training: An Indispensable Therapy").

With regard to **effectiveness**: By good patient selection—how to do this is discussed in chapters "Towards a Clinical Classification System (APOC) for Position-Dependent Obstructive Sleep Apnea", "Retrospective Cohort Analysis with the APOC System", "Correlation Between Calculated/Predicted and Actual AHI After Positional Therapy", "Position-Dependent Sleep Apnea: Implications for Diagnosis and Management" and "Positional Therapy in Obstructive Sleep Apnea: For Whom and for Whom Not"—one can easily identify many excellent candidates for positional therapy.

With regard to **patient friendliness**: Several studies comparing positional therapy to oral device therapy are ongoing. It is yet unclear whether patients prefer positional therapy to oral devices or CPAP, in case all treatment options would be possible.

Wide availability: Presently positional therapy is rapidly becoming available in many Western European countries, while other parts of the world will hopefully follow shortly. While positional therapy presently is only commercially available, it can be envisaged that before long insurance companies will cover its acquisition. There is wide variation among countries in what and what is not insured in diagnosis and treatment of sleep-disordered breathing. For example, some countries cover CPAP, others do not; some countries cover MRA, others do not; other countries cover CPAP but not surgery. Many European countries cover DISE, while (currently) the USA does not. In many countries, only one form of treatment is covered, e.g. once a patient has a CPAP and would like a MRA (for instance, for travelling); this is often not covered. It looks as if insurance companies have to get used to the fact that multimodality treatments might do better than one treatment alone, and that they should accept the short-term financial consequences (with long-term benefit).

Reversibility: CPAP and oral device therapy are reversible; surgery is not. In case a patient cannot tolerate CPAP for one reason or another, the CPAP appliance can be returned. The same holds true for positional therapy. Oral devices, on the other hand, are custom made and can therefore not be used by another patient, if not successful. Surgeries of course are in no way reversible, and treatment outcomes as no effect, or even detrimental effect, unfortunately can happen.

Cost-effectiveness and good compliance: The costs of positional therapy are lower than that of CPAP, oral device and surgery. It is clear that devices only work when they are being used. Short-term compliance—4 weeks—of the sleep position trainer is 92–100 % (92 % when compliance is defined as use of 4 h/7 night/week, 100 % when compliance is defined as 4 h/5 nights/week) and long-term compliance—6 months—is 60 % (chapters "Short-Term (4 Weeks) Results of the Sleep Position Trainer for Positional Therapy" and "Long-Term (6 Months) Effectiveness, Compliance, and Subjective Sleep Outcomes of Treatment with the Sleep Position Trainer in a Large Cohort of Position-Dependent OSA Patients"). It is hoped that compliance can be further improved by stricter positive reinforcement, explanation, training, stimulation and motivation. Further improvement here is in reach. Technological improvements are under way. Compliance is discussed in chapter "Compliance of Various Forms of OSA Treatment", technology in chapter "10 Problems and Solutions for Positional Therapy: Technical Aspects of the Sleep Position Trainer".

Absence of (major) side effects: Surgery has many sometimes serious and often irreversible side effects. Side effects of CPAP comprise mask leakages, skin pressure lesions, nasal breathing problems, sinus diseases, etc. Side effects of oral device therapy include painful jaws muscles in the morning, dry mouth, hypersalivation and in the long run changes in dental occlusion. So far, no major side effects of positional therapy have been reported.

Possibility to combine with other treatments: Positional therapy can be used as stand-alone therapy or combined with surgery (chapters "Positional Therapy and Palatal Surgery", "Positional Therapy and Tongue Base Surgery", "Residual POSA After Maxillomandibular Advancement in Patients with Severe OSA", "Impact of Upper Airway Surgery on Positional Change During Sleep" and "Comparison of Positional Therapy to CPAP in Patients with Positional Obstructive Sleep Apnea") and with oral devices (chapter "Prevalence and Effect of Supine-Dependent Obstructive Sleep Apnea on Oral Appliance Therapy"). Since CPAP is most used in moderate to severe OSA—usually non-positional OSA—the possibility to combine CPAP and positional therapy is less obvious.

Preventive Medicine

Prevention is a major topic in many areas of medicine: oncology, cardiovascular diseases, etc. It is somewhat strangely underrated in OSA. Many caregivers even are of opinion that OSA should only be treated in "clinically relevant" OSA, e.g. AHI>15. Why? Positional therapy, applied in early disease, habitual snoring and mild-to-moderate OSA, has the potential to cure or at least postpone the development of OSA. If the development of the disease is postponed long enough, it automatically becomes prevention. There is no logical reason to wait with treatment until serious comorbidities such as hypertension have appeared.

Index

N. de Vries et al. (eds.), *Positional Therapy in Obstructive Sleep Apnea*,
DOI 10.1007/978-3-319-09626-1

S

MIX
Papier aus verantwortungsvollen Quellen
Paper from responsible sources
FSC® C105338

If you have any concerns about our products,
you can contact us on
ProductSafety@springernature.com

In case Publisher is established outside the EU,
the EU authorized representative is:
Springer Nature Customer Service Center GmbH
Europaplatz 3, 69115 Heidelberg, Germany

Printed by Libri Plureos GmbH
in Hamburg, Germany